Health Services Management

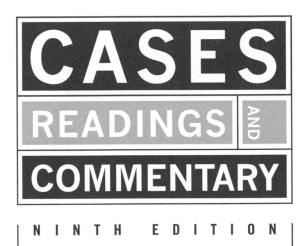

CASES
READINGS AND
COMMENTARY

[NINTH EDITION]

Health Services Management

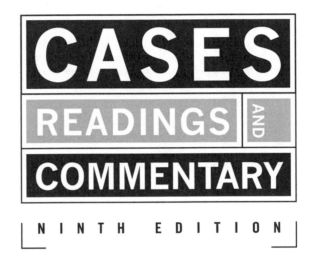

CASES
READINGS AND
COMMENTARY

NINTH EDITION

Anthony R. Kovner,

Ann Scheck McAlearney,

and Duncan Neuhauser

Editors

AUPHA

Your board, staff, or clients may also benefit from this book's insight. For more information on quantity discounts, contact the Health Administration Press Marketing Manager at (312) 424-9470.

15   14   13   12   8   7   6   5

Library of Congress Cataloging-in-Publication Data

Health services management : readings, cases, and commentary / [edited by] Anthony R. Kovner, Ann Scheck McAlearney, Duncan Neuhauser. — 9th ed.
    p. ; cm.
  Includes bibliographical references and index.
  ISBN 978-1-56793-324-6
 1. Health services administration—Case studies. I. Kovner, Anthony R. II. McAlearney, Ann Scheck. III. Neuhauser, Duncan, 1939–
  [DNLM: 1. Hospital Administration—Collected Works. 2. Health Services Administration—Collected Works. 3. Organizational Case Studies—Collected Works. WX 150 H4357 2009]
  RA971.H434 2009
  362.1068—dc22

2009015384

Found an error or typo? We want to know! Please email it to hap1@ache.org, and put "Book Error" in the subject line.

For photocopying and copyright information, please contact Copyright Clearance Center at www.copyright.com or (978) 750-8400.

The paper used in this publication meets the minimum requirements of American National Standard for Information Sciences-Permanence of Paper for Printed Library Materials, ANSI Z39.48-1984. ∞™

Project manager: Eduard Avis; Acquisitions editor: Eileen Lynch; Book designer: Scott Miller; Cover designer: Gloria Chantell

Health Administration Press
A division of the Foundation
  of the American College of
  Healthcare Executives
One North Franklin Street
Suite 1700
Chicago, IL 60606
(312) 424-2800

Association of University Programs
  in Health Administration
2000 14th Street North
Suite 780
Arlington, VA 22201
(703) 894-0940

To Duncan Neuhauser

We have been working together on these management books for 30 years now, and we have never had an argument. I've consistently learned from what you've had to say. Together we have enjoyed beholding the healthcare enterprise, which always amazes me in its latest twists and turns. Duncan, I admire you for your integrity, sense of humor, wisdom and experience, and intellectual courage. You have always been willing to point out but softly (and not unless someone asks you) that the emperor isn't really wearing any clothes.

—Tony Kovner

To Tony Kovner

You have had the wisdom, energy, and willingness to describe your careers in health management in your autobiographical book *Health Care Management in Mind—Eight Careers* (Springer Publishing Co., 2000). You kindly let me write an "afterword" to this book where I tried to describe our successful working relationship lasting over three decades. Here is another way to describe our working relationship: It is like sailing two boats and planning to meet at the same port at the same time. This requires years of learning and a lot of skills, but not much communication once our objective is precisely defined. Done well, there is no need for committee meetings, organizational overhead, or raging arguments. This trip is as enjoyable as the successful arrival. It is clear you have enjoyed the trip of your career as much as your successful arrival to the applause of our peers, as reflected in your receiving the 1999 Gary Filerman Prize for Educational Leadership of the Association of University Programs in Health Administration.

—Duncan Neuhauser

To Ann Scheck McAlearney

You are the next generation to whom we leave our legacy of assembling and writing the ninth edition of *Health Services Management*. We chose you because of your track record of publishing and teaching, with particular success in your book *Population Health Management*, and in your articles on leadership development. You are pleasant, focused, and reliable and have played a leadership role in putting together this ninth edition.

—Tony Kovner
—Duncan Neuhauser

CONTENTS

Preface to the Ninth Edition xiii

A Short History of the Case Method of Teaching xv
Karen Schachter Weingrod and Duncan Neuhauser

Learning Through the Case Method xxiii
Anthony R. Kovner

How to Retrieve Journal Articles from the Internet—A Guide
for Students xxv

Overview xxvii

PART I: THE ROLE OF THE MANAGER

Commentary 3

The Readings 7
    Evidence-Based Management Reconsidered 7
    Anthony R. Kovner and Thomas G. Rundall

The Cases 35
    Case A   A New Faculty Practice Administrator for the
                   Department of Medicine 37
                   Anthony R. Kovner and David M. Kaplan
    Case B   The Associate Director and the Controllers 50
                   Anthony R. Kovner
    Case C   Now What? 58
                   Ann Scheck McAlearney

Short Case 1   Nowhere Job 68
                    David Melman
Short Case 2   Manager Morale at Uptown Hospital 69
                    Sofia Agoritsas
Short Case 3   A Sure Thing 72
                    David M. Kaplan and Anthony R. Kovner
Short Case 4   The First Day 75
                    Ann Scheck McAlearney
Short Case 5   Mid-Career Change 76
                    Jacob Victory

PART II: CONTROL

Commentary 81

The Readings 89
    Taming the Measurement Monster 89
    Patrice L. Spath

The Cases 107
    Case D   An Information Technology Implementation
                    Challenge 108
                    Ann Scheck McAlearney
    Case E   Improving Financial Performance in the
                    Orthopedic Unit... 116
                    Anthony R. Kovner
    Case F   Evidence-Based Quality Management in a Home
                    Health Organization................................. 124
                    Cynthia Struk and Duncan Neuhauser
    Short Case 6   CQI at Suburban Hospital 137
                    Larry K. McReynolds
    Short Case 7   ED at Queens Hospital Center 139
                    Anthony R. Kovner
    Short Case 8   Sparks Medical Center and the Board of Trustees 140
                    Anthony R. Kovner
    Short Case 9   Pay for Performance: Hypertension 140
                    Brook Watts and Duncan Neuhauser
    Short Case 10 Financial Reporting to the Board..........................142
                    Anthony R. Kovner
    Short Case 11 A Purchasing Decision 146
                    Abhi Kasinadhuni and Ann Scheck McAlearney

PART III: ORGANIZATIONAL DESIGN

Commentary 151

The Readings 159
    Convenient Care Clinics: Opposition, Opportunity, and the
    Path to Health System Integration 159
    Dean Q. Lin

The Cases 173
    Case G   Improving Organizational Development in
                 Health Services 175
                 Ann Scheck McAlearney and Rebecca Schmale
    Case H   The Future of Disease Management at
                 Superior Medical Group 183
                 Helen Nunberg
    Case I   Selling an Evidence-Based Design for
                 Waterford Hospital 194
                 Nathan Burt and Ann Scheck McAlearney
    Short Case 12 A Proposal for the Restructuring of Wise
                 Medical Center 202
                 Anthony R. Kovner
    Short Case 13 A Hospitalist Program for Plateau University
                 Hospital 204
                 Jeff Weiss
    Short Case 14 Integrating Rehabilitation Services into the
                 Visiting Nurse Service of America 207
                 Jacob Victory
    Short Case 15 Matrix or Mess? 210
                 Ann Scheck McAlearney

PART IV: PROFESSIONAL INTEGRATION

Commentary 215

The Readings 219
    The Tectonic Plates Are Shifting: Cultural Change vs.
    Mural Dyslexia 219
    Kenneth Cohn, Leonard H. Friedman, and Thomas R. Allyn
    The Revolution in Hospital Management 239
    John R. Griffith and Kenneth R. White

The Cases 261

    Case J   Physician Leadership: MetroHealth System
                 of Cleveland 265
                 Anthony R. Kovner

    Case K   Managing Relationships: Taking Care of
                 Your Nurses 287
                 Anthony R. Kovner

    Short Case 16 Complaining Doctor and Ambulatory Care 292
                 Anthony R. Kovner

    Short Case 17 Doctors and Capital Budget 292
                 Anthony R. Kovner

    Short Case 18 Doctors and a New Medical Day Care Program
                 for the Terminally Ill 292
                 Anthony R. Kovner

    Short Case 19 Average Length of Stay 293
                 Anthony R. Kovner

    Short Case 20 Building the Office of the Medical Director 293
                 Gary Kalkut

PART V: ADAPTATION

Commentary 297

The Readings 299
    Strategic Cycling: Shaking Complacency in Healthcare
    Strategic Planning 301
    Jim Begun and Kathleen B. Heatwole

The Cases 317

    Case L   The Visiting Nurse Association of Cleveland 318
                 Duncan Neuhauser

    Case M   The Piney Woods Hospital Emergency
                 Department 329
                 Julie Anstine, Kyle Dorsey, Nicholas Schmidt,
                 Denise Hamilton, Randa Hall, and Ann Scheck
                 McAlearney

    Case N   An Investment Decision at Central Med
                 Health System 340
                 Emily Allinder, Jason Dopoulos, Breanne
                 Pfotenhauer, David Reisman, Erick Vidmar,
                 Jason Waibel, and Ann Scheck McAlearney

Short Case 21 New Chief of Ob-Gyn: The Next Three Years 346
Anthony R. Kovner
Short Case 22 To Sell or Not to Sell 347
Anthony R. Kovner
Short Case 23 A New Look? 348
Ann Scheck McAlearney and Sarah M. Roesch
Short Case 24 Disparities in Care at Southern Regional
Health System 351
Ann Scheck McAlearney
Short Case 25 Annual Performance Evaluation: Can You
Coach Kindness? 352
Ann Scheck McAlearney

PART VI: ACCOUNTABILITY

Commentary 357

The Readings 363
Transparency—"Deal or No Deal?" 363
Sandy Lutz

The Cases 377
Case O   Letter to the CEO 380
Anonymous
Case P   Whose Hospital? 387
Anthony R. Kovner
Case Q   What Happens When Patients Cannot Pay? 405
Ann Scheck McAlearney and Paula H. Song
Short Case 26 The Conflicted HMO Manager 408
Anthony R. Kovner
Short Case 27 The Great Mosaic: Multiculturalism at
Seaview Nursing Home 409
James Castiglione and Anthony R. Kovner
Short Case 28 No Parity in Behavioral Health Coverage 410
Ann Scheck McAlearney
Short Case 29 Ergonomics in Practice 411
J. Mac Crawford and Ann Scheck McAlearney
Short Case 30 What's in a Name? 413
Ann Scheck McAlearney and Sarah M. Roesch
Short Case 31 Patient Satisfaction in an Inner-City Hospital 415
Claudia Caine and Anthony R. Kovner

Reading List of Books for Healthcare Managers 419

Index 421

About the Editors 439

About the Contributors 441

PREFACE TO THE NINTH EDITION

*H*ealth Services Management: Readings, Cases, and Commentary is distinctive in its overview of management and organizational behavior theory. The book is organized in a framework that begins with those parts of work over which managers have the greatest control—the manager himself or herself and control systems—then extends to cover parts of the work over which managers have a good deal of control (at least over the short run)—organizational design and professional integration—and concludes with those parts of the work over which managers have less control—adaptation, including implementation of strategy, and accountability to interests that supply the organization with resources. Throughout there is an emphasis on the case method approach to teaching healthcare management.

The cases take place in a variety of organizations, including a faculty practice, a neighborhood health center, a small rural hospital, an HMO, a multi-hospital health system, a medical group, an academic medical center, a home health organization, a visiting nurse association, and a number of community hospitals.

An instructor's manual is available online that includes suggested syllabi, approaches for discussing several topics in each part—for example, on the role of the manager, suggested topics include history of the manager's role in healthcare, organizational settings here and abroad, and career planning for managers in healthcare—and teaching notes for the case studies, the great majority of which have been classroom-tested. For information about the online instructor's materials, please email hap1@ache.org.

We wrote and edited *Health Services Management: Readings, Cases, and Commentary* with the idea that it will be used as a stand-alone textbook, but it can also be used as a complement to other textbooks. For this edition, we have again presented a single textbook of readings, cases, and commentary, for the following reasons: (1) less expense for the student; (2) facilitation of course use of other textbooks; and (3) availability of the readings on the Internet, which means they don't have to be included in the textbook (although we include at least one reading for each of the text's six parts). A note for students on how to retrieve journal articles through the Internet is included in the text. This book can still be viewed as a casebook, but also includes suggested readings.

Some things have not changed through the nine editions of this text (this is now the 30th year of writing these books). The first has been the desire to have readings that build on good evidence rather than just opinion. At first, this goal was hard to achieve because of the thinness of the literature. Now it is hard to choose among many good papers. Second has been our goal to link theory with practice—to build a bridge between the social science literature and the actual work of improvement. Third, the text has always been divided into six sections—the role of the manager, control, organizational design, professional integration, adaptability, and accountability—each with a commentary.

We welcome dialogue with our readers and can be reached via e-mail at:

Anthony R. Kovner   anthony.kovner@nyu.edu
Ann Scheck McAlearney   mcalearney.1@osu.edu
Duncan Neuhauser   duncan.neuhauser@case.edu

A SHORT HISTORY OF THE CASE METHOD OF TEACHING

Karen Schachter Weingrod and Duncan Neuhauser

Teaching by example is no doubt as old as the first parent and child. In medicine it surely started with a healer, the first apprentice, and a patient. University education in medicine started about 800 years ago, focused on abstract principles and scholastic reasoning, and was removed from practicality. In the late 1700s in France, medical education moved into hospitals or "the clinic," where patients in large numbers could be observed, autopsies performed, and the physiological state linked back to the patients' signs and symptoms (Foucault 1973). This was one step in the departure from the abstract medical theorizing in universities (often about the "four humours"), which may have had no bearing on actual disease processes.

Education in law also became increasingly abstract, conveyed through the erudite lecture. It built theoretical constructs and was logically well reasoned. The professor spoke and the student memorized and recited without much opportunity for practical experience or discussion. This had become the standard by the late 1850s.

It is only by comparison with what went on before in universities that the case method of teaching represented such a striking change. The historical development of the case method can be traced to Harvard University. Perhaps it is not surprising that this change occurred in the United States rather than in Europe, with the American inclinations toward democratic equality, practicality, and positivism, and the lack of interest in classic abstract theorizing.

The change started in 1870 when the president of Harvard University, Charles William Eliot, appointed the obscure lawyer Christopher Columbus Langdell as dean of the Harvard Law School.

Langdell believed law to be a science. In his own words: "Law considered as a science, consists of certain principles or doctrines. To have such a mastery of these as to be able to apply them with constant faculty and certainty to the ever-tangled skein of human affairs, is what constitutes a good lawyer; and hence to acquire that mastery should be the business of every earnest student of the law" (Langdell 1967).

The specimens needed for the study of Langdell's science of law were judicial opinions as recorded in books and stored in libraries. He accepted the science of law, but he turned the learning process back to front. Instead of giving a lecture that would define a principle of law and give supporting examples of judicial opinions, he gave the students the judicial opinions without the principle and by use of a Socratic dialogue extracted from the students in the classroom the principles that would make sense out of the cases. The student role was now active rather than passive. Students were subjected to rigorous questioning of the case material. They were asked to defend their judgments and to confess to error when their judgments were illogical. Although this dialectic was carried on by the professor and one or two students at a time, all of the students learned and were on the edge of their seats, fearing or hoping they would be called on next. The law school style that evolved has put the student under public pressure to reason quickly, clearly, and coherently in a way that is valuable in the courtroom or during negotiation. After a discouraging start, Langdell attracted such able instructors as Oliver Wendell Holmes, Jr. They carried the day, and now the case method of teaching is nearly universal in American law schools.

The introduction of the case method of teaching to medicine is also known. A Harvard medical student of the class of 1901, Walter B. Cannon, shared a room with Harry Bigelow, a third-year law student. The excitement with which Bigelow and his classmates debated the issues within the cases they were reading for class contrasted sharply with the passivity of medical school lectures.

In 1900, discussing the value of the case method in medicine, Harvard President Charles Eliot (1900) described the earlier medical education as follows:

> I think it was thirty-five years ago that I was a lecturer at the Harvard Medical School for one winter; at that time lectures began in the school at eight o'clock in the morning and went on steadily till two o'clock—six mortal hours, one after the other of lectures, without a question from the professor, without the possibility of an observation by the student, none whatever, just the lecture to be listened to, and possibly taken notes of. Some of the students could hardly write.

In December 1899, Cannon persuaded one of his instructors, G. L. Walton, to present one of the cases in written form from his private practice as an experiment. Walton printed a sheet with the patient's history and allowed the students a week to study it. The lively discussion that ensued in class made Walton an immediate convert (Benison, Barger, and Wolfe 1987). Other faculty soon followed, including Richard C. Cabot.

Through the case method, medical students would learn to judge and interpret clinical data, to estimate the value of evidence, and to recognize the gaps in their knowledge—something that straight lecturing could never reveal. The case method of teaching allowed students to throw off passivity in the lecture hall and integrate their knowledge of anatomy, physiology, pathology, and therapeutics into a unified mode of thought.

As a student, Cannon (1900) wrote two articles about the case method in 1900 for the *Boston Medical and Surgical Journal* (later to become *The New England Journal of Medicine*). He sent a copy of one of these papers to the famous clinician professor Dr. William Osler of Johns Hopkins University. Osler replied, "I have long held that the only possible way of teaching students the subject of medicine is by personal daily contact with cases, which they study not only once or twice, but follow systematically" (Benison, Barger, and Wolfe 1987). If a written medical case was interesting, a real live patient in the classroom could be memorable. Osler regularly introduced patients to his class and asked students to interview and examine the patient and discuss the medical problems involved. He would regularly send students to the library and laboratory to seek answers and report back to the rest of the class (Chesney 1958). This is ideal teaching. Osler's students worshipped him, but with today's division of labor in medicine between basic science and clinical medicine, such a synthesis is close to impossible.

The May 24, 1900, issue of the *Boston Medical and Surgical Journal* was devoted to articles and comments by Eliot, Cannon, Cabot, and others about the case method of teaching. In some ways this journal issue remains the best general discussion of the case method. This approach was adopted rapidly at other medical schools, and books of written cases quickly followed in neurology (1902), surgery (1904), and orthopedic surgery (1905) (Benison, Barger, and Wolfe 1987).

Cannon went on to a distinguished career in medical research. Cabot joined the medical staff of the Massachusetts General Hospital, and in 1906 published his first book of cases. (He also introduced the first social worker into a hospital[1] [Benison, Barger, and Wolfe 1987].) He was concerned about the undesirable separation of clinical physicians and pathologists; too many diagnoses were turning out to be false at autopsy. To remedy this, Cabot began to hold his case exercises with students, house officers, and visitors.

Cabot's clinical/pathological conferences took on a stereotypical style and eventually were adopted in teaching hospitals throughout the world. First, the patient's history, symptoms, and test results would be described. Then an invited specialist would discuss the case, suggest an explanation, and give a diagnosis. Finally, the pathologist would present the autopsy or pathological diagnosis and questions would follow to elaborate points.

In 1915, Cabot sent written copies of his cases to interested physicians as "at home case method exercises." These became so popular that in 1923 the *Boston Medical and Surgical Journal* began to publish one per issue, starting with the October 1923 issue. This journal has since changed its name to *The New England Journal of Medicine*, but the "Cabot Case Records" still appear with each issue.

A look at a current *New England Journal of Medicine* case will show how much the case method has changed since Langdell's original concept. The student or house officer is no longer asked to discuss the case; rather, it is the expert who puts her reputation on the line. She has the opportunity to demonstrate wisdom, but can also be refuted in front of a large audience. Although every physician in the audience probably makes mental diagnoses, the case presentation has become a passive affair, like a lecture.

Cabot left the Massachusetts General Hospital to head the Social Relations (sociology, psychology, cultural anthropology) department at Harvard. He brought the case method with him, but it disappeared from use there by the time of his death in 1939 (Buck 1965). The social science disciplines were concerned with theory building, hypothesis testing, and research methodology, and to such "unapplied" pure scientists perhaps the case method was considered primitive. Further, the use of the case method of teaching also diminished in the first two preclinical years of medical school as clinical scientists came more and more to the fore with their laboratory work and research on physiology, pharmacology, biochemistry, and molecular biology. Today problem-solving learning in medical schools is widespread and replacing the passive learning of traditional lectures.

In 1908, the Harvard Business School was created as a department of the Graduate School of Arts and Sciences. It was initially criticized as merely a school for "successful money-making." Early on an effort was made to teach through the use of written problems involving situations faced by actual business executives, presented in sufficient factual detail to enable students to develop their own decisions. The school's first book of cases, on marketing, was published in 1922 by Melvin T. Copeland.[2] Today nearly every class in the Harvard Business School is taught by the case method.

Unlike the law school, where cases come directly from judicial decisions (sometimes abbreviated by the instructor) and the medical school, where the patient is the basis for the case, the business faculty and their aides must enter organizations to collect and compile their material. This latter mode of selection offers substantial editorial latitude. Here more than elsewhere the case writer's vision, or lack of it, defines the content of the case.

Unlike a pathologist's autopsy diagnosis, a business case is not designed to have a right answer. In fact, one usually never knows whether the business in question lives or dies. Rather, the cases are written in a way that splits a large class (up to 80 students) into factions. The best cases are those that create divergent opinions; the professor becomes more an orchestra leader than a source of truth. The professor's opinion or answer may never be made explicit. Following a discussion, a student's question related to what really happened or what should have been done may be answered, "I don't know" or "I think the key issues were picked up in the case discussion." Such hesitancy on the part of the instructor is often desirable. To praise or condemn a particular faction in the classroom can discourage future discussions.

William Ellet (2007) defines a business school case as describing a real situation with three characteristics: "A significant business issue or issues, significant information on which to base conclusions and having no stated conclusions." A good case allows the reader to construct conclusions, filter out irrelevant information, furnish missing information through inference, and combine evidence from different parts of the case to support the conclusions.

The class atmosphere in a business school is likely to be less pressured than in a law school. Like a good surgeon, a good lawyer must often think very quickly, but unlike the surgeon his thinking is demonstrated verbally and publicly. He must persuade by the power of his logic rather than by force of authority. Business and management are different. Key managerial decisions—What business are we in? Who are our customers? Where should we be ten years from now?—may take months or even years to answer.

The fact that the business manager's time frame reduces the pressure for immediate answers makes management education different from physician education in other ways. Physicians are required to absorb countless facts on anatomy, disease symptoms, and drug side effects. Confronted with 20 patients a day, the physician often has no time, even over the Internet, to consult references. The manager has a longer time horizon for decision making in business. Therefore, managerial education focuses more on problem-solving techniques than does standard medical education.

Not all business schools have endorsed the case method of teaching. Some schools focus on teaching the "science" of economics, human behavior, and operations research. The faculty are concerned with theory building, hypothesis testing, statistical methodology, and the social sciences. Some business schools use about half social sciences and half case method. Each school is convinced that its teaching philosophy is best. Conceptually, the debate can be broken into two aspects: science versus professionalism, and active versus passive learning.

There is little question that active student involvement in learning is better than passive listening to lectures. The case method is one of many approaches to increasing student participation. Student written reports are another form of active learning.

Academic science is not overly concerned with the practical problems of the world, but professionals are and professional education should be. The lawyer, physician, and manager cannot wait for perfect knowledge; they have to make decisions in the face of uncertainty. Science can help with these decisions to varying degrees. To the extent that scientific theories have the power to predict and explain, they can be used by professionals. In the jargon of statistics: the higher the percentage of variance explained, the more useful the scientific theory, the smaller the role for clinical or professional judgment, and the lesser the role for case method teaching as opposed to, for example, mathematical problem solving.

It can be argued that the professional will always be working at the frontier of the limits of scientific prediction. When science is the perfect predictor, then often the problem is solved, or the application is delegated to computers or technicians, or, as in some branches of engineering, professional skills focus on the manipulation of accurate but complex mathematical equations.

Scientific medicine now understands smallpox so well that it no longer exists. Physicians spend most of their time on problems that are not solved: cancer, heart disease, or the common complaints of living that bring most people to doctors. In management, the budget cycle, personnel position control, sterile operating room environment, and maintenance of the business office ledgers are handled routinely by organizational members and usually do not consume the attention of the chief executive officer. In law, the known formulations become the "boilerplate" of contracts.

The debate between business schools over the use of cases illustrates the difference in belief in the power of the social sciences in the business environment. Teaching modes related to science and judgment will always be in uneasy balance with each other, shifting with time and place. Innovative medical schools have moved away from the scientific lectures of the preclinical years and toward a case problem–solving mode. On the other side of the coin, a quiet revolution is being waged in clinical reasoning. The principles of statistics, epidemiology, and economics, filtered through the techniques of decision analysis, cost-effectiveness analysis, computer modeling, and artificial intelligence, are making the Cabot Case Record approach obsolete for clinical reasoning. Scientific methods of clinical reasoning are beginning to replace aspects of professional or clinical judgment in medicine (Barnes, Christensen, and Hansen 1994).

This does not mean that the professional aspect of medicine will be eliminated by computer-based science. Rather, the frontiers, the unknown areas calling for professional judgment, will shift to new areas, such as the development of socio-emotional rapport with patients—what used to be called "the bedside manner."[3]

The cases that make up this book are derived from the business school style of case teaching. As such they do not have answers. The cases can be used to apply management concepts to practical problems; however, these concepts (scientific theory seems too strong a term to apply to them) may help solve these case problems but will not yield the one "right" answer. They all leave much room for debate.

Notes

1. Although not the first hospital-based social worker to work with Cabot, his best-known social worker colleague was Walter Cannon's sister, Ida Cannon.
2. For more on the history of the case method of teaching managers, see Roy Penchansky, *Health Services Administration: Policy Cases and the Case Method* (Boston: Harvard University Press, 1968), pp. 395–453.
3. A proposal to increase the problem-solving content of medical education is found in Association of American Medical Colleges, *Graduate Medical Education: Proposals for the Eighties* (Washington, DC: AAMC, 1980). This is also reprinted as a supplement in *Journal of Medical Education* 56, no. 9 (September 1981), part 2.

References

Barnes, L. B., C. R. Christensen, and A. J. Hansen. 1994. *Teaching and the Case Method*, 3rd edition. Boston: Harvard Business School Press.

Benison, S., A. C. Barger, and E. L. Wolfe. 1987. *Walter B. Cannon: The Life and Times of a Young Scientist* pp. 65–75, 417–18. Cambridge, MA: Harvard University Press.

Buck, P. (ed.) 1965. *The Social Sciences at Harvard*. Boston: Harvard University Press.

Cannon, W. B. 1900. "The Case Method of Teaching Systematic Medicare." *Boston Medical and Surgical Journal* 142 (2): 31–36; and "The Case System in Medicine." *Boston Medical and Surgical Journal* 142 (22): 563–64.

Chesney, A. M. 1958. *The Johns Hopkins Hospital and the Johns Hopkins University School of Medicine*, vol. 11, 1893–1905, 125–28. Baltimore, MD: The Johns Hopkins Press.

Eliot, C. 1900. "The Inductive Method Applied to Medicine." *Boston Medical and Surgical Journal* 142 (22): 557.

Ellet, W. 2007. *The Case Study Handbook*. Boston: Harvard Business School Press.

Foucault, M. 1973. *The Birth of the Clinic*. New York: Vintage.

Langdell, C. C. 1967. *Cases and Contracts* (1871), cited in *The Law at Harvard*, 174. Cambridge, MA: Harvard University Press.

LEARNING THROUGH THE CASE METHOD

Anthony R. Kovner

A "case" is a description of a situation or problem facing a manager that requires analysis, decision, and planning a course of action. A decision may be to delay a decision, and a planned course of action may be to take no action. A case takes place in time. A case must have an issue. As McNair says, "there must be a question of what somebody should do, what somebody should have done, who is to blame for the situation, what is the best decision to be made under the circumstances" (Towl 1969). A case represents selected details about a situation; it represents selection by the case writer.

The case method involves class discussion that is guided by a teacher so that students can diagnose and define important problems in a situation, acquire competence in developing useful alternatives to respond to such problems, and improve judgment in selecting action alternatives. Students learn to diagnose constraints and opportunities faced by the manager in implementation and to overcome constraints such as limited time and dollars.

As Ellet (2007) points out, "you have to read a case actively and construct your own meaning." Students should consider what the situation is, what the manager has to know about the situation, and what the manager's working hypothesis is. Can the problem be defined differently? What's the biggest downside of the recommended decision? Has the student been objective and thorough about the evaluative findings that do not jibe with the overall assessment?

Students often have difficulty adjusting to a classroom without an authority figure, without lectures from which to take notes, and in which little information is offered by the teacher, at least until the class discussion has ended. Some students find it irritating to have to listen to their peers when they are paying to learn what the teacher has to say.

Students must learn to take responsibility for their own view of a case, to develop an argument that they can explain, and to listen to others who disagree. Students should speak up early. To learn to be a good participant, students must participate. When students go to the classroom, they should be familiar with the information in the case, have a conclusion about the main issue, have evidence explaining why their conclusion is reasonable, and show they have thought about other conclusions. It is suggested that students spend at least two hours preparing for case discussion.

In a case course, students are often asked to adopt the perspectives of certain characters in the case, to play certain roles. To deny someone or persuade someone requires an understanding of the needs and perceptions of others. Role-playing can promote a better understanding of viewpoints that otherwise may seem irrational. Students can better understand their own values and underlying assumptions when their opinions are challenged by peers and teachers.

To conclude, it is important to understand what a case is not and what case method cannot teach. Cases are not real life—they present only part of a situation. Writing or communicating a case may be as difficult as or more difficult than evaluating someone else's written case. Like many a consultant, the student can never see the results—what would have happened if the case participants had followed his advice.

Some aspects of management can be learned only by managing. How else can one understand when someone says one thing but means another? How else can one judge whether to confront or oppose a member of the ruling coalition when that member's behavior appears to threaten the long-range interests of the organization? Students and managers have to form and adopt their own value systems and make their own decisions. A case course can give students a better understanding of the nature of the role they will be playing as managers—an understanding that can help them to manage better, if not well.

References

Ellet, W. 2007. *The Case Study Handbook*. Boston: Harvard Business School Press.

Towl, R. 1969. *To Study Administration*, 67. Boston: Graduate School of Business Administration, Harvard University.

HOW TO RETRIEVE JOURNAL ARTICLES FROM THE INTERNET—A GUIDE FOR STUDENTS

Many of the journal articles referenced in this text may be easily accessed and printed from the Internet free of charge, presupposing the publisher has granted your school library access to its electronic archives. The following steps are intended to guide one through the process of locating, viewing, and printing journal articles from the Internet.

1. Access your school library homepage. If you do not know the web address of your school library homepage, you can probably find a link to it on your school's homepage.
2. Locate the directory of electronic journals to which your school library subscribes. Many library homepages display a link to "Electronic Journals and Texts" or "E-Journals and Texts" or the like. If so, click on this link. If the link is not on the homepage, try searching for the directory in areas such as "research," "databases and catalogs," or "journals."
3. Locate the directory that is likely to contain the journal you are looking for. The journal directories are often stratified according to broad subject areas. For instance, if you are looking for an article in the *Harvard Business Review,* click on the "Business" directory heading. Likewise, an article in *Health Care Management Review* would be found by clicking on the "Medicine and Health" directory heading.
4. Locate and click on the journal title in the directory. Some directories offer an option to search for the journal using a key word in the title. Otherwise, find the journal title according to the first letter in the title. If you do not see the journal title you are looking for, either the publisher has not made an electronic version of the journal available or your school's library does not subscribe to the journal. (However, this does not mean that the paper version is not available in the library.)

5. Choose and click on the volume and issue number of the journal that contains the article. A table of contents of that issue will appear. Occasionally, issues may not be included in the archive because they are either too old or too new.

6. Choose and click on the article you wish to print. The article will appear.

7. Print the article by clicking on your web browser's Print button or by choosing "Print" from the File menu.

OVERVIEW

> Why do we do what we do?
> How do we know it works?
> How can we do it better?
> —*John Bingham, Twin Falls, Idaho*

Creating and maintaining a health services organization in which these three questions are constantly asked and answered is the role of the health services manager. This book, in its nine editions, has attempted to select from the best current literature on health services management to help learners understand the role of the manager, organizational design and control, the blending of organization and health professionals, change (adaptation), and responsiveness (accountability). The central focus is on the role of health services managers and how they modify and maintain an organization within its context. The organizations described include hospitals, nursing homes, ambulatory care, HMOs, and integrated delivery systems, which may combine many of these components.

Levels and Issues

The role of managers can be conceptualized in many different ways according to what they need to know and what they do.

The manager's role can be categorized by listing knowledge areas for the general managers, as seen in Figure 1, which lists 12 areas (Boyatzis et al. 1995). This general knowledge needs to be applied in a specific management context, in this case health services.

An organization such as a hospital, a group practice, or a nursing home can also be conceptualized in many different ways. One can use an organization chart; draw sociometric diagrams; indicate the flow of production based on inputs, process, and outputs; write its history; describe its key policies; and so forth. Each of these is appropriate, depending on the questions being asked. We use the following conceptualization.

The organization can be viewed as a set of concentric rings (see Figure 2). At the center is the senior manager and his or her role, in the immediate managerial context (the manager). In the second ring going outward, the

FIGURE 1
Knowledge
Areas for
General
Management

Knowledge Area	Relevant Part of This Book
1. Organizational behavior 2. Labor and human resource policy	I. Role of the Manager
3. Accounting 4. Management statistics 5. Information and decision systems 6. Operation research 7. Operations management	II. Control
8. Organization design theory	III. Organizational Design
9. Marketing 10. Finance 11. Economics	IV. Professional Integration V. Adaptation
12. Policy, law, ethics	VI. Accountability

All the above need to be used within the specific features of health services.

SOURCE: Modified from Boyatzis et al. (1995).

manager works to design the structure of the organization, to specify procedures, to use resources, and to provide a feedback mechanism to evaluate performance (control and organizational design). The third ring (professional integration) represents the interaction between management and professional members of the organization, including physicians. The fourth ring (adaptation) is concerned with how the organization can and must respond to fit its present and future environments. The fifth ring (accountability) signifies how the environment imposes requirements for responsiveness on the organization (Sutermeister 1969).

Figure 2 makes the manager the "sun" in a heliocentric view of the organization. Although another diagrammatic perspective would be used if this were a book for patients, physicians, or trustees, we use this particular conceptualization because our book is written for those who are, or wish to be, health services managers. However, we do not deny the usefulness of other ways of viewing the organization.

The outline of this book follows the form of Figure 2, starting from the center and moving outward. The parts, described below, focus on key problems and issues at each level in the organization.

Part I, "The Role of the Manager," is concerned with the immediate context within which managers work, how they spend their time, the importance of judgment, the kinds of problems they are challenged by, and the opportunities and constraints they face in implementing change and sustaining the organization.

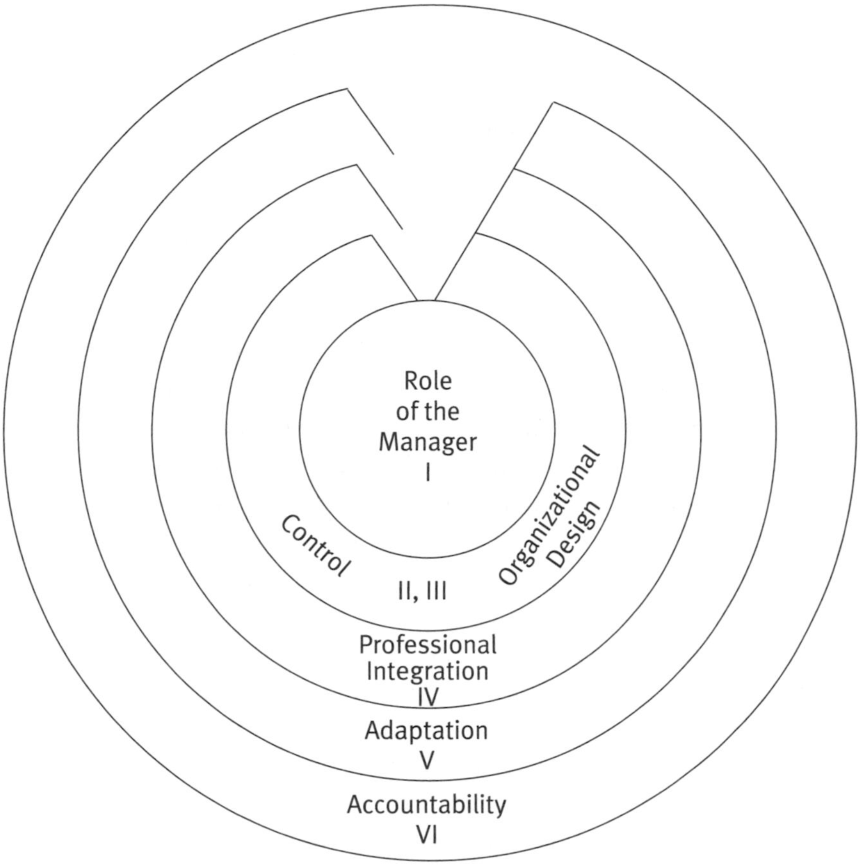

FIGURE 2
Manager,
Organization,
and
Environment

Role
of the
Manager
I

Control

Organizational
Design

II, III

Professional
Integration
IV

Adaptation
V

Accountability
VI

Part of Book	Key Issues	Organizational Space	Activity and Mind-Set
I	Role of the Manager	The manager	Managing self (reflection)
			Managing relationships (collaborative)
II, III	Control, Organizational Design	Management, internal organization	Managing the organization (analytic)
IV	Professional Integration	Internal organization	
V	Adaptation	Organization, environment	Managing change (action)
VI	Accountability	Environment, organization	Managing external (worldly) context

SOURCE: Mintzberg and Gosling (2002).

Parts II and III cover "Control" and "Organizational Design." In large organizations, managers cannot work face-to-face with all employees. Rather, they must specify their activities indirectly, relying on other managers, formal rules, hierarchy, budgets, information systems, and impersonal techniques for control and evaluation. Managers will be successful to different degrees in structuring and monitoring the organization to achieve their view of organizational purpose.

Similarly, organization members will respond to these efforts in various ways with independent actions, resistance, or cooperation. A critical problem is the degree to which professionals, especially physicians, are integrated into the organization. This is addressed in Part IV, "Professional Integration."

Managers must adapt both to changes in the organization's internal structure and function and to the organization's specific environment, as discussed in Part V, "Adaptation." Managers must be accountable to the community or publics served, as indicated in the readings in Part VI, "Accountability." These last two parts are concerned with the health services organization's interface with suppliers of needed resources such as manpower, funding, legitimacy, and information.

At the center of the circle, managers are able to influence what happens. Moving toward the periphery, their influence steadily declines and is replaced by other forces. This is shown schematically in Figure 3, where managers' influence flows in diminishing strength from left to right. The influence of others (government, patients, professionals, employees, co-managers, and so on) flows with diminishing strength from right to left. The slope and height of the diagonal line, reflecting the balance of these forces, should be viewed as variable through time and dependent on the manager, the organization, and the environment.

Figure 4 presents, in an oversimplified way, examples of issues and problems at various levels of the organization that are within or outside the manager's sphere of influence. A more accurate representation would indicate

FIGURE 3

The Flow of Influence Within a Health Services Organization

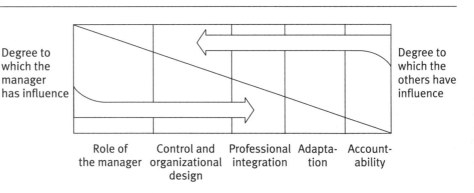

Degree to which the manager has influence

Degree to which the others have influence

Role of the manager | Control and organizational design | Professional integration | Adaptation | Accountability

FIGURE 4

Degree to which manager can influence activities →

Level	Can influence	Cannot influence
I Role of the Manager	Leadership style How the manager spends his or her time What the manager does Whom the manager talks to The management team Who they are What they do	Manager's personality and previous experience Limits of the manager's capacity Authority of office Actions of trustees
II, III Control, Organizational Design	Structure of organization Procedures Resources Information systems Incentive systems Scope of services provided	Resource limits Technological imperatives Information overload Delays, distortions
IV Professional Integration	Labor relations Morale Skill mix of staff Personnel policies Level of conflict	Values of staff Historical organizational structure Professional organizations, unions Informal groups
V Adaptation	Community perception Funding Workforce supply	Social history Competition Government regulations
IV General environment (accountability)	Health behavior	Socioeconomics Prevalence of illness Value systems

← Degree to which manager cannot influence activities →

Examples of Issues and Problems Associated with Different Levels of the Organization

that each of these issues and problems is more or less influenced by the manager at different times and to varying degrees in certain types of organizations facing certain types of environments.

Managers have most control over the structure and function of their own office (the role of the manager). They also exert some control over the authority of their office and the actions of their co-managers and trustees. They can, to a considerable extent, decide how to spend their time, what problems to address and in what order, who should be on the management team and what they should do, and so forth. However, managers' experience, work background, physical capacity, and personality are to some degree fixed and beyond their ability to change.

At the next level, managers can impose structure and specify control and information systems, but only within the limits of resource availability and technological imperatives. Information and control systems cannot be complete, exhaustive, or immediate in their effects; they are not error-free and are often costly in terms of money and managerial time.

Managers' design and control efforts will be met with different levels of acceptance by workers, professionals, and patients, all of whom sometimes act independently of, and are at odds with, managers. Often managers can do little to change the attitudes of physicians, union officials, and patients.

At the environmental level, managers have some modest influence on legislation, regulation, third-party financing, community values, and other organizations' actions. However, much of the specific behavior of groups and organizations in their environment, and most of the general environment as well, is beyond the control or influence of a manager.

Skills representative of a good manager are summarized in Figure 5. Boyatzis and colleagues (1995) list these as "subthemes" under the overall leadership goal of "creating economic, intellectual, and human value." These subthemes have been reorganized in Figure 5 to align them with the six parts of this book.

The role all managers have is to directly supervise a team of people. This requires supervisory skills at a face-to-face level. A list of these skills is shown in Figure 6 (McConnell 1992).

Griffith and White (2007), in their book *The Well-Managed Health-care Organization*, create another classification of health services management knowledge and skills. They organize this book under three large managerial objectives of governing, caring, and learning. For Griffith and White, governing consists of making the health services organization responsive to its environment. Caring means building a high-quality clinical service, and learning inte-

FIGURE 5
Skills of the
Good Manager

Part	Issue	Skills of the Good Manager
I	Role of the Manager	Understand oneself Be a leader and team member
II	Control	Innovate in the use of information
III	Organizational Design	Innovate in the use of technology
IV	Professional Integration	Stimulate professional integrity
V	Adaptation	Manage change in a complex, diverse, and interdependent world
VI	Accountability	Show integrity and social responsibility

FIGURE 6
The Role of
the Manager

Supervisory Skills	
Supervisory Skills and Domains	*Relevant Content*
Leadership style	Self-awareness, delegation, participatory management, constancy of purpose
Communication	Verbal, non-verbal, written
Time management	
Continuing education	For self and team members
Motivation	
Measurement and appraisal of team-member performance	Performance reviews
Human resource policies	Hiring, pay raises, dismissed union agreements, coping with the problem or troubled employee Personnel rules
Creating a positive work environment	Morale, praise, criticism, motivation, justice, fairness
Running effective meetings	
Budgeting	
Knowledge of relevant laws	
Ability to use relevant technology appropriately	Knowledge of the work of the department
Management of change	Understanding customer needs, planning, quality improvement
Decision making, analytic reasoning	System thinking, quantitative analysis, social objectivity

grates meeting, planning, marketing, finance, and information needs. Griffith and White's typology is matched to the structure of this book in Figure 7.

The terms continuous quality improvement (CQI), total quality management, and quality improvement are often used interchangeably in North America, although they mean different things to some people. These ideas are defined in at least three ways. One is by the writings of Walter Shewhart, W. Edwards Deming, Joseph Juran, and like-minded thinkers, which concern reducing variation in standard operations processes. A second way defines CQI as a way to answer these three questions: Why do we do what we do? How do we know it works? How can we do it better? The third definition is very similar to the second, promoting customer-mindedness, statistical-mindedness, and organizational transformation.

Customer-mindedness (accountability) focuses on meeting customer needs and desires. In the health field this has led to asking such questions as, "What is good care for people with high blood pressure or asthma in the population we serve?" It has led to increased use of patient satisfaction

FIGURE 7
Organizational
Conceptual
Frameworks

Griffith/White	Kovner/McAlearney/Neuhauser
Governing, Relating to the Environment	Accountability, Role of the Manager
The Caring Organization	Organizational Design, Professional Integration
Learning: Meeting Support Needs	Control, Adaptation
Quality Improvement	

surveys and their comparison across hospitals. Statistical-mindedness is concerned with measurement throughout the organization to understand processes, outcomes, and variation in those outcomes. What percent of inpatient meals are cold when eaten and why? Reducing variation (fewer cold meals) is an example of process improvement by reduction in variation, which can be seen as improving organizational control through improved design.

Organizational transformation occurs through managerial leadership (adaptation). Leading this change is central to the role of the manager and requires defining a clear mission, encouraging everyone to work on improvement, and creating a climate free of fear. How can everyone in a health services organization join in this common effort (professional integration)? The answer is related to what Peter Senge (1990) describes as a learning organization in which people change behavior after reflecting on their experience.

CQI is also described by reference to Deming's (1982) 14 points (see Figure 8). Behind these points are a number of assumptions. Production is a process with inherent variation. Understanding the causes of variation and changing the process to reduce variation will result in improved quality. Changing the way meals get from kitchen to patient rooms could reduce the number of cold meals. Inspection, fear, quotas, and slogans will not help—education, pride of workmanship, teamwork, participation, and leadership will. All this transformation is intended to better meet the needs and wishes of those we serve.

Despite the fact that the active use of CQI methods in health services is less than 25 years old, it is now a worldwide movement.

Performance Requirements

All organizations can be described as having four performance requirements: goal attainment, system maintenance, adaptive capability, and values integration (Mouzelis 1971).

Goal attainment is the requirement that organizations achieve at least enough of their goals to justify their support. The care has to be good enough for patients to come. The earnings have to be large enough to replace capital over time and to ensure money to meet the payroll.

FIGURE 8

Deming's 14
Points

Book Part	Issue	Deming's Points
I	Role of the Manager	(1) Create constancy of purpose for improvement of product and service (2) Adopt the new philosophy of quality improvement (7) Institute leadership
II	Control	(3) Cease reliance on inspection (10) Eliminate slogans and (11) quotas (4) Do not award business on price alone
III	Organizational Design	(5) Improve constantly and forever the process for planning, production, and service
IV	Professional Integration	(6) Institute on-the-job training (continuing education) (8) Drive out fear (9) Break down barriers between staff areas (teamwork) (12) Encourage pride of workmanship
V	Adaptation	(5) Improve constantly (13) Promote education and self-improvement for everyone (14) Put everyone in the organization to work to accomplish this transformation
VI	Accountability	All 14 points drive to better meeting the needs and wishes of those we serve.

System maintenance concerns organizational performance in self-renewal. Are the organization's members and suppliers stable over time, or are these relationships in the process of disintegrating? System maintenance includes the degree to which revenues match expenses, new staff match departing staff, deteriorating equipment is replaced, and incentive systems are appropriate to the level of effort required. It includes the maintenance of rules, procedures, and information systems. Alternative terms for system maintenance are *integration*, *structure*, *stability*, and *homeostasis*.

Adaptive capability involves organizational performance in changing to meet and cope with new conditions. Organizations must be innovative (proactive) and responsive (reactive). One indicator of adaptive capability is the presence or absence of specialized units that are primarily concerned with this function, such as strategic planning groups. Change is necessary for the organization to continue to survive and achieve its goals. Other terms specifying adaptive capability include *change orientation* and *organizational responsiveness*.

Values integration deals with organizational performance relative to congruence of the values of organizational members with the organization's goals and of organizational values with larger societal values—for example, the extent to which management and health services professionals are committed to the ideals of high-quality care, team effort, compassion, and continuing education. To the extent that the values of personnel are consistent with organizational goals, there may be less misuse of organizational resources. To the extent that organizational goals are consistent with societal goals, the organization may find it has higher prestige and access to more resources (Etzioni 1961). The concept of "corporate culture" has received a lot of attention. The specific cultures of different organizations have been described, in particular how they relate to goal attainment and innovation. Hospitals and medical centers often have strong cultures built on long histories, religious traditions, and notable individuals.

Conclusion

Organizations and their management can be described in many ways. Good management practices and organization survival skills are such perennially popular topics that new books fill whole shelves in local bookstores. This book uses several classifications. The first defines the six parts of this book: the role of the manager, control, organizational design, professional integration, adaptation, and accountability. Of these, professional integration is a distinctive emphasis for the health field because of the prominent semi-independent nature of the many highly skilled professionals who play important roles in care.

A second classification used here is goal attainment, system maintenance, adaptive capability, and values integration.

A third way of looking at organizations is through quality improvement, which focuses on systems thinking. Customer-mindedness, statistical-mindedness and organizational transformation are concepts that can focus our understanding.

This overview has introduced these classifications and linked them to others, particularly in the figures. With these ways to organize one's thoughts about health services organizations, the reader is ready to proceed to the readings, cases, and commentary that follow in this ninth edition of this book.

References

Boyatzis, R. E., S. S. Cowen, D. A. Kolb, and Associates. 1995. *Innovation in Professional Education*. San Francisco: Jossey-Bass.

Deming, W. E. 1982. *Out of the Crisis.* Cambridge, MA: Massachusetts Institute of Technology, Center for Advanced Engineering Study.

Etzioni, A. 1961. *A Comparative Analysis of Complex Organizations.* New York: Free Press.

Griffith, J. R., and K. R. White. 2007. *The Well-Managed Healthcare Organization,* 6th edition. Chicago: Health Administration Press.

McConnell, C. 1992. *The Effective Healthcare Supervisor.* Rockville, MD: Aspen Publishers.

Mintzberg, H., and J. Gosling. 2002. "Educating Managers Beyond Borders." *Academy of Management Learning and Education* 1 (1): 64–76.

Mouzelis, N. 1971. *Organization and Bureaucracy.* Chicago: Aldine.

Senge, P. 1990. *The Fifth Discipline.* New York: Doubleday.

Sutermeister, R. A. 1969. *People and Productivity,* 2nd edition. New York: McGraw-Hill.

Selected Bibliography

Argyris, C. *Knowledge for Action: A Guide to Overcoming Barriers to Organizational Change.* San Francisco: Jossey-Bass, 1993.

Barnard, C. *Functions of the Executive.* Cambridge, MA: Harvard University Press, 1964.

Bass, B. M. *Leadership and Performance Beyond Expectations.* New York: The Free Press, 1985.

Becker, S., and D. Neuhauser. *Organizational Efficiency.* New York: Elsevier, North Holland, 1975.

Berwick, D. M., A. B. Godfrey, and J. Roessner. *Curing Health Care.* San Francisco: Jossey-Bass, 1990.

Bolman, L., and T. Deal. *Modern Approaches to Understanding and Managing Organizations.* San Francisco: Jossey-Bass, 1990.

Boyatzis, R. E., S. S. Cowen, D. A. Kolb, and Associates. *Innovation in Professional Education.* San Francisco: Jossey-Bass, 1995.

Caplow, T. *Principles of Organization.* New York: Harcourt, Brace & World, 1964.

Deal, T. E., and A. A. Kennedy. *Corporate Cultures.* Reading, MA: Addison-Wesley, 1982.

Deming, W. E. *Out of the Crisis.* Cambridge, MA: Massachusetts Institute of Technology, Center for Advanced Engineering Study, 1982.

Drucker, P. F. *Managing the Non-Profit Organization.* New York: Harper Collins, 1990.

Feldstein, P. *Health Policy Issues: An Economic Perspective,* 4th edition. Chicago: Health Administration Press, 2003.

Glouberman, S., and H. Mintzberg. "Managing the Care of the Health and the Cure of Disease—Part I: Differentiating." *Health Care Management Review* Winter 2001, pp. 56–59.

Glouberman, S., and H. Mintzberg. "Managing the Care of the Health and the Cure of Disease—Part II: Interjection." *Health Care Management Review* Winter 2001, pp 70–84.

Greenberg, J., and R. A. Baron. *Behavior in Organizations,* 7th edition. Upper Saddle River, NJ: Prentice Hall, 2000.

Griffith, J. R., and K. R. White. *The Well-Managed Healthcare Organization*, 6th edition. Chicago: Health Administration Press, 2007.

Guillen, M. F. *Models of Management.* Chicago: University of Chicago Press, 1994.

Handy, C. *Understanding Organizations.* New York: Oxford University Press, 1993.

Institute of Medicine. *To Err Is Human: Building a Safer Health System.* Washington, DC: National Academies Press, 2000.

Institute of Medicine. *Crossing the Quality Chasm.* Washington, DC: National Academy Press, 2001.

Joint Commission. *Striving Toward Improvement: Six Hospitals in Search of Quality.* Oakbrook Terrace, IL: Joint Commission, 1992.

Juran, J. M., ed. *A History of Managing for Quality: The Evolution, Trends and Future Directions of Managing for Quality.* Milwaukee, WI: ASQ Quality Press, 1995.

Kelly, D. *Applying Quality Management in Healthcare.* Chicago: Health Administration Press, 2003.

Langley, G. J., K. M. Nola, T. W. Nolan, C. L. Norman, and L. P. Provost. *The Improvement Guide: A Practical Approach to Enhancing Organizational Performances.* San Francisco: Jossey-Bass, 1996.

Lawrence, P., and J. Lorsch. *Organization and Environment.* Cambridge, MA: Graduate School of Business Administration, Harvard University, 1972.

Meyer, M. *Environments and Organizations.* San Francisco: Jossey-Bass, 1978.

Mick, S. S., and M. E. Wyttenbach, eds. *Advances in Health Care Organization Theory.* San Francisco: Jossey-Bass, 2003.

Morgan, G. *Images of Organization.* Beverly Hills, CA: Sage Library of Social Research, 1986.

Nystrom, P. C., and W. H. Starbuck. *Handbook of Organization Design.* New York: Oxford University Press, 1981.

Parsons, T. *Structure and Process in Modern Societies.* Glencoe, IL: Free Press, 1960.

Parsons, T. "Suggestions for a Sociological Approach to the Theory of Organizations." *Administrative Science Quarterly* June 1956, 1: 63–85, 224–39.

Peters, T. J. *Thriving on Chaos.* New York: Knopf, 1987.

Quinn, R. E. *Beyond Rational Management.* San Francisco: Jossey-Bass, 1985.

Schein, E. H. *Organizational Culture and Leadership.* San Francisco: Jossey-Bass, 1985.

Scott, W. R. "The Organization of Medical Care Services: Toward an Integrated Theoretical Model." *Medical Care Review* Fall 1993, 50 (3): 271–303.

Scott, W. R. *Organizations, Rational, Natural and Open Systems*, 2nd edition. Englewood Cliffs, NJ: Prentice-Hall, 1987.

Selznick, P. *Leadership in Administration.* Evanston, IL: Row Peterson, 1957.

Senge, P. M. *The Fifth Discipline.* New York: Doubleday, 1990.

Shortell, S. M., and A. D. Kaluzny. "Organizational Theory and Health Services Management." In *Health Care Management*, 4th edition. Albany, NY: Delmar, 2000, pp. 4–33.

Shortell, S. M., R. R. Gillies, and D. A. Anderson. *Remaking Health Care in America*. San Francisco: Jossey-Bass, 1996.

Slee, D. A., V. N. Slee, and H. J. Schmidt. *Slee's Health Care Terms*, 5th Comprehensive Edition. St. Paul, MN: Tringa Press, 2008.

Sloane, R., B. Sloane, and R. Harder. *Introduction to Healthcare Delivery Organizations*, 4th edition. Chicago: Health Administration Press, 2003.

THE ROLE OF THE MANAGER

A leader is best
When people barely know that he exists
Not so good when people obey
And acclaim him,
Worst when they despise him.
Fail to honor people,
They fail to honor you;
But of a good leader, who talks little,
When his work is done, his aim fulfilled,
They will say, 'we did this ourselves.'
—*Lao Tzu*

COMMENTARY

What's unusual about managing healthcare organizations (HCOs)? Most HCOs are not-for-profit and small, and most health services managers are generalists rather than specialists. The goals of HCOs—patient care, research, teaching, and community service—are more complex than the goals of car manufacturers or police forces. Translating such goals into measurable objectives is difficult, as the objectives of most healthcare organizations cannot be reduced to greater profits or market share. Healthcare is labor intensive, the work is often complex, and it involves many professionals working together. The health services manager must gain at least tacit consent from a variety of stakeholders—including board members, patients, the community, doctors, nurses, other workers, payers, regulators—some of whom may not agree with the organization's goals and often unstated objectives.

What Do Healthcare Managers Do?

Managers do what they are supposed to do, what they want to do, and what they can do. Managers confront reality, develop agendas and networks, think strategically about their work, and learn how to manage themselves effectively to accomplish organizational goals. Because they generally lack ownership of the firm, healthcare managers are often risk averse. They worry about their own survival as well as goal attainment. They make trade-offs between improving patient care, breaking even financially, and keeping clinicians content.

Key internal stakeholders may not want nor see the need for strategic interventions, yet managers may be facing important external stakeholders demanding change. Healthcare managers must help their organizations respond to the demands of those external stakeholders while mobilizing the support of, or placating, internal interest groups.

The healthcare enterprise is increasingly concerned with measuring results, but healthcare is difficult to measure. Managers must have patience and show creativity in applying quantitative measures, which are often more relevant to process than outcomes of care.

Another important aspect of the healthcare manager's job is finance. Managers must understand and generate funds from various payers and contributors.

Complicating the manager's job is the fact that doctors and nurses may see managers primarily as support staff for their work. This image may contrast with a manager's view of herself as "relating the organization to its environment," or "coordinating processes of care to achieve measurable objectives." Managerial work is accomplished in part through e-mails and meetings that some clinicians may regard largely as a waste of their time; they feel they could be more usefully involved in providing patient care.

The role of the health services manager has changed substantially over time. Medicare and Medicaid, introduced in 1965, fostered the growing complexity and increasing costs of healthcare. New organizations have appeared, such as health maintenance organizations, preferred provider organizations, skilled nursing homes, ambulatory surgery centers, neighborhood health centers, and minute clinics. Healthcare management is no longer primarily hospital acute care management, and many hospitals provide a range of services extending far beyond acute care.

Different Organizational Settings

The work of healthcare managers varies by the type of organization. Healthcare organizations include academic medical centers, neighborhood health centers, small rural community hospitals, Medicaid-focused health maintenance organizations, large public hospitals, visiting nurse services, Veteran's Administration hospital networks, and health departments, among others. These organizations are large or small; rural, suburban, or urban; financially well-endowed or struggling. They face different challenges and can respond to different opportunities.

Expectations for Managerial Performance

The healthcare manager's work is being transformed by an information revolution and a revolution in performance expectations. Healthcare managers are expected to support quality improvement, lead revenue generation, contain costs, and manage relationships with important stakeholder groups. Managers are challenged by situations such as having inadequate resources to provide high-quality care. Greater performance expectations are being placed on managers in the face of limitations as to what HCOs can charge for their services, while costs may be increasing at a faster rate.

Top management gets excellent performance by hiring great people, creating a performance culture that links rewards with results, demanding shared values, and believing that everyone counts. This is how General Electric does it. GE wants managers with high energy who can energize the people around them, who have an "edge" so they can make tough decisions, and who can execute decisions (Hogan 2001).

Ullian says that being a successful manager means picking the right boss. Effective managers can communicate the "bad" news, are accountable for performance, respect others, have the courage to take action, and can learn from their mistakes and weaknesses. Successful managers are self-confident and cheerful (Ullian 2001).

Managers should ask themselves: who are the key stakeholders impacting on goal achievement? What do these stakeholders expect? How satisfied are they with current performance?

Managerial interventions should always be financially and politically feasible. The manager should know where the money is coming from before he suggests an initiative and where the buy-in is going to come from for successful implementation.

Managers should reflect on what they intend to accomplish over the next 12 months, and determine whose support they need to achieve these goals. Every manager should consider her resume as her lifeline and keep it current. She should ask herself: what results did I achieve last year? Will I achieve results this year that make for a convincing track record of accomplishment?

Thinking Strategically About the Job

Managers should understand the flexibility of their positions. Each managerial job has three characteristics: (1) the demands of the job that the manager must actively carry out; (2) the constraints on the position, or those activities that the manager is not allowed to carry out; and (3) the options or choices the manager can make concerning how she is going to spend her time and presence (Steward and Fondas 1992).

Goleman (1998) stresses the importance of emotional intelligence for management success, suggesting that it is more important than a high IQ and great technical skills, and that it can be learned. The five components of emotional intelligence are:

- Self-awareness (how managers see themselves being seen by others)
- Self-regulation (thinking before speaking)
- Motivation (the drive to achieve results)
- Empathy (seeing others as they see themselves), and
- Social skills (in listening and responding)

All managers make decisions based on evidence. How can they obtain better evidence to make more effective decisions? Managers should be able to:

- identify emerging opportunities;
- precisely define management challenges or opportunities;

- collect data;
- find and critically appraise relevant information from published and non-published sources;
- understand the process of change; and
- be able to conduct and evaluate experiments in which new methods are piloted (Kovner, Elton, and Billings 2000).

McCall, Lombardo, and Morrison (1988) have suggested the following framework for management development:

- Find out about shortcomings.
- Accept responsibility for any shortcomings that result because of a lack of knowledge, skills, or experience, or because of personality, limited ability, or being a situational misfit.
- Decide what to do about it accordingly. Either build new strengths, such as finding ways to get help and support while learning; anticipate situations, such as seeking advice or counsel; compensate, for example, by avoiding certain situations; or change yourself (which is very difficult to do), either through intensive counseling and coaching or through personal change effort.

References

Goleman, D. 1998. "What Makes a Leader?" *Harvard Business Review* 76 (6): 93–102.

Hogan, J. 2001. "Thriving in Healthcare—Learning Every Day." *Journal of Healthcare Administration Education* (Spec. No.): 63–67.

Kovner, A. R., J. Elton, and J. Billings. 2000. "Transforming Health Management: An Evidence-Based Approach." *Frontiers of Health Services Management* 16 (4): 3–24.

McCall, M. W., M. M. Lombardo, and A. M. Morrison. 1988. *The Lessons of Experience: How Successful Executives Develop on the Job*. Lexington, MA: Lexington Books.

Steward, R., and N. Fondas. 1992. "How Managers Can Think Strategically About Their Jobs." *Journal of Management Development* 11 (7): 10–17.

Ullian, E. 2001. Presentation at the National Summit on the Future of Education and Practice in Health Management and Policy. Orlando, FL, February 8–9.

THE READINGS

The required reading for Part I is "Evidence-Based Management Recon-sidered" by Kovner and Rundall. The authors suggest that the sense of urgency associated with improving the quality of medical care does not exist with respect to improving the quality of management decision making. A more evidence-based approach would improve the competence of the decision makers and their motivation to use more scientific methods when making de-cisions. To aid the manager in understanding and applying an evidence-based approach to decision making, the authors provide practical tools, techniques, and resources for immediate use.

Evidence-Based Management Reconsidered

Anthony R. Kovner and Thomas G. Rundall
From *Frontiers of Health Services Management* 22: 3–46, Spring 2006

> "What we do for and with patients and *how we organize* those efforts should, to the extent possible, be based on knowledge of what works. Put differently, both the application of clinical medicine and the application of organizational behavior should be evidence based."
>
> Stephen M. Shortell, Ph.D., FACHE (Shortell 2001)

> "What discourages our use of research is something that is typical of all health systems. That is, we are on a rapid cycle…We don't have two years to study some-thing. Sometimes having 40 percent of the information on something may be enough. We make a decision and change it if it doesn't work."
>
> Health system manager (Kovner 2005)

The numerous developments in evidence-based decision making over the past decade should influence health organization leaders and managers to explicitly incorporate such decision making in their management processes. For example, the considerable use of evidence-based decision making by physicians has resulted in the proliferation of patient care guidelines and related decision-support materials for physicians (Sackett et al. 1996; Fried-land 1998; Sackett et al. 2000; Geyman, Deyo, and Ramsey 2000; Eddy 2005; AHRQ 2006a). Acceptance of the evidence-based approach has been growing in nursing, public health, health policy making, and other specialty areas in the health sciences (Lomas 2000; Donaldson, Mugford, and Vale 2002; Lavis et al. 2002; Stewart 2002; Lavis et al. 2003; Brownson et al 2003; Muir Gray 2004; Shojania and Grimshaw 2005; Hatcher and Oakley-Browne 2005; Fox 2005). As Muir Gray suggests (2004) an evidence-based approach would improve the competence of decision-makers and their motivation to use more scientific methods when making a decision. In their recent book, *Management Mistakes in Healthcare*, Paul Hofmann and Frankie Perry call for the identification, correction, and prevention of management mistakes in healthcare (Hofmann and Perry 2005). Moreover, articles have appeared in health management and health services research journals urging health services managers to examine the nature of decision making in their organizations and to consider adopting an evidence-based approach (Axelson 1998; Davies and Nutley 1999; Kovner, Elton, and Billings 2000; Walshe and Rundall 2001; Greenhalgh et al. 2004; Muir Gray 2004; Clancy and Cronin 2005). Web-based sources of evidence for managers have emerged, including compendiums of primary research studies and research syntheses developed by the Agency for Healthcare Research and Quality (http://www .ahrq.gov/research/), the Cochrane Effective Practice and Organization of Care Group (http://www.epoc.uottawa.ca/) and others. Federal agencies have supported research to improve quality, safety, and efficiency in the organization and delivery of health services (AHRQ 2006b). For example, since 2000 the Agency for Healthcare Research and Quality (AHRQ) has funded the Integrated Delivery System Research Network (IDSRN), now "Accelerating Change and Transformation in Organizations and Networks" (AC-TION), which was explicitly designed to create, support, and disseminate scientific evidence about what works and what does not work. Since 1991 the Center for Health Management Research (http://depts.washington .edu/chmr/about/), a National Science Foundation–funded Industry-University Research Collaborative, has been facilitating collaborative research among university-based health services researchers and health system managers. Finally, evidence-based decision making has been increasingly incorporated into lists of competencies necessary for effective management of modern health services organizations. The management competencies proposed by the Healthcare Leadership Alliance (2005) include acquiring, appraising, and applying research findings to management decisions.[1] Similarly, the Health Leadership Competency Model, developed by the National Center for Healthcare Leadership (2004), incorporates competencies supporting evidence-based decision making, most notably the competency referred to as "analytical thinking":

> The ability to understand a situation, issue, or problem by breaking it into smaller pieces or tracing its implications in a step-by-step way. It includes organizing the

parts of a situation, issues, or problem systematically; making systematic comparisons of different features or aspects; setting priorities on a rational basis; and identifying time sequences, causal relationships, or if-then relationships.

Similar developments are unfolding in the health systems of other developed countries. Indeed, if anything, countries with national health insurance and/or a public delivery system have developed more resources than the United States for evidence-based health services management. For example, the United Kingdom National Health Service has established the NHS Service Delivery and Organization Programme (http://www.sdo.lshtm.ac.uk/), the U.K. National Library for Health (http://www.nelh.nhs.uk/), and the Health Management Online resource within the National Health Service in Scotland (http://www.healthmanagementonline.co.uk/), and the Canadian government has established the Canadian Health Services Research Foundation (http://www.chsrf.ca/).

Recent research in the United Kingdom and in Canada suggests that health managers and policy makers make little use of the evidence-based approach to decision making and, indeed, reveals a wide gap between the health services research and health policy and management communities (Lavis, et al. 2002; Canadian Health Services Research Foundation 2000; 2004). In those countries, a number of steps have been identified that could increase the uptake of evidence-based health services management (EBHSM). For example, the Canadian Health Services Research Foundation (2000, 7) suggests:

> [D]ecision makers need to find more effective ways to organize and communicate their priorities and problems, while researchers and research funders must develop mechanisms to access information on these priorities and problems and turn them into research activity. . . . Researchers need to learn how to simplify their findings and demonstrate their application to the health system in order to communicate better with decision makers and knowledge purveyors. . . . The knowledge purveyors have to improve their ability to screen and appraise information—to sort the facts from the stories. . . . Decision makers and their organizations need to improve their capacity to receive such appraised and screened information and to act upon it.

Moreover, studies in Canada and the United Kingdom have noted the substantial differences between health services managers and health services researchers in their understandings of what is considered evidence, what type of systematic review of evidence is helpful to decision makers, and the extent to which management and policy decision making can and should be evidence based (Canadian Health Services Research Foundation 2005; Sheldon 2005; Mays, Pope, and Popay 2005; Pawson et al. 2005; Lavis et al. 2005).

No study of U.S. health services managers' perspectives on evidence-based decision making exists, hence, we have little evidence to guide us in developing strategies to strengthen understanding and use of EBHSM among health services managers. The purposes of this article are fourfold: (1) to briefly describe the evidence-based management approach; (2) to describe the questions to which EBHSM can be applied; (3) to report on a recent study conducted by one of the authors (Kovner 2005) to understand better the use of evidence in decision making by health services managers; and (4) to suggest a number of practical strategies that U.S. health services organizations can use to implement or strengthen an evidence-based approach to decision making in their organization.

What Is Evidence-Based Health Services Management?

Evidence-based health services management applies the idea of evidence-based decision making to business process, operational, and strategic decisions in health services organizations. Simply put, EBHSM is the systematic application of the best available evidence to the evaluation of managerial strategies for improving the performance of health services organizations. What distinguishes EBHSM from other approaches to decision making is the notion that whenever possible, health services managers should incorporate into their decision making evidence from well-conducted management research. It must be emphasized that other sources of information and knowledge, such as personal experience, experiences of others in similar situations, expert opinion, and simple inspection of data trends and patterns, can and should be used if such information is the best available evidence for a given decision. As is the case with evidence-based medicine, the research evidence one uses in EBHSM does not replace but rather complements other types of knowledge and information.

The EBHSM approach recognizes that decision making is a process rather than a simple act of choosing among alternatives. Under ideal circumstances, this process involves a number of steps. Figures 1 and 2 depict the contribution of the EBHSM approach to two frequently used decision-making processes in health organizations.

The decision-making process begins with the identification of a problem (step 1), or more specifically, identification of the discrepancy between an existing and a desired state of affairs. The decision maker(s) uses various techniques, types of information, analyses, and actions to complete the cycle, with information gained from an evaluation of the decision (step 8) helping to determine whether the problem continues to exist in the future. Of special interest to the field of EBHSM are steps 5 and 6. The promise of EBHSM is that by incorporating the best evidence available at the time that alternatives must be assessed and a decision must be made will result in better decisions, thereby improving organizational performance.

Figure 2 depicts the familiar Shewhart PDSA cycle frequently used in quality improvement efforts in health organizations (Kelly 2003: Institute for Healthcare Improvement 2003; Juran 1989). Although research evidence can be useful in making decisions throughout this cycle, the knowledge base created by the Plan and Study steps—understanding the nature of the

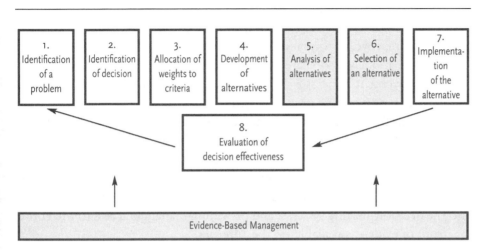

FIGURE I.1
The Eight Step Decision-Making Process

Adapted from Robbins and DeCenzo (2004, 106).

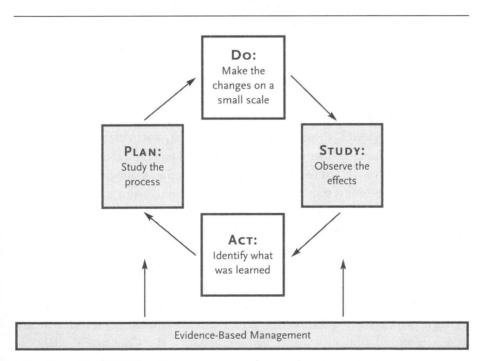

FIGURE I.2
The Shewhart PDSA Quality Improvement Cycle

Adapted from Kelly (2003, 32).

problem, the process in which it is embedded, and the effects of any given intervention—can be greatly increased by comparing local data with studies of other organizations.

The generic eight-step decision-making model and the PDSA decision-making approach for improving quality share several strengths. The models help managers systematically identify causes of problems. They provide insights necessary for designing and implementing interventions to improve performance. Each encourages monitoring and evaluation of decisions to continually improve performance over time.

These models also share some important weaknesses. They tend to make improvement processes "inward looking," focusing on information and data that are available or can be generated within the organization. The models place little emphasis on systematic research in other organizations. Neither model makes use of modern electronic resources to help managers solve problems. Hence, the use of evidence-based management techniques can strengthen these decision-making processes by extending the vision of decision makers beyond their organization's walls, bringing existing evidence into the decision-making process, and providing managers access to the entire spectrum of evidence available on the Internet.

To What Types of Management Questions Can EBHSM Be Applied?

Evidence-based health services management can be applied to three types of management issues: core business transaction management, operational management, and strategic management. Management questions include those that directly influence the way in which patient care is financed, organized, and delivered, as well as those that are supportive to patient care and those that involve external arrangements among non-clinical personnel (See Table 1).

Although EBHSM techniques can be applied to management decisions regarding core business transactions, research on these issues is not easily available to health services managers. Management decisions regarding core business transactions may be made by trial and error, copying successful processes in other organizations, or seeking technical consultation. On the other hand, considerable research is available to address many (but not all) operational and strategic issues confronting health services managers. Indeed, systematic reviews exist that summarize research evidence on each of the operational and strategic management questions listed in Table 1 at the Agency for Healthcare Research and Quality (www.ahrq.gov/research/), the Cochrane Collaboration Effective Practice and Organization of Care Group (www.epoc.uottawa.ca), and the Cochrane Consumers and Communication Review Group (www

TABLE I.1

Examples of
Management
Questions to
Which EBHSM
Can Be Applied

Type of Management Issue	Management Questions
Core Business Transactions	• How can the payer process MD claims for payment more quickly? • How can the health system's information on patient eligibility for benefits be made more accurate? • What methods for paying physician claims achieve speed, convenience, and accuracy requirements?
Operational Management	• How can nurse absenteeism be reduced? • Will decreasing the patient/nurse ratio improve patient outcomes? • Does hospital discharge planning and follow up improve patients' outcomes? • Does hand washing among healthcare workers reduce hospital-acquired infections? • Does basing part of employees' compensation on achievement of unit or team goals improve teamwork and coordination?
Strategic Management	• How do hospital mergers affect administrative costs? • Do hospital-physician joint ventures, such as orthopedic surgery centers, have negative effects on in-hospital surgery? • Does the implementation of an electronic medical record improve the quality of patient care? • Do pay-for-performance incentives substantially improve targeted care processes?

.latrobe.edu.au/cochrane) websites. These sites also provide a considerable amount of research regarding organizational structures and processes that may influence patient care processes and patient outcomes.

Applying evidence to the assessment of alternatives and the selection of a "best" alternative is itself a five-step process:

1. Formulating the research question
2. Acquiring the relevant research findings and other types of evidence
3. Assessing the validity, quality, and applicability of the evidence
4. Presenting the evidence in a way that will make it likely that it will be used in the decision process
5. Applying the evidence in decision making

The brief exposition of each step below will illuminate the main features of the approach. (For other more detailed discussions of evidence-based decision making see Muir Gray 2004; Mack, Crawford, and Reed 2004; and Mays, Pope, and Popay 2005).

Formulating the Research Question

The first step is to turn the management question into a research question, framing the issue in a way that will increase the probability of locating useful research studies. This task requires more thought than one may first believe. Often, a very specific management question will have to be broadened to find relevant research, but overly broad, vague, or highly abstract research questions must be avoided. For example, if a manager is interested in knowing the likely effect of implementing a hospitalist program on the cost and quality of care for patients treated for cardiac problems in a suburban Arizona hospital, finding even one study that meets all the inclusion criteria implied by such a narrow, specific question is unlikely. Broadening the management question somewhat (e.g., What is the impact of a hospitalist program on the cost and quality of inpatient care in U.S. community hospitals?) makes it more likely that studies will be found that will be of some value to the hospitalist program implementation decision. However, broadening the question too much (e.g., What is the impact of hospitalists on the healthcare delivery system?) makes it likely that many studies included will not be relevant to the specific issue of interest to the manager. A good guideline for formulating the research question is to incorporate into the question statements that clarify the technique, the setting, and the outcome of interest (see sidebar).

Acquiring Research Evidence

Evidence relevant to the management research question can be obtained from a wide array of sources; colleagues, consultants, and known experts are frequent sources of evidence. Many managers will find it helpful to use the Internet to locate research articles. Health organizations that have made significant investments in knowledge management may have libraries, trained librarians and webmasters, intranet information resources, or an in-house management decision-support system. The vast majority of managers will not have such resources, but will be limited to what they can find on the open Internet.

Guidelines in Formulating an Appropriate Research Question

1. What management tool or technique is being considered?
2. What is the setting in which the technique would be applied?
3. What is the desired managerial process or outcome?

Two general approaches can be used to acquire research evidence via the open Internet:

1. Searching websites that provide access to systematic reviews or meta-analyses. For example, the Effective Practice and Organization of Care (EPOC) group within the Cochrane Library as mentioned above may provide insight.
2. Searching bibliographic databases such as MEDLINE, PubMed, or Google Scholar for published and unpublished primary studies of relevance to the research question (see sidebar). For example using the search terms "hospitalist," "cost," and "quality" to search the Scholar Google database produced over 60 citations, many of which appeared to be qualitative or quantitative research studies. One of those articles was co-authored by one of us (Coffman and Rundall 2005).

A research synthesis of a large number of primary research articles is especially useful to decision makers since the authors of the synthesis have already made an attempt to assess the quality of the evidence and to draw out the conclusions that are supported by the evidence. Once relevant articles have been found, they may be electronically stored and, if desired, printed out to make them easier to read and assess.

What types of evidence can be incorporated in evidence-based management? This issue has caused considerable debate in the EBHSM literature. Some analysts have argued that EBHSM should follow the lead of evidence-based medicine and rely upon evidence syntheses, which are systematic

---

SIDEBAR I.1
Resources for Health Services Management Research

Agency for Healthcare Research and Quality: www.ahrq.gov/
    research/
Effective Practice and Organization of Care Group: www.epoc
    .uottawa.ca/
Consumers and Communication Review Group: www.latrobe.edu
    .au/cochrane/
Center for Health Management Research: http://depts.washington
    .edu/chmr/research/
PubMed: www.ncbi.nlm.nih.gov/entrez/query.fcgi?db=PubMed
MEDLINE: www.nlm.nih.gov/databases/databases_medline.html
Google Scholar: http://scholar.google.com

reviews of the evidence from studies of the effects of a particular policy or managerial intervention.

Critics of this rather restrictive definition of evidence point out that relatively few evidence syntheses are available on issues of concern to health services managers, that the standard procedures for carrying out systematic reviews dismiss many useful studies as methodologically weak, and that from a managerial perspective the knowledge and insights gained from qualitative case studies, expert opinion, and personal experience should be considered evidence (Davies and Nutley 1999; Bero and Jadad 1997; Mays, Pope, and Popay 2005; Pawson et al. 2005). This issue is far from resolved as it involves the age-old debate over the need for balance between rigor and relevance in applied research.

As Ham recently pointed out, dismissing the relevance of systematic reviews and giving personal experience and other kinds of intelligence equal standing with the evidence generated by formal research studies runs the risk of "throwing the baby out with the bath water" (Ham 2005). A compromise approach may be to relax the criteria for the inclusion of studies and extend search strategies beyond established databases (Ham 2005). Moreover, researchers and managers must remember that the principles of EBHSM as described at the outset of this article explicitly incorporate both rigorous research as well as experiential judgment and research studies conducted with smaller samples and weaker designs than would be desirable. The point of the EBHSM approach is to create an expectation that managers will seek the best research evidence available at the time a decision is made, and to incorporate this evidence with other sources of information, such as expert opinion and personal experience in the decision-making process.

Assessing the Quality of the Evidence

Managers must have some minimal competency in assessing management research, critical appraisal skills that will enable them to judge the quality of the evidence available. Ideally, managers should have, or have available to them, competency to assess:

- Strength of the research design
- Study context and setting
- Sample sizes of the study groups
- Control for confounding factors
- Reliability and validity of the measurements
- Methods and procedures used
- Justification of the conclusions
- Study sponsorship
- Consistency of the findings with other studies

In many cases, these issues will be addressed in the research report itself. For example, in the Coffman and Rundall evidence synthesis of studies of the effect of hospitalists on hospital costs and quality of care, 21 studies were identified that met minimal inclusion and exclusion search criteria. Still, these studies varied significantly in their overall research designs (e.g., experimental design with randomized control group versus quasi-experimental designs without randomization); types of comparison groups used in the quasi-experimental studies (e.g., concurrent versus historical); the size of the intervention and control/comparison groups; the statistical control for confounding factors; and the length of time over which the intervention was operative before evaluation data were collected. To understand the findings from these studies, these important differences in the strengths of the studies, and hence in the quality of the evidence, were incorporated in the synthesis. At a minimum, managers should be aware of the importance of assessing these aspects of research studies and be able to evaluate the extent to which they have been addressed in any given primary research study or research synthesis.

Presenting the Evidence

Managers and researchers should present evidence to the decision-making process in a way that is timely, brief, avoids technical jargon, provides clear descriptions of the questions addressed, incorporates the context of the research and findings, offers an assessment of the strength of the evidence, gives the results and implications for practice, and is easy to access (see sidebar). The Coffman and Rundall (2005) synthesis attempted to present the evidence found in multiple studies in a way that would be understandable to managers and other nonspecialists in the field. The 21 studies were organized into groups based on strength of research design and methods.

SIDEBAR I.2
Guidelines for Presentation of Evidence

Present timely evidence.
Be brief.
Avoid technical jargon.
Provide clear descriptions of the questions addressed.
Incorporate the context of the research and findings.
Offer an assessment of the strength of the evidence.
Give the results and implications for practice.
Make the presentation easy to access.

Simple tables were used showing how many of the 21 studies in each group demonstrated reduction in resource use (e.g., lower total costs or charges), improvement in measures of quality of care (e.g., lower readmission rate), and increase in patient satisfaction (e.g., self-reported satisfaction with patient care experience).

The Coffman and Rundall article is not offered as a "best practice" of how to present evidence to health services managers. Indeed, publishing a briefer version in a journal explicitly marketed to managers would have increased its reach. However, we believe that managers, clinicians, and patients who searched for and found this article would have understood the findings. Managers and clinicians in hospitals and physician organizations could have easily incorporated these findings, including the qualifications proposed by the authors, into their assessment of the likely effects of adopting a hospitalist program.

Applying the Evidence to the Decision

Getting health services organization decision makers to use evidence may be the most challenging step. Most organizations today do not have the incentives or capabilities necessary for routinely using evidence in decision making. Substantial staff time is often required to ensure an adequate deliberative process. Opportunity costs are associated with disseminating and discussing the implications of research findings for a particular decision in a given organization. Ego costs to managers and others who feel their preferences are challenged by the evidence might be incurred.

The multiple ways in which research evidence assist the decision-making process are poorly understood. Many users demand that the available evidence have immediate, instrumental use for a particular decision, but often the available research evidence cannot be used in that way. Rather, the evidence is better used to increase the decision maker's enlightenment regarding the decision issue by increasing the manager's understanding of the nature of a problem; opening up communication among managers and other stakeholders; enabling the manager to generate creative solutions; and enhancing the manager's ability to estimate the likely effects of each alternative solution to a problem. These are important, but under-appreciated, contributions of the evidence-based approach to decision making.

In fact, the same body of evidence can be used for instrumental and enlightenment purposes by organizations in different stages of a decision process. For example, the Coffman and Rundall evidence synthesis on the effects of hospitalists on hospital costs and quality of care was presented to representatives of several health systems that are members of the Center for Health Management Research (CHMR). This presentation increased the representatives' awareness of the availability of the various studies and their findings. More instrumental use was made of the synthesis by one of the CHMR member health systems who invited a coauthor of the study to present the results to over 60 middle- and senior-level managers as part of a seminar on evidence-based management. The findings from the synthesis were incorporated in on-going discussions about whether and how to implement hospitalist programs in the system's hospitals. At another CHMR health system, the results of the synthesis were presented at a board of directors' meeting and contributed directly to the system's decision to implement hospitalist programs in two of its hospitals.

A Study of the Use of Evidence in Decision Making by Health Services Managers in the United States

Kovner (2005) recently conducted a study designed to identify and explore factors associated with knowledge transfer between researchers and managers of health systems. The research focused on managers of five health systems and four types of decisions. The decision issues were: selecting the indicators for assessing the success of diabetes management programs; strengthening the relationship between budgeting procedures and strategic priorities; selecting the operational metrics to include in managerial dashboards, and adapting compensation systems for managers of physician performance. The study methodology included 68 interviews of managers of 17 non-profit health systems located in regions throughout the United States. Of these interviews, 56 were with managers of five health systems that were members of the Center for Health Management Research (CHMR). The other 12 interviews were with managers in 12 health systems similar in size and sponsorship to one or more of the five CHMR health systems. In each interview, each manager was asked a series of questions to gain an understanding of whether they used evidence in decision making about each of the four issues described above, and how evidence was used to make decisions in their organization. Specifically, the managers were asked:

- Can you tell us about a recent decision that you are or were part of making?
- What process did the team working on the decision use to find evidence?
- In what respect was this a typical process, or not, for this type of decision?
- How do you assess if the evidence is of high quality, relevant, and applicable?
- What are three professional journals, websites, or other publications you find most useful in making decisions?

As in the Canadian and United Kingdom studies of evidence use by health services managers, U.S. managers reported little use of the evidence-based approach as described above for decision making. None of the 68 managers interviewed mentioned using evidence from management research to make strategic decisions. The journals that managers found useful were not research journals, or if they were research journals, they were not management journals. Journals cited included the *Harvard Business Review*, *Modern Healthcare*, *Health Affairs*, and *The New England Journal of Medicine*. Twenty-two websites were mentioned as useful, including those of the Agency for Health Care Research and Quality (www.ahrq.gov), Centers for Medicare & Medicaid Services (cms.hhs.gov), the Institute for Healthcare Improvement (www.ihi.org) and the Joint Commission on the Accreditation of Healthcare Organizations (www.jcaho.org). The data from this study suggest that there is a good deal of similarity between U.S. health services managers and their Canadian and British counterparts.

Interestingly, when asked, "How do you feel that your organization's culture promotes your use of evidence in decision making?" respondents gave generally positive comments. All 15 of the 15 respondents in the five health systems that were specifically asked this question spoke positively that their system's culture promoted the use of evidence in decision making. The apparent contradiction between the reported non-use of EBHSM and organizational cultures favorable to the use of evidence in decision making is rooted in the managers' working definition of "evidence." As in Canada and the United Kingdom, the definition of evidence among health services managers differs from that used by most health services researchers (Canadian Health Services Research Foundation 2004). Many respondents indicated that they used evidence in making decisions, but what they referred to as evidence was frequently their own experience, anecdotes that had been communicated to them, information from Internet sites, and advice from consultants and advisory organizations such as the Health Care Advisory Board. None of the managers interviewed reported that in their organizations the evidentiary process for strategic decision making was regularly reviewed or that there was formal oversight of the deliberative process.

In further analyzing the data to identify ideas and strategies that might be used to increase the use of EBHSM, Kovner (2005) identified four factors that respondents suggested may influence use of management research in health systems:

1. External demands for performance accountability
2. An accountability structure for knowledge transfer
3. A questioning organizational culture
4. Participation in management research

From these findings, we recommend strategies for increasing the use of evidence-based decision making among health services managers.

Strategies to Increase the Use of EBHSM

External Demands for Performance Accountability

The increasing demands for accountability by external organizations have conflicting effects on the use of evidence-based management. Managers reported that their systems were increasingly expected and/or required to meet process and outcome performance targets set by purchasers, quality improvement organizations, and public and private regulatory groups. These external organizations, such as the Joint Commission on Accreditation of Healthcare Organizations, the Centers for Medicare and Medicaid Services, the National Quality Forum, the Leapfrog Group, and national and regional pay-for-performance programs, are increasingly identifying healthcare patient care process and outcome criteria and setting performance standards for health systems. Health system managers clearly recognize the strategic importance of the recognition and rewards offered by these external organizations, and in many cases such external pressures for accountability increase the use of evidence-based management. However, in other cases managers are concerned that motivation to search for and use research evidence in their quality improvement efforts is undermined by the focus on quality improvement processes, outcomes, and performance targets set by external agencies. One health system manager expressed this concern in the following way:

> In the past, before there were so many requirements for data reporting, we had a different process for setting performance indicators. We looked at the literature for the right thing to do, and then we met with committees of physicians and nurses and asked them what was important. . . . Today, however, there is so much demand for publicly reported data that we don't choose which areas to try to develop and improve dashboards and scorecards. We respond to demand.

In environments where external stakeholders are setting health systems' performance criteria and standards, we suggest that managers clearly link evidence searching and application to the development of organizational structures and processes that improve organizational performance on the externally set criteria, in effect marrying evidence-based medicine and evidence-based management to deliver the right treatment to the right patient, for the right condition, at the right time. In this way the strategic importance of evidence-based management can be established and enhanced over time as the use of research evidence is seen to contribute to the design of more effective processes for delivering care that meets externally set performance targets. If evidence-based management is not perceived to be strategically important to a health system, few resources will be devoted to it.

An Accountability Structure for Knowledge Transfer

Formalizing the responsibility structure for dissemination and use of evidence focuses and increases the impact of knowledge transfer. If no one is responsible for a function, it is unlikely that the function will be performed effectively in a complex, large healthcare organization. To be a priority goal, dissemination and use of management research must be seen as consistent with and as contributing to the organizational goals of the leadership. On the other hand, the lack of an accountability structure contributes to a casual approach to searching for evidence that typically relies on convenient sources and minimal effort. For example, one health system manager reported:

> I get evidence from two sources: conversations with other people in the healthcare industry, and my past professional experience.

Unfortunately, health systems do not designate managers as being responsible and accountable for knowledge transfer or for assessing research evidence as part of their decision-making process. Moreover, at the present time metrics are lacking to assess the benefits of obtaining better evidence for management decision making. Clearly, the use of evidence-based management would increase if health systems assigned responsibility for knowledge management to individuals or teams within the organization. A parallel strategy is to fix management responsibility for review of deliberative processes as part of the regular process of strategic decision making.

A Questioning Organizational Culture

A questioning culture affects the amount and speed of knowledge transfer between producers, disseminators, and targets of evidence-based management research. Health systems that support evidence-based decision making have cultures that recognize that encouraging questioning behavior among managers can lessen future problems that arise out of hasty and insufficiently considered decisions. However, challenging decisions and introducing research evidence into problem-solving discussions can cause anxiety among managers, creating a sense that managerial judgment and expertise is perceived by colleagues as inadequate or not trustworthy. As a health system respondent put it:

> On a philosophical basis, people tend to agree [about the desirability of evidence-based management]. When it comes to actually doing the work though, you start getting push back.

We suggest several strategies for building a questioning culture. Managers can participate in research "rounds," management research journal clubs,

SIDEBAR I.3
Building a Questioning Culture

- Organize research rounds, management research journal clubs, and research seminars
- Analyze the results of past operational and strategic decisions, including comparing the systems' performance with findings from research on other organizations
- Conduct staff development programs to enhance managers' abilities to find, assess, and apply research findings
- Link compensation to metrics related to obtaining and using relevant evidence in decision making and sharing evidence with key stakeholders
- Develop guidelines for decision making that require an assessment of research evidence

or research seminars led by internal managers or researchers from academic or other research institutions. Managers can routinely be asked by senior leaders to analyze the results of past operational and strategic decisions, including comparing their systems' performance with findings from research on other organizations. Staff development programs can be conducted to help institutionalize evidence-based decision making and enhance managers' abilities to find, assess, and apply research findings. Manager's compensation can be linked to metrics related to obtaining and using relevant evidence in decision making and sharing evidence with key stakeholders. Finally, we suggest that health systems develop organizational guidelines for decision making that require an assessment of available research evidence.

Participation in Management Research

Research dissemination, use, and impact will be affected by the level of participation of health system management in knowledge transfer. Lavis and colleagues (2003) found that research transfer often required interactive engagement, as it is a very time-consuming and skill-intensive process. They stress the importance of developing uptake skills for research among target audiences. In the Kovner study, managers who conducted their own studies, focus groups, or market assessments were more supportive of evidence-based decision making. However, these managers had limited evidence-searching and appraisal skills. None of the health systems employed specialists in knowledge management. Access to resources such as the Cochrane Collaboration website or even management journals was limited. Clearly, familiarity with research and with the skills and technologic apparatus associated with health services research are important factors driving the use of evidence in decision making. In some cases, these shortcomings can be overcome through the use of consulting or specialized research services. In the case of one health system:

> We developed a strategic plan for our heart services. Part of that was gaining an understanding of the minds of consumers in the local market. . . . We used a national company to do a random study. . . . This was an empirical work; it was a conjoint study. It gave us longitudinal ideas and information about our primary market. The national company asked questions that were our questions. We hired a company that does consumer research and we told them what we wanted to know.

Several strategies can increase health systems managers' research capability and actual participation in management research:

- Management training in evidence-based management;
- Investing internal funds in management research projects;
- Partnering with research organizations, such as survey firms and academic research centers; and
- Implementing information technology and knowledge management systems.

To put in perspective the findings reported above, we introduce some key ideas from the work of Shortell and his colleagues (Shortell et al. 2000) on the key success factors for clinical integration in health services. Shortell and his colleagues identified four organizational dimensions (strategic, structural, cultural, and technical) that influence delivery systems' ability to achieve significant organizational change, such as clinical integration. We adapted their framework and have applied it to our findings about the use of evidence-based management in health systems.

The Strategic Dimension

The strategic dimension emphasizes that significant organizational change—such as the adoption of evidence-based management practices—must focus on strategically important issues facing the health system. The implication is that to be widely used in health systems, evidence-based management must be seen by health system managers as a core strategic priority of the system. Our finding regarding the influence of external demands for performance accountability—a key strategic issue for health systems—on managers' support for evidence-based management is consistent with this dimension.

The Structural Dimension

The structural dimension refers to the overall structure of the system to support evidence-based management, including the use of designated committees, task forces, and individuals identified as responsible for implementing and diffusing evidence-based management practices. Our finding about the need for an accountability structure for knowledge transfer fits well within this dimension.

The Cultural Dimension

The cultural dimension refers to the beliefs, norms, values, and behaviors of people in the health system who may either support or oppose evidence-based management. Our findings regarding the importance of having a questioning culture as a precondition for evidence-based management are consistent with this dimension.

The Technical Dimension

The technical dimension refers to the extent to which people have the necessary knowledge, training, and skills to practice evidence-based management and the extent to which they have access to information technology and other technological assets. Again, our findings with regard to the importance of managers' having research skills, experience in performing research, and the critical appraisal skills necessary to assess research evidence performed by others is consistent with this dimension.

As Shortell, et al. (2000) argue, to achieve a high degree of organizational change in core processes such as the integration of clinical services or the use of research evidence in management decision making, health systems "must attend to all four dimensions simultaneously and attempt to align them with each other" (p. 140). In Figure 3 we have suggested what happens when one or another dimension is missing.

When the strategic dimension is missing, no important decisions are made using research evidence. When efforts are made to practice evidence-based management, they have little effect because they are not directed at the strategic priorities of the system.

When the structural dimension is missing, sporadic, isolated efforts to incorporate research evidence in decision making may occur, but little system-wide use of evidence-based decision making is present. This is because no one is accountable for diffusing these practices throughout the system and few appropriate committees or task forces train and disseminate the concepts and techniques of evidence-based decision making.

When the cultural component is missing, efforts to introduce evidence-based decision making quickly wither and fade away because the organizational culture does not support evidence-based management. People do not believe evidence-based decision making will produce better decisions, and it is not rewarded by the organization.

Absence of the technical dimension results in frustration and false starts in attempts to implement evidence-based management because managers do not have the necessary training in the principles of evidence-based decision

FIGURE I.3

Effect of
Organizational
Components
on Use of
EBHSM

External Demands for Performance Accountability (Strategic Dimension)	Accountability Structure for Knowledge Transfer (Structural Dimension)	Questioning Culture (Cultural Dimension)	Participation in Management Research (Technical Dimension)	Result
	✔	✔	✔	No significant use of research evidence on anything really important
✔		✔	✔	Inability to acquire research evidence and disseminate it throughout the system
✔	✔		✔	Small, intermittent use of evidence in decision making; no lasting impact
✔	✔	✔		Frustration and false starts in attempts to incorporate evidence in decision making
✔	✔	✔	✔	Lasting systemwide adoption of evidence-based management

✔ = Present   ☐ = Absent

Adapted from Shortell et al. (2000).

making, evidence searching, and research appraisal, and they may not have access to needed Internet and other resources.

This interpretation of the findings may indicate why evidence-based management is so little used, and suggests that a concerted effort will be required to change the situation. Only when all four dimensions are simultaneously made more supportive of evidence-based management and aligned with each other will sustainable progress occur.

Conclusion

The extent to which evidence-based decision making remains outside the repertoire of many health services managers is reflected in the way management mistakes are handled in most organizations and by instances of major decisions being made without regard to existing evidence that bears on the issue.

The rationale for using an evidence-based approach to managing health services organizations mirrors the rationale for evidence-based medicine. The movement toward evidence-based clinical practice was prompted by the observation of unexplained wide variations in clinical practice patterns, by the poor uptake of therapies of known effectiveness, and by the persistent use of treatments and technologies known to be ineffective. These problems are also common in managerial practice in healthcare organizations.

The sense of urgency associated with improving the quality of medical care does not exist with respect to improving the quality of management decision making. One reason for this complacency is that instances of overuse, underuse, and misuse of management tactics and strategies receive far less attention and are much more difficult to document than their clinical equivalents. Surely, mistakes of judgment that result in irrefutable harm to people, significant financial loss, or profound organizational change may motivate public and private inquiries into "how could this have happened?" For example, the failed merger of the hospitals owned by Stanford University and the University of California at San Francisco cost both institutions a combined $176 million over a 29-month period and stimulated considerable public discussion of the reasons for the failure of the merger (Russell 2000). However, the visibility of the Stanford–UCSF hospital fiasco stands in stark contrast to the way most management mistakes are handled. Relatively few ineffective or harmful management decisions are acknowledged, examined, and used as the source of organizational learning (Hofmann 2005; Jones 2005; Russell and Greenspan 2005). Moreover, the fact that a merger of two highly rated hospitals with close ties to world-renowned universities could proceed in spite of a substantial body of research that was available at the time that raised serious concerns about that type of merger (Bogue et al. 1995; Alexander, Halpern, and Lee 1996; Brooks and Jones 1997; Conner et al. 1997) serves as a vivid and painful reminder of a management quality chasm in health services organizations. A substantial gap exists between what is known about many management questions and what health managers do. We *must* close this gap.

Note

1. The Healthcare Leadership Alliance comprises the American College of Healthcare Executives, American College of Physician Executives, American Organization of Nurse Executives, Healthcare Financial Management Association, Healthcare Information and Management Systems Society, Medical Group Management Association, and American College of Medical Practice Executives.

Acknowledgment

The authors gratefully acknowledge the assistance of Chris Kovner, Juliana Tilemma, and Erica Foldy, and of course the managers whom Kovner interviewed in the collection of information used in the preparation of this article. We would also like to acknowledge the financial support of the Center for Health Management Research in conducting the research reported here.

References

AHRQ. 2006a. National Guideline Clearinghouse. [Online resource; modified 10/10/05; retrieved 10/13/05]. www.guideline.gov

AHRQ 2006b. Research Findings. [Online resource; retrieved 10/21/05]. www.ahrq .gov/research/

Alexander, J. A., M. T. Halpern, and S-Y. D. Lee. 1996. "The Short-Term Effects of Merger on Hospital Operations." *Health Services Research* 30 (6): 827–47.

Axelson, R. 1998. "Towards an Evidence-Based Health Care Management." *International Journal of Health Planning and Management* 13: 307–17.

Bero, L. A., and A. R. Jadad. 1997. "How Consumers and Policymakers Can Use Systematic Reviews for Decision Making." *Annals of Internal Medicine* 127 (127): 37–42.

Bogue, R. J., S. M. Shortell, M.-W. Sohn, L. M. Manheim, G. Bazzoli, and C. Chan. 1995. "Hospital Reorganization After Merger." *Medical Care* 33 (7): 676–86.

Brooks, G. R., and V. G. Jones. 1997. "Hospital Mergers and Market Overlap." *Health Services Research* 31 (6): 701–22.

Brownson, R. C., E. A. Baker, T. L. Leet, and K. N. Gillespie. 2003. *Evidence-Based Public Health*. Oxford: Oxford University Press.

Canadian Health Services Research Foundation. 2000. *Health Services Research and Evidence-Based Decision Making*, 7. Ottawa, Canada: Health Services Research Foundation.

———. 2004. *What Counts? Interpreting Evidence-based Decision-making for Management and Policy*. Ottawa, Canada: Health Services Research Foundation.

———. 2005. *Conceptualizing and Combining Evidence for Health System Guidance*. Ottawa, Canada: Health Services Research Foundation.

Clancy, C., and K. Cronin. 2005. "Evidence-based Decision Making: Global Evidence, Local Decisions." *Health Affairs* 24 (1): 151–62.

Cochrane Effective Practice and Organization of Care Group. 2006. [Online resource; updated 5/24/04; retrieved 10/13/05]. http://www.epoc.uottawa.ca/

Cochrane Consumers and Communication Review Group. 2006. [Online resource; updated 10/12/05; retrieved 10/21/05]. http://www.latrobe.edu.au/ cochrane/

Coffman, J., and T. G. Rundall. 2005. "The Impact of Hospitalists on the Cost and Quality of Inpatient Care in the United States: A Research Synthesis." *Medical Care Research and Review* 62 (4): 379–406.

Conner, R. A., R. D. Feldman, B. E. Dowd, and T. A. Radcliff. 1997. "Which Types of Hospital Mergers Save Money?" *Health Affairs* 16 (6): 62–74.

Davenport, T. H., and L. Prusak. 1998. *Working Knowledge*, 144–61. Boston: Harvard Business School Press.

Davies, H. T. O., and S. M. Nutley. 1999. "The Rise and Rise of Evidence in Health Care." *Public Money and Management* (Jan–Mar): 9–16.

Donaldson, C., M. Mugford, and L. Vale. 2002. *Evidence-Based Health Economics*. London: BMJ Books.

Eddy, D. M. 2005. "Evidence-Based Medicine: A Unified Approach." *Health Affairs* 24 (1): 9–17.

Friedland, D. J., ed. 1998. *Evidence-Based Medicine: A Framework for Clinical Practice*. Stamford, CT: Appleton & Lange.

Fox, D. 2005. "Evidence of Evidence-based Health Policy: The Politics of Systematic Reviews in Coverage Decision." *Health Affairs* 24 (1): 114–22.

Geyman, J. P., R. A. Deyo, and S. D. Ramsey. 2000. *Evidence-Based Clinical Practice: Concepts and Approaches*. Boston: Butterworth and Heinemann.

Greenhalgh, T., G. Robert, F. Macfarlane, P. Bate, and O. Kyriakidou. 2004. "Diffusion of Innovations in Service Organizations: Systematic Review and Recommendations." *The Milbank Quarterly* 82 (4): 581–629.

Ham, C. 2005. "Don't Throw the Baby Out With the Bath Water" (commentary). *Journal of Health Services Research and Policy* 10 S1: 51–52.

Hatcher, S., and M. Oakley-Browne. 2005. *Evidence-Based Mental Health*. London: Churchill Livingston.

Healthcare Leadership Alliance. 2005. *Competency Directory*. [Online document; retrieved 12/13/05]. http://www.healthcareleadershipalliance.org/directory.cfm.

Hofmann, P. B. 2005. "Acknowledging and Examining Management Mistakes." In *Management Mistakes in Healthcare: Identification, Correction, and Prevention*, edited by P. B. Hofmann and F. Perry, 3–27. Cambridge: Cambridge University Press.

Hofmann, P. B., and F. Perry. 2005. *Management Mistakes in Healthcare: Identification, Correction, and Prevention*. Cambridge: Cambridge University Press.

Institute for Healthcare Improvement. 2003. "Breakthrough Series Collaboratives." [Online information; retrieved 06/06/02]. http://www.ihi.org/ihi.

Jones, W. J. 2005. "Identifying, Classifying and Disclosing Mistakes." In *Management Mistakes in Healthcare: Identification, Correction, and Prevention*, edited by P. B. Hofmann and F. Perry, 40–73. Cambridge: Cambridge University Press.

Juran, J. M. 1989. *Juran on Leadership for Quality: An Executive Handbook*. New York: The Free Press.

Kelly, D. L. 2003. *Applying Quality Management in Healthcare: A Process for Improvement*. Chicago: Health Administration Press.

Kovner, A. R. 2005. "Factors Associated with Use of Management Research by Health Systems." Unpublished report for the Center for Health Management Research, University of Washington, Seattle.

Kovner, A. R., J. J. Elton, and J. Billings. 2000. "Transforming Health Management: An Evidence-Based Approach." *Frontiers of Health Services Management* 16 (4): 3–25.

Lavis, J., H. Davies, A. Oxman, J.–L. Denis, K. Golden-Biddle, and E. Ferlie. 2005. "Towards Systematic Reviews That Inform Health Care Management and Policy-Making." *Journal of Health Services Research and Policy* 10 (S1): 35–48.

Lavis, J. N., D. Robertson, J. M. Woodside, C. B. McLeod, J. Abelson, and The Knowledge Transfer Group. 2003. "How Can Research Organizations More Effectively Transfer Research Knowledge to Decision Makers?" *The Milbank Quarterly* 81 (2): 221–48.

Lavis, J. N., S. E. Ross, J. E. Hurley, J. M. Hohenadel, G. L. Stoddart, C. A. Woodward, and J. Abelson. 2002. "Examining the Role of Health Services Research in Public Policy Making." *Milbank Quarterly* 80 (1): 125–53.

Lomas, J. 2000. "Using 'Linkage and Exchange' to Move Research into Policy at a Canadian Foundation." *Health Affairs* 19 (3): 236–40.

Mack, K. E., M. A. Crawford, and M. C. Reed. 2004. *Decision Making for Improved Performance.* Chicago: Health Administration Press.

Mays, N., C. Pope, and J. Popay. 2005. "Systematically Reviewing Qualitative and Quantitative Evidence to Inform Management and Policy-Making in the Health Field." *Journal of Health Services Research and Policy* 10 (S1): 6–20.

Muir Gray, J. A. 2004. *Evidence-Based Health Care: How to Make Health Policy and Management Decisions.* New York: Churchill Livingston.

National Center for Healthcare Leadership. 2004. *Health Leadership Competency Model,* version 2.0, 1–9. Chicago: National Center for Healthcare Leadership.

Pawson, R., T. Greenhalgh, G. Harvey, and K. Walshe. 2005. "Realist Review—A New Method of Systematic Review Designed for Complex Policy Interventions." *Journal of Health Services Research and Policy* 10 (S1): 21–34.

Robbins, S. P., and D. A. DeCenzo. 2004. *Fundamentals of Management: Essential Concepts and Applications*, 4th edition. Upper Saddle River, NJ: Pearson Prentice Hall.

Russell, J. A., and B. Greenspan. 2005. "Correcting and Preventing Management Mistakes." In *Management Mistakes in Healthcare: Identification, Correction and Prevention*, edited by P. B. Hofmann and F. Perry, 84–102. Cambridge: Cambridge University Press.

Russell, S. 2000. "$176 Million Tab on Failed Hospital Merger." *San Francisco Chronicle*, December 14.

Sackett, D. L., W. M. Rosenberg, J. A. Gray, R. B. Haynes, and W. S. Richardson. 1996. "Evidence-Based Medicine: What It Is and What It Isn't." *British Medical Journal* 312 (7023): 71–72.

Sackett, D. L., S. E. Straus, W. S. Richardson, W. Rosenberg, and R. B. Haynes. 2000. *Evidence-Based Medicine: How to Practice and Teach EBM,* 2nd ed. New York: Churchill Livingston.

Sheldon, T. 2005. "Making Evidence Synthesis More Useful for Management and Policy-Making." *Journal of Health Services Research and Policy* 10 (S1): 1–4.

Shojania, K. G., and J. M. Grimshaw. 2005. "Evidence-Based Quality Improvement: The State of the Science." *Health Affairs* 24 (1): 138–50.

Shortell, S. M., R. R. Gillies, D. A. Anderson, K. M. Erickson, and J. B. Mitchell. 2000. *Remaking Health Care in America*, 2nd ed. San Francisco: Jossey-Bass.

Shortell, S. 2001. "A Time for Concerted Action." *Frontiers of Health Services Management* 18 (1): 33–46.

Stewart, R. 2002. *Evidence-Based Management: A Practical Guide for Health Professionals*. Abingdon, UK: Radcliffe Medical Press.

Walshe, K., and T. Rundall. 2001. "Evidence-Based Management: From Theory to Practice in Health Care." *The Milbank Quarterly* 79 (3): 429–47.

Discussion Questions on Required Reading

1. How can you tell whether a major medical center is or is not using evidence-based management?
2. Develop an action plan for implementing evidence-based management in a large academic medical center.
3. Make the business case for using evidence-based management.
4. How do the incentives under which healthcare managers function constrain the implementation of evidence-based management?

Required Supplementary Readings

Christensen, C., R. Bohmer, and J. Kenagy. 2000. "Will Disruptive Innovations Cure Healthcare?" *Harvard Business Review* (September–October): 102–12.

Dye, C. F., and A. N. Garman. 2006. *Exceptional Leadership: 16 Critical Competencies for Healthcare Executives*. Chicago: Health Administration Press.

Griffith, J. R., and K. R. White. 2005. "The Revolution in Hospital Management." *Journal of Healthcare Management* 50 (3): 170–90.

———. 2007. "Managing the Healthcare Organization." In *The Well-Managed Healthcare Organization*, 6th edition, 109–54. Chicago: Health Administration Press.

Discussion Questions for Required Supplemental Readings

1. What kinds of skills and experience should graduates of master's programs in healthcare administration have prior to seeking employment in a large healthcare organization?

2. What are some of the differences in managing the following organizations: large suburban non-profit hospital, large urban physicians' group practice, small urban for-profit nursing home, small rural non-profit hospital?
3. What are the risks and rewards to healthcare managers undertaking to implement "disruptive innovations"?
4. How should boards of trustees evaluate management performance?

Recommended Supplementary Readings

Collins, J. 2001. "Level 5 Leadership: The Triumph of Humility and Fierce Resolve." *Harvard Business Review* (January): 67–76.

Dreachslin, J. L. 1996. *Diversity Leadership*. Chicago: Health Administration Press.

Evashwick, C. and J. Riedel. 2004. *Managing Long-Term Care*. Chicago: Health Administration Press.

Griffith, J. R. 1993. *The Moral Challenges of Healthcare Management*. Chicago: Health Administration Press.

———. 2007. "Improving Preparation for Senior Management in Healthcare," *Journal of Health Administration Education* (Winter): 11–32.

Katz, R. L. 1974. "Skills of an Effective Administrator." *Harvard Business Review* 52 (5): 90–102.

Kovner, A. R. 2000. *Healthcare Management in Mind: Eight Careers*. New York: Springer.

———. 2006. "Healthcare Management Education 2007: Stirring the Pot." *Journal of Health Administration Education* (Winter): 59–69.

Kovner, A. R., J. J. Elton, and J. Billings. 2000. "Transforming Evidence-Based Management: An Evidence-Based Approach." *Frontiers of Health Services Management* 16 (4): 3–25.

McAlearney, A. S. 2006. "Leadership Development in Healthcare Organizations: A Qualitative Study." *Journal of Organizational Behavior* 27 (7): 967–82.

———. 2008. "Using Leadership Development Programs to Improve Quality and Efficiency in Healthcare." *Journal of Healthcare Management* 53 (5): 319–31.

Peace, W. H. 2001. "The Hard Work of Being a Soft Manager." *Harvard Business Review* (December): 99–104.

Shortell, S. M., T. G. Rundall, and J. Hsu. 2007. "Improving Patient Care by Linking Evidence-Based Medicine and Evidence-Based Management." *Journal of the American Medical Association* 298 (6): 673–76.

Wenzel, F. J., and J. M. Wenzel. 2005. *Fundamentals of Physician Practice Management.* Chicago: Health Administration Press.

THE CASES

Personnel decisions, critical to managerial effectiveness, are often postponed by healthcare managers or not handled with sufficient care. For example, considerably more time may be spent on the decision to purchase or lease a piece of valuable equipment costing $900,000 with a useful life of seven years than on the decision to hire a registered nurse earning $60,000 a year who may work for the organization for 20 years.

Even more important than the hiring decision is the continuous evaluation and motivation of subordinates and colleagues, many of whom may have been hired by a manager's predecessors. If the managers do not perform at an expected level of competence, what are the supervisor's options? What are the manager's options if she disagrees with her boss's expectations or evaluation? If the boss does not fire or transfer a manager being evaluated, her own effectiveness may suffer because she lacks a key aide to implement her strategy and support her politically. Ineffective managers may have been working loyally for an organization for many years. Searching for and training a new manager costs time and money; in addition, the risk exists that a new hire's performance will not be as anticipated.

Managerial personnel decisions become even more complicated when, as in "The Associate Director and the Controllers," the healthcare manager is dealing with a functional specialist who is line responsible to the top manager and staff responsible to the chief controller in a multi-unit medical center. The straight and dotted lines of authority on the organizational chart become fuzzy and difficult to agree upon in practice, especially when the associate director's boss and the medical center director of finance distrust each other. In this case study, key staff of the two recently merged units have different value orientations—the base hospital primarily serving attending physicians in their private practices, and the ambulatory health services program emphasizing the provision of respectful patient care to low-income patients residing in the local community.

The manager's job is often a lonely one. Important decisions are seldom made on an either-or basis, and often involve personal as well as organizational risks and benefits. In "A New Faculty Practice Administrator for the Department of Medicine," the weighing of risks and benefits is different for Sam Bones, the chief of medicine, than it is for Sandra Compson, the group practice administrator, or for Compson's eventual successor. Similarly, in "The Associate Director and the Controllers," the stakes of the game are higher for James Joel, the ambulatory health service program manager, and for Percy Oram, its controller, than for Milton Schlitz, the medical center director of finance, and for Miller Harrang, the chief executive officer of the ambulatory health services program.

Why must Joel decide to do anything at all? In "A New Faculty Practice Administrator," Bones must choose a new group practice administrator. But in "The Associate Director and the Controllers," Joel can decide not to get involved and allow Harrang and Schlitz to deal with the consequences of Oram's ineffectiveness. How much should it matter to Joel whether Oram remains on the job or not, so long as Joel can protect his own job? On the other hand, Joel is being paid to manage, not to observe or to protect himself. Good management generally makes a difference to the patient, as well as to an organization's ruling coalition. How much of a difference is open to question. But who will look after the manager's interest if she doesn't look after it herself? This is the first rule of managerial survival. Looking after one's own interest does not mean that the manager should lock her office door, read reports, and sit there telling subordinates what to do. Instead, there are opportunities to strategically plan one's professional development, as considered in the case, "Now What?"

Healthcare managers often face tremendous pressures from government to move in certain directions and resistance from physicians who do not wish to move one step further than that required by law. How much value do managers add to organizational performance? Not much, according to Pfeffer and Salancik (1978), who argue that the contribution of managers accounts for about 10 percent of the variance in organizational performance, and who agree with the sportscaster's cliche, that "managers are hired to be fired." An increasing amount of evidence, however, indicates that managers *do* make a difference in organizational performance, if only as they play a key role in obtaining the resources necessary for organizational survival and growth.

If the healthcare manager can never meet all the expectations of key organizational stakeholders, she can at least be seen as taking stakeholder interests into account in policy formulation and implementation. This requires regular communication, which takes valuable time. What makes for an effective healthcare manager? The answer depends on stakeholder perceptions as well as on any given manager's actual behavior or motivation. Sometimes—as in the short case of "Nowhere Job"—the right thing for the manager *is* to resign. Clearly healthcare managers must acquire information, learn skills, and have values consistent with an organizational context and its ruling coalition. It is not always easy to decide what actions to take after the manager receives disquieting information, such as that shown in the short case of "Manager Morale at Uptown Hospital." Similarly, the realities faced by new managers in "A Sure Thing," "The First Day," and "Mid-Career Change" all create challenges for these individuals to manage their own expectations as well as their new jobs.

Evaluating managerial effectiveness or contribution carries a cost. All pertinent information may not be available at a reasonable cost. Reliance on measurement may divert attention inappropriately away from what can be easily measured. Evaluating managers, like management itself, involves judgment, which in Ray Brown's (1969) phrase, is "knowledge ripened by experience."

For management students, case discussions are an excellent way to get safe experience in forming managerial judgments.

References

Brown, R. 1969. *Judgment in Administration,* 9. New York: McGraw-Hill.
Pfeffer, J., and G. R. Salancik. 1978. *The External Control of Organizations,* p. 17. New York: Harper & Row.

Case A
A New Faculty Practice Administrator for the Department of Medicine

Anthony R. Kovner and David M. Kaplan

Sandra Compson was leaving her position as faculty practice administrator at Wise Medical Center to raise a family. Dr. Sam Bones, chief of medicine, asked Compson to become involved in the selection of her replacement before leaving.

Wise Medical Center is regarded as one of the largest and best-managed hospitals in Eastern City. The CEO, Dr. Worthy, was appointed in 2003. He has captained the dramatic growth of the medical center, its financial success, and the improvement of its medical teaching programs. Over the last five years, almost all the clinical chiefs have been replaced. Internal medicine is the largest department in the medical center. Dr. Bones is a specialist in cardiovascular disease and has an excellent reputation as a clinician.

His department has grown very large, and Bones has difficulty in staffing the large number of beds with medical residents. Bones is praised for his leadership skills, his intelligence, and his caring for those who work with him. He has been criticized for his unwillingness to make tough decisions regarding the economics of the department and for not getting rid of physicians who don't or won't meet his own and the department's high standards of quality. The medical center and the department face stiff financial pressures, and Dr. Worthy and others are trying to determine what the medical center's response to managed care should be. The medical center currently relies heavily upon referrals from its managed care panel, its network hospitals and clinics, and community physicians.

The faculty practice plan (FPP) in the department of medicine was formally launched upon the arrival of Dr. Worthy in 2003, as were the faculty practices in various other departments. The FPP in the department consists of 16 subspecialties and 100 providers who all share the faculty practice suite. The suite, which is 10,450 square feet, consists of 40 exam rooms, 10 consultation rooms, a reception and waiting area, a small laboratory, a technician's area, a billing office, and an office for the practice administrator.

The FPP staff for the department of medicine consists of six secretaries, two registered nurses, three midlevel providers, one medical technician, and one practice administrator. Larger physician practices including general internal medicine, neurology, and hematology/oncology bring additional staff with them when they are holding their sessions.

Compson, the practice administrator, is responsible for scheduling the subspecialty clinic sessions for each division within the department of medicine. Each provider is assigned a session with dedicated rooms. The medical center utilizes an electronic scheduling system, where all the providers have dedicated blocks of time to schedule patient appointments. It has been estimated that several of the physicians do not have enough volume to fill their sessions, while other physicians have a large backlog of patients and a long wait time to be seen.

The FPP suite currently operates from 9 a.m. to 5 p.m., Monday through Friday. Visits have increased by 15 percent over a three-year period from 15,000 to 17,250. Demand is such that if more staff and space were available volume might be able to increase by an additional 7 percent with little or no additional investment.

Compson has limited access to the financial information such as revenue, expense, and billing records for the faculty practice since an outsourced company performs all of the faculty practice outpatient billing. (It is important to note that the medical center's patient accounts department handles the inpatient billing.) The billing system ties directly into the scheduling system. Dr. Worthy and his leadership team selected both the billing/scheduling system and the billing company in 2003. The systems are outdated and the subspecialties have limited knowledge of their financial standing. Historically, this hasn't been a tremendous issue because all of the physicians are salaried and do not have any financial incentives to increase productivity.

The original operating concept of the faculty practice suite was to create a place with an upscale ambiance where physicians could see their patients.

The purpose for creating the suite was to recover scattered examination space throughout the medical center and to take advantage of economies of shared space. Based on these concepts, decisions were made early to maximize treatment space at the expense of chart storage space, which is limited. In fact, many providers are forced to bring their charts to and from other locations to each clinic session. The practice had evaluated an electronic medical record system in 2005, but it was deemed too expensive.

Recently, the division of cardiology wanted to create a heart failure program and approached Dr. Worthy and Compson with a proposal that would have generated an additional 600 patients and 200 additional heart valve surgeries a year, bringing an additional $1.2 million in revenue to the medical center. But with no space available to accommodate this demand, and no capital to build a new facility, the proposal was denied.

Bones's final interview with Compson follows:

Bones: Sandra, as you know, you've done a splendid job here this past year and we'll be sorry to lose you. The situation of the departmental faculty practice as I see it is this: During the past few years the practice has been organized and it has grown dramatically. We seem to be having a lot of operating problems, such as limited space, poor support for the physicians, and antiquated billing and scheduling systems. The question now is, what skills and experience should the ideal practice administrator possess to enhance the practice? What do you think?

Compson: Well, Dr. Bones, as you know, I've enjoyed tremendously the opportunity to work with you and with the members of the department and I will be sorry to leave, although I am looking forward very much to raising a family. I think the kind of person you need is not necessarily the type of person you needed back in 2003. Then you needed someone who could "put out fires" and try to keep the place running. Now I think you need a systems person who can make the place run more effectively, while simultaneously keeping up the morale of the staff and communicating with the physicians.

Bones: I agree with you. I want someone personable and energetic, who isn't afraid of work, who can get along with the doctors and the hospital administration. I think the most important thing is getting our physicians the kind of support they need to run a first-class faculty practice. The systems aren't working down there. According to the reports I've seen (see Tables I.2 and I.3), the department isn't making the kind of money that it should be making, and we should be making it much more efficient and productive for our physicians to practice here.

Compson: As you know, per your instructions, I've started the interviewing process and will send you all the good candidates. I have spoken to

TABLE I.2

Faculty
Practice Suite
Billings and
Collections,
Fiscal Year
2005

Month	Billings	Collections	Contractual Allowances	Gross Collection Rate	Net Collection Rate
September	$ 3,241,151	$ 1,199,226	$ 1,296,460	37%	62%
October	$ 3,213,040	$ 1,349,477	$ 1,285,216	42%	70%
November	$ 2,864,251	$ 859,275	$ 1,145,700	30%	50%
December	$ 2,203,564	$ 1,013,639	$ 881,426	46%	77%
January	$ 3,514,687	$ 1,827,637	$ 1,405,875	52%	87%
February	$ 2,647,159	$ 952,977	$ 1,058,864	36%	60%
March	$ 3,268,573	$ 1,830,401	$ 1,307,429	56%	93%
April	$ 3,358,751	$ 1,612,200	$ 1,343,500	48%	80%
May	$ 3,046,892	$ 1,736,728	$ 1,218,757	57%	95%
June	$ 2,781,441	$ 1,668,865	$ 1,112,576	60%	100%
July	$ 2,813,332	$ 1,153,466	$ 1,125,333	41%	68%
August	$ 2,215,116	$ 863,895	$ 886,046	39%	65%
Total	**$35,167,957**	**$16,067,788**	**$14,067,183**	**46%**	**76%**

TABLE I.3

Faculty Practice
Suite Quarterly
Statistics:
Departmental
Key Indicators,
Fiscal Year
2004–Fiscal
Year 2005

	2004	2005	% Variance
Total Number Providers	80	100	25%
Percent Utilization	72%	68%	−6%
Visits	15,000	17,250	15%
Total Provider Sessions	9,600	12,000	25%
Revenue	$15,599,794	$16,067,788	3%
Expenses	$12,703,456	$13,338,629	5%
Net Profit/(Loss)	**$2,896,338**	**$2,729,159**	**−6%**

several directors of programs of healthcare administration and to the hospital human resources department. There aren't a lot of good people available with systems and management experience in healthcare. I don't want someone who is strictly a systems person. The manager must be in touch with the needs, wants, requirements, and expectations of the customers. I see the customers of the faculty practice as both the physicians and the patients.

Bones: Sandra, I agree with you there. I know you'll excuse me, but I have to attend an important strategic planning meeting for the hospital. I still don't quite understand what they're going to do, but I wish they'd give more emphasis in the plan to building up the medical center's research capabilities.

Compson: All right. Then I'll be getting back to you soon. I will make appointments with Renee, your secretary, for all the promising candidates.

One month after Sandra Compson's interview with Bones, she has completed interviews with 11 candidates for the position. She has eliminated from consideration four graduates from health administration programs who lack appropriate work experience and three medical center employees in the finance department who she feels would not relate well to the physicians in the group. Compson made tape recordings of her interviews with the remaining four promising candidates and has had difficulty in choosing among them.

Compson's first interview was with David O'Brien, currently an assistant director for patient accounts in the finance department. The patient accounts area is responsible for all inpatient billing within the medical center. The second interview was with Sal Sorrentino, a recent graduate from the City University program in health policy and management. Prior to attending the program Sal was the assistant director of a neighborhood health center. The third interview was with Marcia Rabin, a classmate of Sorrentino's at City University and director of human resources at a large multispecialty practice. The final candidate was Bonnie Goldsmith, who recently completed two years with the U.S. Department of Health and Human Services in Washington, D.C., after graduating with a master's in health administration (MHA) from City University. Compson has elected to review the tapes with Tim Brass, the senior vice president of clinical operations, before forwarding her recommendations to Dr. Bones.

David O'Brien

Compson (to Brass): The first interview is with David O'Brien. He is approximately 25 years old, and dresses very conservatively. When I spoke with Barbara Karen, Wise Medical Center's senior vice president of finance, she said David was energetic and conscientious, and that he gets things accomplished. She gave him a very positive reference for this position. When asked about his weaknesses she did say that he was a bit intense, and sometimes intimidates and antagonizes others. She continued to say that David has no problems, it seems, in getting along with his superiors, but has limited experience in working with physicians. (Compson plays a tape of the interview.)

Compson: David, can you tell me in a few words something about your background and experience?

O'Brien: Sure, Ms. Compson. I attended Upstate College, where I was a business major. After graduation I started working in the hospital finance department, specifically patient accounts as a biller. Just last year I was promoted as the assistant director within patient accounts. My eventual goal is to receive my master's degree at City University, in its MHA program.

Compson: Going at night?

O'Brien: Well, I don't think there will be any problem. Others have done it here at the medical center, and I want to get out of finance and into management.

Compson: Dave, what would you say has been your greatest accomplishment in patient accounts?

O'Brien: I would say that I've really improved the system for inpatient billing and collections, starting with getting the bills out on time, all the way through to collections, and in refining and improving the data system that indicates how well we are performing. Performance has improved since I've taken the job—in speed, in accuracy, in the percentage collected, and in the time it takes for the hospital to get its money.

Compson: Dave, that does sound impressive. If you were faculty practice administrator, what would you consider to be your greatest asset?

O'Brien: I would say it's my ability to get a job done. There are too many people in this field who are just willing to go along with the way things have always been done until there's pressure from leadership to change, and then it's often too late to do something, or to do it the right way.

Compson: And what would you say is your greatest liability?

O'Brien: Well, you know, in every organization some people are against change, because either it affects their own interest or because they just don't like change. After all, every change in somebody's department has to affect everyone involved in a relative, if not in an absolute, way. As my teacher used to say, "You don't make an omelet without breaking eggs." And I guess as I look for ways to implement change I must rub some people the wrong way.

Compson: What aspect of the job in the faculty practice do you think is most important?

O'Brien: I think it's improving the net revenues. I've spoken with the billing clerk in the practice and she thinks the doctors could vastly improve utilization of the facility by making changes in the scheduling, so that docs aren't allocated time slots if they're not using them effectively. Also, the reports generated by the practice could be greatly improved. I'd like to track physician productivity in dollars relative to the opportunity costs involved in their using examining room space.

Compson: Before you go, is there anything you would like to ask me about the job?

O'Brien: As a matter of fact there is. We've talked about the salary and the benefits, but if I perform as expected, what is the likelihood of a decent increase after the first year? You know I have a wife and two young children.

Compson: Well, I'd say the chances are pretty good. Dr. Bones is fair and I think he would be generous if the practice results improved significantly. (She turns off the tape recorder.)

Brass: He seems like a fine candidate.

Salvatore Sorrentino

Compson (to Brass): Sal Sorrentino is the next candidate. Sal is 27 years old. He is presentable—although he dresses a bit on the flashy side—and is fast talking and enthusiastic. When I spoke to his reference, Dr. Plotkin of the neighborhood health center, he highly recommended Sal for the position. He said Sal was idealistic, energetic, and pleasant. If there was any weakness, Dr. Plotkin thought that Sal has a tendency to initiate or implement new policies and procedures without understanding the implications. I asked him to clarify, or to provide an example, and he said Sal had decided to change the way patients were scheduled without getting any input from the physicians, nurses, or secretarial staff. The result was that patients were being triple booked, and having in some cases to wait for over two hours for their appointment. The issue was quickly resolved, and Dr. Plotkin believed that Sal had learned his lesson. Dr. Plotkin did reiterate that he highly recommends Sal for this position. (Compson plays a tape of the interview.)

Compson: Sal, can you tell me in a few words something about your background and experience?

Sorrentino: Yes, I can. I was a political science major at City University, then I got involved with various community and non-profit groups. While working with St. Angelo's Church, I was active in trying to improve the availability of maternal and child health services to the Latino population; as a result, I met the assistant director for community relations at the neighborhood health center. It turns out that we were both vitally concerned with helping patients, and helping to provide needed services to the community. Before long I was offered a position as an administrative assistant at the health center. Shortly after starting this job, I was able to secure a scholarship to the City University graduate program in health policy and management.

Compson: And what would you say, Sal, was your greatest accomplishment at the neighborhood health center?

Sorrentino: Well, one of the things I am proudest of is the community health fair I planned and organized. We involved community groups of all ethnic and work-related backgrounds and got the health professionals to staff the booths at the fair. We worked with business corporations to get prizes and literature on, for example, proper nutrition. We conducted screening examinations for eye problems and provided tuberculosis and

Pap tests. We followed up with all patients who needed help after the fair was over. The fair was well-attended and many people learned for the first time about the services the center had to offer. Of course, I accomplished a lot of other things, such as implementing a new billing system at the satellite of the neighborhood health center.

Compson: Tell me more about that.

Sorrentino: It wasn't so much really. We needed to get more information than we were getting about patients coming for service. We had to make an effort to collect from those patients who could pay something and to have records that were suitable for reporting purposes. It was hard to implement because the staff was more interested in the patients getting service than in collecting the money.

Compson: I see. In the position we have been talking about, what do you think would be your greatest asset?

Sorrentino: Well, I see the highest priority for the group as that of attracting more patients. As my father told me, the way you make money in a business is primarily by increasing revenue rather than cutting back on expenses. I think the practice could improve rapport with patients and make changes in the suite so that the setting would be more attractive and comfortable for them. I think the practice would probably need an attractive brochure. The waiting area should be spruced up. I think the patients should know in advance how much services will cost. I'd like to devote part of my time to developing relationships with HMOs and managed care plans to negotiate enhanced rates to help increase receipts. In addition, I believe that the practice could benefit by extending the hours of operation, such as opening on Saturday mornings, or starting extended evening hours.

Compson: That sounds like an excellent idea. I've been pushing for Saturday hours also, but we aren't using our full capacity during the week as it is now. Another question, Sal, what do you think would be your greatest liability, if any, if you were chosen for the position?

Sorrentino: I don't know. I want to get things done in a hurry, I guess. I'm eager for results. Maybe I have a tendency to move a little too fast. Not really. It's hard to talk of one's faults. I really think that I would excel in this position and I'd like the opportunity to do so. I'm not always that good at following through on all the little details of an operation. But I'm excellent at working with people who will see to all the details.

Compson: I'm a little sorry to hear that because I think a lot of details are involved in this work.

Sorrentino: I didn't mean to say that I didn't like detail work or that I wasn't good at it. I would just say that it's a relative weakness—I really prefer the other kind of work I was describing rather than doing the billing clerk's work for him or her.

Compson: I see. What do you think is the most important aspect of the job we've been talking about in terms of the work that needs to be done?

Sorrentino: I guess first you have to get all your systems working properly, such as billing and reporting, and I think next the most important thing is to increase your revenues. Based on your description it sounds like Dr. Bones's plan for the department is for the faculty practice to generate enough revenue to help support faculty member salaries.

Compson: You're right there. Is there anything now you want to ask me about the job, before you go up and talk to Dr. Bones?

Sorrentino: Two things really. First, what kind of person is Dr. Bones to work for? And, second, do you think there are good opportunities in management to further advance from this position?

Compson: In answer to your first question, I think Dr. Bones is an excellent person to work for, so long as you produce for him. He's loyal, and gives you enough autonomy. Perhaps my only complaint is that it is sometimes difficult to see him, because he is such a busy man and I don't want to bother him with things I would like to discuss. I have recommended to him that he appoint another physician within the department as head of the faculty practice, a plan that I know Dr. Bones is considering. As to your second question, yes, the medical center is a large employer of people like yourself and you can make a lot of useful contacts here. Also I feel ambulatory care is the place to be in health-care management in the future. (She turns off the tape.)

Brass: Well, these first two candidates have quite contrasting backgrounds. Yet it seems clear to me that either of them might do a perfectly respectable job, although of course the outcomes resulting from their work might be quite different.

Marcia Rabin

Compson (to Brass): Yes, that's so. The third candidate is Marcia Rabin. Marcia is 24 years old, attractive, and energetic. Les Carson, the CEO of Partner's Health Group, highly recommended her for the position. Ms. Rabin was the director of human resources for the Group, which consisted of 50 physicians and 20 support staff. Carson said she was hard working, and got along well with both professional and non-professional staff. If there is any fault to find with her, Carson said that Rabin takes her work too seriously, drives herself too hard, and as a result may be absent for a few days, largely because she has difficulty determining priorities. But Carson stressed that Rabin has performed very well on all the big jobs that he has given her to do, that she was reliable and competent. (Compson plays a tape of the interview.)

Compson: Ms. Rabin, can you tell me in a few words something about your background and experience?

Rabin: Certainly, I guess you don't want me to go back to high school, but I was president of my student government at Suburban High. In college I majored in psychology, and for a while I thought I would like to be a psychologist. But my father works in a hospital; he is director of housekeeping at Sisters Hospital, and encouraged me to go into healthcare management. After attending the City University master's program, I was hired as the director of human resources at Partner's. Previously they didn't have a department of human resources, but when the Group bought two additional practices and expanded from 10 to 50 physicians a department was established. While at Partner's I worked under the tutelage of Mr. Les Carson, the CEO.

Compson: What would you say was your greatest accomplishment as director of human resources?

Rabin: Really, I think it was my ability to fill all the entry-level jobs, or rather to keep filling them. Also, we started and finished a job classification system under my supervision, and inaugurated an annual pay increment schedule that I think worked more fairly than the previous system. I think my real accomplishment was in legitimating the department of human resources in the group practice, where such a department had never existed before. This meant being able to service other departments and to accomplish jobs for them that used to take up a lot of their time or that they couldn't do as well before.

Compson: That sounds interesting. In terms of the present position with Dr. Bones, what would you say is your greatest asset?

Rabin: I don't know exactly how to answer that question. My first response would be to say I like and am good at doing systems work—creating order out of chaos and working effectively with people so that they feel it is their system, not something that I pushed on them. Of course, this is difficult to do because, in my case, the departments had to accept the human resources system we established; it's the only way to do things as part of a large organization. But at least the pacing and some of the details were left to them, and first we proved that we really could be of help to them.

Compson: And what, if you'll pardon my asking, would you say is your greatest liability?

Rabin: Well, if you must know, Ms. Compson, I'm not aggressive enough. Sometimes I think my efforts aren't properly appreciated, and I don't push myself to the front the way some people do. I work hard and I work well and it annoys me, sometimes more than it should, that others who don't work so hard and do so well push themselves forward and move ahead faster.

Compson: What aspect of the job, as I have tried to outline it to you, would you say is the most important, I mean at this time in the history of the faculty practice?

Rabin: I think you have to set up more clearly defined ways of doing things, *systems* if you prefer the word. I noted in the materials that you shared with me that your collection rate isn't what it should be and that your utilization of examining rooms is well below capacity also. I don't think that this kind of systems work is so different from my work in human resources, plus I have taken a few courses in quantitative analysis and feel pretty comfortable with numbers.

Compson: Are there any questions that you would like to ask me?

Rabin: Well, one question is how have the physicians, most of them men, related to having a woman in this position? Second, when can you let me know if you are offering me the job? I have been offered a job as assistant director of human resources at King Hospital, and although they aren't pressing me that hard, I would like to be able to tell them something soon.

Compson: With regard to the first question, sure, some of the physicians don't give you the respect as a manager that you would like to have, but I don't know to what extent this has to do with my being a woman. I think being a woman also has its advantages, with some of the docs. To answer your second question, I think it will take about a month for Dr. Bones to decide on a candidate. I can't tell you what you should say to the King people. You are one of the four candidates whom I am sending on to see Dr. Bones. (She turns off the tape.)

Bonnie Goldsmith

Compson (to Brass): Permit me to introduce our last candidate, Bonnie Goldsmith. She dresses conservatively and gives the impression of a modest, unassuming, kindly, young woman of 27. Her boss, Dr. Muldoon, who recently left the Centers for Medicare and Medicaid Services (CMS), recommended Bonnie as hard working, modest, and reliable. He said Bonnie gets along with people, but tends to lack drive as well as the ability to think independently. However, Dr. Muldoon says that once a task is clearly outlined, Bonnie is thorough, dedicated, and relentless. As an example he praised Bonnie's work on a recent Task Force on the Aging report. (She plays a tape of the interview.)

Compson: Bonnie, can you tell me a few words about your background and experience?

Goldsmith: Yes, I was a zoology major at City University. Originally I wanted to be a physician. In fact, I attended medical school for one year, then decided it just wasn't for me. I didn't know what I wanted to do. I don't know why but I thought that working in a hospital admitting department might be interesting, and I did that for a while. My father is a psychiatrist. The administrator is a good friend of my father's, and he talked to me and convinced me to apply to City University's graduate program in health policy and management. Back in school I really enjoyed the coursework related to quality improvement, information systems, and statistical analysis. A whole new world opened up to me, although I must confess I had a bit of difficulty with some of the heavy reading and writing courses. After graduation, I was fortunate to get a position with the CMS. Once again, my father's connections helped to open some doors for me. For the past two years at the CMS I have been working to help complete a Task Force on the Aging report, which was finally published three months ago.

Compson: What would you say has been your greatest accomplishment at CMS?

Goldsmith: I would say it was the staff work I did on the President's Task Force on the Aging. I went into a lot of nursing homes and other chronic care institutions and saw what a lousy deal most of our aged get. It isn't so much this way in Europe, which I visited a couple of years ago with my father. In Europe, the homes are more like residences and fewer people go into homes. When they do go, they can take their furniture with them, and it doesn't cost as much.

Compson: What kind of solutions did you come up with?

Goldsmith: Well, it's a pretty difficult problem. I mean the part about making it possible not to have to institutionalize the elderly. I guess there are tax incentives that could be passed to allow people to keep their relatives at home. Also, more people should be able to bring their relatives into homes for day care activities and to institutionalize them for a week or two each year if necessary, either because the aged member of the household is sick or because other members of the household want a rest. Of course, we need better regulation of nursing homes to set standards for care and to establish closer relations between homes and hospitals.

Compson: I see. What do you think would be your greatest asset in the position that exists here within the department of medicine?

Goldsmith: I don't know. Perhaps it's my ability to get along with and to understand the needs and problems of the medical profession. I don't have a big ego. I like analytical work, solving operations problems, and I think I'm pretty persistent in trying to solve them.

Compson: And your greatest liability?

Goldsmith: Well, some people think I'm not aggressive enough. I don't know what this means, really, unless it is forcing your opinions on others. I guess I'm not a great innovator, and I don't like to work that much. I mean I work hard, but I don't want work to be an obsession, like it is for my father. I mean that I'm married, with a nice husband and a young son, and I want to enjoy my work and do well, but I also want to enjoy my family. I guess you could call it a lack of ambition. But I think this country needs more people like me, people whose satisfaction comes from a job well done rather than striving for money, status, and power. I'm intellectually committed to group practice as a better way to deliver healthcare, and I'd like to do my part to see that primary care is improved in this country. So this may be a liability or an asset, I don't know.

Compson: I'm not sure either. But certainly if you do the job well, what you say makes sense. Well, enough of that. What aspects of the job strike you as most important?

Goldsmith: Well, I don't know. Certainly, the practice has to be organized systematically, and billing has to be improved. I'd like to track these processes scientifically, see what the standards are and should be, track the variance from standards by analyzing all the steps in these processes, and then work with all the individuals involved from physicians to receptionists in improving these systems. This might require a number of meetings, and I don't know how feasible such meetings would be because of people's time requirements. There are a few questions I would like to ask you.

Compson: Please go ahead.

Goldsmith: My first question is, do you think the faculty practice is going to grow? The second is incidental, but I would like to know more about the benefits, such as tuition remission, as I was thinking of furthering my education at City, perhaps taking some more courses in statistical analysis.

Compson: I think the faculty practice will continue to grow. Space is our key constraint now, and the medical center will have to figure out how we are going to better deal with managed care. Also, should we eventually combine the faculty practice plans in the various departments into one multidisciplinary group practice that is also in the managed care business? Of course this all has to be squared with the department's ambitious goals in teaching and research. Sometimes, despite the excellent reputation of the medical center and the quality of its leadership, I wonder if we can possibly excel in all these different areas as well as in all of the leading areas of clinical medicine. With respect to your second question, yes, I believe tuition remission for such purposes is available, although I don't see where you will have the time to fit everything in with the demands of this job, which are quite considerable, and with your family obligations. (She turns off the tape.)

The Recommendation

Brass: Well, Sandy, now all you have to do is tell Dr. Bones whom you recommend for the job.

Compson: I need to sleep on it. This selection process is much more difficult than I had envisioned, but that's what makes it so much fun.

Brass: I agree with you there. Sorry, but I've got to leave now. I will also mull this over and I'll give you my opinion tomorrow.

Case Questions

1. What criteria would you use in evaluating the four candidates?
2. What are the strengths and weaknesses of each candidate?
3. What are Bones's criteria in evaluating the four candidates?
4. Whom would you recommend to Bones as your selection for the position?
5. What is the evidence that you used in making this recommendation?

Case B
The Associate Director and the Controllers

Anthony R. Kovner

Fortunately for Jim Joel, he didn't lose his temper often. Otherwise, he might not have been able to function as associate director of the Morris Healthcare Program of the Nathan D. Wise Medical Center (NWMC) (see Figure I.4). But now, he had become so enraged at the Morris program controller, Percy Oram, that he had to concentrate hard to keep from yelling. Joel had just been informed by Felix Schwartzberg, an assistant director, that the accounting department was not collecting cash from the billing assistants in the family health units as previously agreed. Unfortunately, Oram did not usually keep Joel informed of his actions. But in any case, Joel knew his own reaction was excessive—an aspiring health services executive did not throw a tantrum, which is what he now felt like doing.

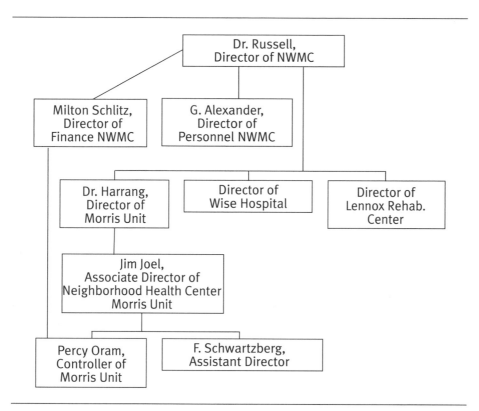

FIGURE I.4
Organization
Chart:
Nathan D. Wise
Medical Center

Joel was 30 years old, ambitious, and a recent graduate from Ivy University's master in healthcare administration program. Before returning to school, he had worked as a registered representative on Wall Street, where he had found the work remunerative but uninteresting. The director of the Ivy program, Dr. Leon Russell, assumed the post of director of the Nathan D. Wise Medical Center three years ago. Joel, one of his best students, asked to join Russell toward the end of that year, and he was hired shortly thereafter as an assistant hospital administrator. The Nathan D. Wise Medical Center is located in New York City and comprises three large programs: the Nathan D. Wise Hospital, the Lennox Rehabilitation Center, and the Morris Healthcare Program. The hospital and the rehabilitation center are owned by the Wise Medical Center, but the Morris Healthcare Program is operated by the Wise Medical Center under contract with the city of New York and is located in a city-owned facility.

Russell had been impressed with his former student's drive and promise and had originally created a job for Joel. This included half-time as a staff assistant at Wise Hospital and half-time as an evaluator at the Morris Unit, where new methods of delivering ambulatory medical care were being developed and demonstrated. Eventually Russell offered Joel the position of associate director of the Morris Unit. The director of the Morris Unit was Dr. Miller Harrang, a 45-year-old physician.

Joel felt ambivalent regarding Russell's offer. He knew he would take the position, even before requesting a night to think it over, but at the same time he had certain reservations. Joel enjoyed his work at the hospital. He had submitted an in-depth plan for increasing efficiency of the operating room, which had been enthusiastically accepted by the medical staff executive committee, and he was just starting an evaluation of patient transport in the hospital. His key interest was implementation of his master's thesis on nurse staffing. Joel believed that by assigning rooms to patients on the basis of their nursing needs, one-third fewer registered nurses would be required. Joel wished to be director of a large general hospital within ten years. He wasn't sure how working at the Morris Unit would advance him toward that goal, nor how comfortable he would feel working in a facility serving the poor in a slum section of the city.

However, after taking the job, Joel found before long that he liked working at the Morris Unit immensely. Morris was rapidly expanding—in the past year, the number of physician visits had increased 25 percent to 215,000. Through a generous grant from the Office of Economic Opportunity (OEO), the budget had increased from $15 million to $25 million. Joel worked 65 to 70 hours a week. There was so much to do. He liked Harrang and the others who worked at Morris. The atmosphere was busy and informal, a nice change of pace from Wise Hospital, where things happened more slowly. Dramatic change was the norm at Morris, whether this was conversion of the medical and pediatric clinics to family health units, or confrontations with a community health council resulting in increased participation in policymaking by the poor.

There was no formal division of responsibility between Harrang and Joel. Harrang spent most of his time in community relations (time-consuming and frustrating), in individual conversations with members of the medical staff at Morris, and in working out problems with Wise Hospital. Harrang also took responsibility for certain medical units such as the emergency room, obstetrics-gynecology (ob-gyn), and psychiatry. Joel's primary responsibility lay in the area of staff activities such as finance, personnel, and purchasing. He also supervised several departments or units, including laboratory, x-ray, pharmacy, dental, housekeeping, and maintenance. Responsibility for the family health units was shared by the two top administrators.

Before Harrang became director, the Morris Unit had been run as a unit independent from Wise Hospital. The unit was decentralized, with departments such as laboratory and internal medicine handling their own personnel and often their own purchasing. It was Russell's wish to create a more integrated medical center, and Joel saw an important part of his job as creating staff departments (such as personnel and purchasing) and upgrading these functions with the help of medical center experts.

When Joel arrived, the controller's department consisted of four individuals: Bill Connor, the controller, who promptly resigned (Joel never met this individual, whom he was told had personal problems of an unspecified nature); Peter Stavrogin, an industrious bookkeeper, who was a 55-year-old Eastern European refugee with a limited knowledge of English; a payroll clerk; and a secretary. This was the staff for an organization of more than 400 employees that was funded by five different agencies under five different contracts. The accounting department had heavy personnel responsibilities as well, at least so far as payroll was concerned, because no personnel department as such existed. One of the first things Joel did was hire Connor's replacement. In doing so—and to conform with Russell's policy of an integrated medical center—Joel enlisted the help of the medical center staff: Milton Schlitz, the director of financial affairs, and Grover Alexander, the director of personnel. Alexander volunteered to place the ads and check the references of applicants for the controller position, and Schlitz suggested that he screen the applicants. The best three or four would then be reviewed by Joel and Harrang who, between them, would select the new controller. Joel was pleased with this arrangement, although he thought the recommended salary for the position was too low. He agreed to go along, however, based on the recommendations of Alexander and Schlitz, who had considerably more experience in these matters.

However, because of what Schlitz and Alexander believed to be a shortage of qualified accountants, and the undesirable location of Morris, they found only two prospective applicants. Albert Fodor, a 55-year-old certified public accountant (CPA), with no hospital experience but good references, was the obvious first choice to be Morris's new controller. Fodor was pleasant and industrious. It took him six months to learn the job. Fodor then resigned, citing that the tremendous pressure and workload were too great for a man of his years. The payroll clerk also resigned at this time for a higher-paying job at another hospital.

During the next three months, Joel employed three new billing clerks as well as a personnel assistant and a purchasing agent. Most of the accounting department's work, which would have been done by the controller, was performed by Joel, who handled the budgetary aspects, while Stavrogin covered the accounting aspects. This system was unsatisfactory, however, because both felt Joel should spend less time troubleshooting financial problems and more time on the programmatic aspects of the job. Also, Joel wanted to conduct and supervise a variety of special studies for contract purposes and cost comparisons, an undertaking hardly feasible under the present setup.

So Joel went back to Schlitz and Alexander, insisting that the salary for the controller job be raised $3,000 per year because of the complexity of the job and the distance from Schlitz's direct supervision. Schlitz agreed reluctantly; he knew he would have to raise salaries or face morale problems in the accounting department at Wise Hospital.

After an intensive advertising program, eight to ten candidates had been screened by Schlitz, and three candidates were sent to Joel and Harrang, of whom Perry Oram seemed the best. Oram was 40 years old, without a CPA but with solid accounting experience in a medium-sized business firm. Oram had no hospital or healthcare experience. Schlitz and Joel did not feel that such experience was necessary for the job, although, of course, they would have preferred it. Oram was physically attractive, well-dressed, and married with no children. He said he was interested in advancing himself in the expanding hospital field. Joel went over the Fodor experience with Oram, stressing the work pressures. Oram responded that he was looking for a job where he would have more autonomy, where he was in charge and responsible, and where he knew he would be rewarded (or blamed) based on his performance. Of course, he would like to spend a lot of time at first learning the ropes with Schlitz. Joel told Oram he would let him know later that week if the job was his. Afterward, Joel and Harrang agreed that Oram was the best of the three candidates. However, Harrang had a vague feeling of unease—Oram seemed too good, too qualified for the job. Independently, Schlitz also agreed that Oram was the best of the three candidates. Alexander checked Oram's reference, who confirmed the high opinion of Schlitz and Joel. Oram was then offered the job as controller of the Morris Unit, which he accepted.

From Joel's point of view, things went fairly well at first, perhaps because Joel was busy with other matters and because Oram was spending a lot of time at Wise Hospital with Schlitz. The first sign of trouble was the lateness of the monthly statement that Joel had instituted and required. The statement included detailed categories of departmental costs, comparing costs (Joel hoped eventually to compare costs with performance as well) for this month, last month, and this month last year, as well as cumulative totals for this year. Joel had reviewed with Oram how he wanted the statement done (in what categories), with a cover sheet that would suggest the reasons for any large variances. Oram agreed to furnish such a report, but one month after the month in question, Joel still hadn't received it. When asked, Oram said that he was too busy, and that he was working on it. When the statement finally did arrive on Joel's desk, there was no cover letter about variances, and there were large variances caused by sloppy accounting (items in one category last year, for instance, that were in another this year, causing large discrepancies). Even some of the amounts were incorrect, such as salaries of certain individuals that had not been counted in the proper categories. Joel, patiently but with irritation, explained that this was not what he wanted. He told Oram why he wanted what he wanted, and when he wanted the report—15 days after the end of the month. Timeliness, he emphasized, was especially important because, although the city contract remained at the same sum every year, changes in the OEO budget had to be individually approved by Washington, and OEO funds had to be spent by the year's end. This meant that a lot of shuffling had to be done (e.g., transfer of city positions because of increased salary costs to the OEO budget) based on correct information. Oram apologized and agreed to improve performance.

At the same time, Joel had begun to hear complaints about Oram from other staff members. Linda Lee, the personnel assistant, and Felix Schwartzberg, the assistant director, complained about his rudeness, arrogance, and insensitivity to the poor—like his repeated statements about "welfare chiselers." Such terminology was at odds with the philosophy of the unit. When changes in employee paychecks had to be made because of supervisory mistakes or because of inadequate notice concerning an employee's vacation, Oram reluctantly did the extra work. He warned those involved, without clearing it with Joel, that eventually checks would not be issued on this basis.

Joel had been approached by Oram two weeks previously about a personal matter. Oram explained that he had to come to work an hour and a half late twice a week because of an appointment with his psychiatrist. The psychiatrist couldn't see him before or after work, and he hoped Joel would be sympathetic. Oram was willing to stay late to make up the time. Joel said he wanted to think it over before responding, and then discussed Oram's situation with Schlitz and Harrang. They all agreed that they would have liked to have known this before Oram was hired, but that if the work was done and he made up the time, it would be permitted. It was agreed that Joel would check occasionally in the accounting office, which was located in a separate building a block away from the health services facility, to see if Oram was indeed putting in the extra time.

For about the next six months, Oram's performance remained essentially the same. The cover letter was superficial and the statements were late and often contained mistakes. (The statements did, however, eventually arrive and were eventually corrected.) The special studies requested of Oram were done late and Joel often had to redo them. In checking on Oram, Joel never found him in the office after 5:00 p.m., but he did not check every day. The routine work of the accounting department was being done effectively, but this had been the case before the current situation with Oram, when no controller had been present. Oram had added another clerk, and Joel suspected that Stavrogin was still performing much of the supervisory work as he had been previous to Oram's arrival. Joel was not happy. He discussed the situation with Harrang, who agreed that the statements were less than acceptable. Harrang told Joel to do as he liked, but to clear it first with Schlitz.

Soon after, Joel went to Wise Hospital to discuss Oram with Schlitz. Schlitz, a CPA, had been controller of Wise Hospital, now Wise Medical Center, for 27 years. Schlitz was talkative but often vague, hard-working, basically conservative, and oriented primarily to the needs of Wise Hospital (at least in Joel's opinion) rather than to the medical center at large. This was reflected in the allocation of overhead in the Morris contracts (administrative time allocated was greater than that actually provided) and in the high price of direct services, such as laboratory, performed for Morris by the hospital. More important, Schlitz saw his job almost exclusively as worrying about "the bottom line"—whether the hospital or the Morris Unit ran a deficit or broke even—rather than in terms of performance relative to costs. Nevertheless, Joel thought he had established a cordial relationship with Schlitz, and their discussion about Oram was indeed cordial for the most part. Schlitz agreed that Oram's performance left something to be desired. He was particularly unhappy about the time Oram put in. On the other hand, Schlitz felt that the Morris Unit was in good financial shape and that there was nothing to worry about. In view of the experience with the previous controller, Fodor, Schlitz wondered if indeed they could find a better man for the salary. Schlitz urged that they talk to Oram together but said that he would go along with whatever Joel wanted to do.

Acting on Schlitz's recommendation, Joel set up a meeting with Schlitz, Oram, and Harrang to discuss his dissatisfactions. During the course of the meeting Joel did admit that the monthly statements were improving, but only after extensive prodding. Oram remarked that the reason for this meeting surprised him; he had thought, on the basis of previous meetings with Joel and Schlitz, that they were pleased with his work. He then asked, in fact, to be included in more top-level policy meetings, as he felt that controllers should be part of the top management group. Oram said he felt isolated, which resulted in part from the location of the accounting department in a separate building. Joel responded that he would welcome Oram's participation in policy meetings after the work of the accounting department had been sufficiently upgraded, and that Oram would be kept informed of and invited to all meetings that concerned his department.

Returning to the Morris facility, Joel discussed his perplexity with Harrang. Actually, he asserted, he did not understand what was going on here. Oram never gave him what he wanted. He had no way of knowing how busy Oram actually was. Lately, Oram had said that he couldn't produce certain studies by the stipulated dates because he was busy doing work for Schlitz or attending meetings at the hospital with Schlitz and the controllers of the other units of the medical center.

Harrang replied that he believed that Schlitz was indeed responsible in part for Oram's lack of responsiveness. Schlitz had probably told Oram not to listen to Joel but to do what he, Schlitz, recommended, because Oram's salary and benefits were largely determined by Schlitz rather than by Joel. Schlitz didn't want the accounting department at Morris to use more sophisticated techniques than the hospital because this would reflect badly on Schlitz. Moreover, Schlitz wanted his "own man" at the Morris Unit so that the hospital benefited in all transactions with Morris (e.g., there should be enough slack in the city budget to meet any contingency, with as many staff as possible switched to the OEO budget).

Joel had to agree with Harrang's observation. On the other hand, Harrang had become increasingly bitter toward Russell over the last six months. This concerned a variety of matters, most specifically Harrang's salary. Harrang was working much harder than he had bargained for at Morris, and he didn't feel he was getting the money or the credit he deserved. Nevertheless, Joel did think that Schlitz might be part of the problem; he had never been particularly impressed with Schlitz.

Several weeks later, a new state regulation was passed stating that for city agencies to collect under Medicaid, all efforts must be made to collect from those who, by state edict, could afford to pay. This was in conflict with Morris's philosophy of providing free service to all who said they couldn't pay, and there was much opposition to implementation of the policy by the professionals at Morris. The professional staff felt that no special effort should be made to collect from those who had formerly received free services. Oram disagreed with this philosophy and said that Morris should make every effort to collect.

When it came to implementing collections, Oram requested that the registration staff who were to collect the money be made part of his department, or that a separate cashier's office be set up on the first floor of the health facility. Otherwise his department didn't wish to be involved. Schwartzberg, the assistant director in charge of registration, argued that the registration staff should continue as part of the family health units because of other duties, that no space was available on the first floor for a cashier's office, and that it was not fair to patients to make them stand in two lines, as they would have to under Oram's arrangement, before seeing a health professional. Joel and Harrang sided with Schwartzberg and discussed with Oram a plan under which he would be responsible for the cash collection aspects of the registrar's work. It was agreed that Oram would devise, within a week, a plan for implementation. After two weeks, Schwartzberg reported to Joel that Oram had not devised a plan and was unwilling to cooperate with the plan Schwartzberg and the chief registrar had devised.

Joel pounded his desk. What concerned him was not so much this specific matter, which he knew he would resolve, but what to do in general with Oram. Joel was working Saturday mornings with a militant community group over next year's OEO budget and was still working 60 to 65 hours per week. He didn't think Oram's performance would improve unless Schlitz agreed with Joel's priorities and, even in that event, sufficient improvement was unlikely. On the other hand, Joel did not look forward to hiring a fourth controller in the two years he had worked at Morris. Moreover, the routine work of the accounting department was being performed to the satisfaction of Schlitz. Joel decided to go for a walk by the river and make his decision.

Case Questions

1. What is the problem from Joel's point of view? From Oram's point of view? From Schlitz's point of view? From Harrang's?
2. In what ways should Oram be accountable to Joel and Schlitz?
3. Given that Oram's performance is not acceptable to Joel, what options does Joel have to affect Oram's performance?
4. What do you recommend that Joel do now? Why?
5. What is the evidence that you used in making the above recommendation?

Case C
Now What?

Ann Scheck McAlearney

Kelly Connor had been working at West Liberty Health System for four years, and she was starting to wonder about what was next for her career. She remembered her graduate school experience in health administration fondly, especially now that she had been in the same position for three full years since her first promotion. The excitement of learning new things—and the terror of exams and presentations—were seemingly distant memories. Instead, she felt stuck in her present job as manager of operations for the Division of Cardiology.

While West Liberty was a multi-hospital health system, Connor's expectation that she could grow and learn within the health system was not becoming a reality. She found that the real day-to-day existence of this operations management position was about as un-glamorous as she could imagine, and she was unable to envision a promotion in her near future. Connor had tried to continue to read and learn on the job, but there just wasn't enough time in the day. The firefighting of operations and real-time crises was always first priority, and she was afraid that she would soon be unable to remember how to analyze the business case for a new venture or how to think strategically about just about anything.

As Connor returned home at the end of the week, she decided things had to change. Even though West Liberty seemed like a good and caring employer when she had interviewed all those years ago, they now seemed much better at talking about caring about employees than actually doing something about it. When Connor looked back on the past three years, she realized that she had yet to successfully participate in any seminar or educational class offered by the health system because she could never seem to get away from her job. Yet she also realized that she was not alone. Her friends in other departments had similar complaints, and it seemed that the only way they were able to take a break was to leave the country—but nobody had enough time or money to do that very often.

Feeling burned out and disappointed, Connor knew she needed to do something different, but she didn't know what to do. She wanted to take the educational programs West Liberty offered, but she needed to find some protected time, and she needed to figure out how to navigate the politics and chaos of West Liberty.

Connor set up a meeting with her boss, Patricia Miller, director of cardiology, to voice her concerns. While she told Miller that the reason for the meeting was "professional development," she wasn't sure that Miller understood what Connor meant by that term, and she wasn't confident that Miller would feel capable of providing the guidance Connor sought. Connor, though, knew that she had to get Miller's support before she could reallocate her time to focus on her own professional development. And, since she knew Miller was only swayed by evidence and data, Connor knew she had to do her homework before the meeting.

Considering Her Options

Connor's first step was to investigate the professional development opportunities provided through West Liberty Health System. Looking at the online course catalog, she was amazed at the long list of courses. As she started to look at the individual course titles, though, she found that most of the courses seemed focused on the needs of frontline staff and new managers. Courses with titles such as "Avoiding Needle Stick Injuries" and "Compliance Education" weren't really appropriate for her role, and the management classes such as "Skills for New Managers" and "How to Motivate Your Nursing Staff" seemed too basic. She was encouraged when she found a list of course offerings "under development" in the areas of quality management and performance improvement, but didn't know when the courses would be available or whether they would be appropriate for her when they were rolled out. For now, Connor felt she needed to find courses geared toward mid-level managers, especially those focused on people management skills, but these didn't appear on the West Liberty list.

Expanding her search outside the health system, Connor pulled up websites from organizations such as the American College of Healthcare Executives

(ACHE) and the American Management Association to see if their offerings were any more appropriate. She was delighted to find titles such as "Managing Conflict" and "Improving Your Negotiation Skills" that were offered through some of the professional conferences and meetings. Given her latest performance evaluations, she knew that Miller felt she had opportunities to improve in these areas in particular, and the course descriptions sounded fantastic. However, finding the courses themselves was only the first step. In order to take these courses, she had to gain support from Miller in the form of both financial resources and free time.

Strategically Planning Her Professional Development

Connor knew that the best approach to obtaining Miller's endorsement for her professional development was to develop a plan. By creating a formal plan, Connor would be able to outline her professional development goals and build a case for why achievement of her goals would be important. Further, development of a formal plan would force her to build the evidence case for her professional development, drawing from the available research literature she knew Miller respected.

Determining the Perspective

Connor's project management skills came in particularly handy as she began to sketch out a plan for her professional development. As she remembered from her strategic management course in graduate school, she knew that one of the first decisions she needed to make was about the time horizon of the plan. While she was certainly concerned with both long-term and short-term goals, she decided to focus on two specific time frames for this plan: a two-year horizon for short term, and a five-year horizon for a mid-range term. Another immediate decision she needed to make concerned the perspective of the plan. Despite seeming a bit unorthodox, she decided that she would frame this strategic planning process with herself as the "entity" to be planned, and use her own perspective to base considerations about other stakeholders and so forth.

An Environmental Analysis

Immersing herself in the planning process, Connor began to consider how an environmental analysis would look from the perspective of an individual. She decided that a good next step would be to perform a stakeholder analysis for her professional development. Sketching on a piece of paper, she put herself in the center box, and began to consider other stakeholders in her development. Clearly, West Liberty Health System as an employer could be listed as an important stakeholder, as well as her own division and her professional colleagues. She also considered the perspectives of stakeholders outside the health system

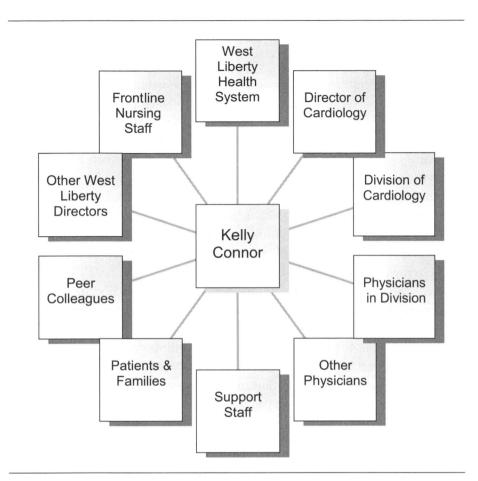

FIGURE I.5
Stakeholder
Map for
Connor's
Professional
Development

such as members of the community, members of her professional community, and so forth, but decided it would be better to focus on the West Liberty environment as a start. Figure I.5 shows her preliminary stakeholder analysis.

Internal Analysis

Satisfied that this stakeholder analysis would help make her case for how her own professional development could impact others within the health system, she then turned to an internal analysis, using her own ideas and hopes to guide her planning process. She was aware of research in management and leadership development, and selected a framework from McCall and colleagues that recommended three particular action steps: (1) learn about personal shortcomings; (2) accept responsibility for shortcomings that result due to lack of knowledge, skills, or experience, or because of personality, limited ability, or situational misfit; and (3) decide what to do about shortcomings (McCall, Lombardo, and Morrison 1988). While none of these three steps was easy, she knew there were several available sources of information to help in her personal analysis.

Connor first reviewed the feedback she had received in her performance evaluations, highlighting patterns that showed opportunities for development. She remembered the uncomfortable moments of each past review when she and the director had come to the sections of "Managing Conflict" and "Building Professional Teams." She had never been comfortable with conflict, and was acutely aware of taking the "easy way" out of most conflicts by capitulating to the other person or referring the issue to her director. Not surprisingly, this tendency was reflected fairly clearly in her last two evaluations. However, she also noted a disturbing pattern in her annual reviews with respect to her ability to work with established nurses in Cardiology. With this group, in particular, she never felt comfortable asserting authority, and, as a result, typically let them walk all over her, often bullying her to get their way. This trend had resulted in several difficult situations over the past year when this group of long-term nurses presented strong resistance to the introduction of a new electronic health record system with electronic medication administration records embedded in the system. Reflecting on a number of examples, Connor realized that this was certainly an area in which she could improve.

Connor also took some time to do a more formal evaluation of her strengths and weaknesses with respect to professional development, and used a competency assessment tool she found available on the web to assess her capabilities for leadership in health administration (Robbins, Bradley, and Spicer 2001). This tool had been developed, tested, and published in the peer-reviewed *Journal of Healthcare Management*, thus offering the kind of credibility Miller appreciated. The tool assessed 52 competencies that were categorized into four different domains: (1) technical skills; (2) industry knowledge; (3) analytic and conceptual reasoning; and (4) interpersonal and emotional intelligence. Completing the assessment, Connor found that she seemed to have an appropriate level of competency in the technical skills areas of operations, finance, and information resources, but had technical skills gaps in the areas of human resources and external affairs. Further, she noted several areas in the domain of interpersonal intelligence where her competence level could be improved.

This Competency Assessment Tool was even more helpful than Connor had anticipated, though, because it provided suggestions about how she could develop different competencies through either on-the-job experience or formal graduate training. For example, in the area of human resources technical skills, one competency area she lacked was the ability to "Demonstrate understanding of the governance function including structure and fiduciary responsibility and impact on management decisions (for both for-profit and not-for-profit organizations)" (Robbins, Bradley, and Spicer 2001). To address this deficiency, the assessment tool suggested the straightforward work-based experience of "attend board and board committee meetings" (Robbins, Bradley, and Spicer 2001). Connor knew that while access to board meetings at West Liberty might not be easy to obtain, evidence about the effectiveness of the work-based experience would help convince Miller and others that this type of experience might be worth arranging to support Connor's professional development.

Goal Planning

Armed with the results of her first personal internal analysis, Connor decided a good next step would be to develop a personal mission statement and several goals for her professional development in the coming years. While this process was also difficult, it helped her to focus her own goals so that she could be clear and compelling when she presented her case to Miller. By focusing on the two- and five-year time horizons she had established, she was able to keep herself from feeling completely overwhelmed. Knowing that the best goals were those that were measurable, Connor outlined her professional development goals and their associated metrics as a start for her discussion with Miller. This preliminary outline is presented in Box I.1.

BOX I.1
Professional Development Goals

Two-Year Goals
- Improvement in conflict management skills, reflected in improvement on Annual Performance Evaluation section of "Managing Conflict"
- Improvement in team-building skills, reflected in improvement in Annual Performance Evaluation section of "Building Professional Teams"
- Successful completion of cross-system project, involving collaboration outside Division of Cardiology
- Expanded professional network to include at least two West Liberty executives
- Higher personal job satisfaction (personal perspective)
- Promotion of at least one direct report to manager at West Liberty

Five-Year Goals
- Promotion to director at West Liberty
- By year three, Annual Performance Evaluation strong in all areas
- High job satisfaction of direct reports, reflected in Annual Employee Work-Life Survey
- Promotion of at least two direct reports to manager at West Liberty in years 3–5

Strategic Options

Once Connor had outlined her goals, she saw that the next step in her strategic professional development planning process was to highlight specific areas of development necessary to achieve her goals. Several areas of needed focus jumped out at her in particular: (1) conflict management; (2) building professional teams; (3) internal networking; (4) cross-system collaboration; (5) leadership development; and (6) employee development.

Considering each of these areas, she was aware that they could be addressed by a variety of approaches, so she built a list of alternative tactics by which she could develop skills and competencies in each area. Connor's preliminary list for the first three focus areas is shown in Table I.4.

A Scenario Analysis

Finally, Connor recognized that Miller, similar to many others, was a visual thinker. One tool she knew of that might help both her and Miller envision alternative professional development options for Connor was a scenario analysis exercise that described what success might look like if things did or did not go as planned. Connor got herself a glass of iced tea and imagined how things might happen for good or bad, considering whether she was able to enlist the support and make the personal and behavioral changes she believed were necessary. Box I.2 shows how she envisioned these three scenarios for the 2-year time horizon.

TABLE I.4
Alternative
Professional
Development
Approaches

Focus Area	Approach
Conflict Management	• External course offering (e.g., ACHE) • Internal course offering (when developed) • Reading and discussion • Structured assignment and feedback • Coaching
Building Professional Teams	• External course offering (e.g., ACHE) • Internal course offering (when developed) • Reading and discussion • Action learning project requiring team development • Structured assignment and feedback • Coaching
Internal Networking	• Attendance at system-wide meetings • Assignment to system-wide task force or project • Invite interested directors, other executives, to lunch, to help mentor informally

BOX I.2
Scenario Analysis of Professional Development Achievements

Scenario 1: Stormy Weather

Unable to enlist sufficient support for her own professional development, Connor was forced to continue the development process on her own. She signed up for multiple class offerings through West Liberty's education division, but was limited by both the course catalog and her own schedule. While she successfully completed several online courses that introduced her to focused topics, she was unable to complete any courses that required in-class sessions due to her inability to get away from her job. The director of cardiology was supportive of Connor's efforts, but unable to provide additional resources to enable her to travel to off-site conferences, or participate in courses that required time away from operations. Connor's performance evaluations continued to be positive, but the director's comments consistently indicated room for improvement in her people skills. The director was particularly concerned about Connor's ability to work with established nurses, and her inability to create and sustain productive teams that involved clinicians. On Connor's part, she remained frustrated about her lack of free time, and about a seemingly endless career as a manager who would never be promoted. She started to look outside West Liberty for new positions, but realized her lack of professional development had limited her job possibilities to lateral moves.

Scenario 2: The Long and Winding Road

While initially frustrated by the incessant demands of her job to be continually available, Connor began to see windows of opportunity for her development. With her director's support, she was able to sign up for a new mentoring program at West Liberty, and developed an interesting professional connection with the director of food services in the health system. This director had been at West Liberty for her entire career, and was able to provide advice about important topics such as negotiating the politics of the health system and using the performance evaluation process as an opportunity for shameless self-promotion. As she pointed out to Connor, West Liberty did not like to lose good people, so building one's professional image as one of the "stars" of the system was an excellent first step toward getting promoted. In addition, through her mentor, Connor was able to find a similarly minded manager of operations in Food Services who was interested in learning more about West Liberty. With the help of both directors, Connor and her colleague negotiated a job

(continued)

Box I.2 (*continued*)

switching arrangement whereby the managers would spend two hours each day in the other's role for a three-month period. During these three months, the managers also agreed to have lunch together at least twice per week in order to ensure that they had direct opportunities to coordinate with each other so that their job rotation hours would not result in lost productivity for either department. While the job rotation itself did not directly lead to a promotion, this creative arrangement helped reduce Connor's frustration with West Liberty, and enabled her to see opportunities throughout the system for the coming years.

Scenario 3: Sunny Side of the Street

Connor's meeting with the director went better than she could have hoped. The director was in complete agreement about the need for Connor to focus on her professional development, and offered to provide whatever resources she could to help Connor succeed. After reviewing Kelly's professional development plan, the two agreed upon a plan of attack for the coming year, and were able to identify two specific off-site conferences that would be well-aligned with Connor's need to develop her conflict management and negotiation skills. In the meantime, the director suggested that Connor read several books related to these topics, and offered to serve as a sounding board to discuss the books at a series of monthly lunches they would schedule. The director also offered to recommend that Connor be placed in the new program that was being developed at West Liberty for "high potentials," ensuring that she would receive executive-level attention to her leadership development in the coming two years. At the end of the meeting, the director handed Connor a copy of one of her recommended books, *Crucial Conversations*, and they agreed upon a date for the first book lunch meeting in the coming month. Nine months flew by, and at Connor's annual performance evaluation meeting, she had her next formal opportunity to discuss professional development with the director. They agreed that the book discussion lunches were both productive and fun, and listed the next three books they would plan to read and discuss. However, their frank discussion about Connor's ability to apply what she had learned from the external courses she had taken at a recent professional meeting highlighted several opportunities for Connor to further develop her leadership skills and practice new behaviors over the coming months. While the new West Liberty Leadership Development program was yet to begin, the director suggested that Connor seek other

(*continued*)

> **Box I.2** *(continued)*
>
> leadership development opportunities within and outside the health system, in order to continue making progress toward her own professional development goals. In particular, the director recommended that Connor enroll in a course through the Center for Creative Leadership focused specifically on leadership development for women, and promised to provide Connor with her full support to attend. Together, they laid out a plan for the next year, and highlighted a possible promotion for Connor within the coming year as a goal toward which to strive.

Preparing for the Meeting

In getting everything together for her meeting with Miller, Connor considered what she should forward to Miller ahead of time and what she should leave for the actual meeting. Knowing Miller hated to be surprised or caught off guard, Connor decided to compile all of her preliminary planning ideas in a "for your eyes only" document that she could send Miller a week in advance of the meeting. This document contained the results of all her analyses, as well as brief paragraphs introducing the various sections and analytic approaches. She knew Miller's time was limited, but she wanted to make sure Miller understood how important this was to her future at West Liberty. Connor was dependent on Miller's buy-in to help her achieve her professional development goals, and felt that her personal strategic plan would provide a solid framework with which she could guide the discussion.

Case Questions

1. What constraints does Connor face within her position? What options does she have to overcome those constraints?
2. What can Connor do within her present job to learn on the job?
3. How has Connor's strategic planning exercise built or weakened her case for spending time away from operations to develop her professional skills?
4. How much of professional development is one's personal responsibility, and how much is the responsibility of the employer?

References

McCall, M. W., M. M. Lombardo, and A. M. Morrison. 1988. *The Lessons of Experience: How Successful Executives Develop on the Job*. Lexington MA: Lexington Books.

Robbins, C. J., E. H. Bradley, and M. Spicer. 2001. "Developing Leadership in Healthcare Administration: A Competency Assessment Tool." *Journal of Healthcare Management* 46 (3): 188–202.

Short Case 1
Nowhere Job

David Melman

John Ernest works for a young and growing healthcare company. The company has successfully developed a market niche by contracting with colleges and universities to manage and operate their campus health centers. Ernest has been hired to develop the operational structure for a new product that will link students' managed care health insurance coverage to services provided by their campus health centers. This new product will result in cost savings as well as improved service delivery. It is a new concept in the industry and while Ernest does not have significant healthcare experience, he does have a great deal of energy and enthusiasm and is expected to learn on the job.

Ernest has not been given a formal job description. He was originally given a list of performance objectives verbally, but these objectives have been subsequently changed without his input, and there have been no new objectives put in place. Ernest's work environment is unusual in that he mostly works out of a home office, with occasional trips to the corporate office 70 miles away. Ernest reports directly to the corporate medical director of the company, but this director is located in Miami, 1,200 miles away. Communication with his boss occurs almost exclusively by e-mail, telephone, or fax.

Ernest has made progress toward achieving organizational objectives, but he is now facing obstacles that are largely due to his isolation from others in the company. He is not informed when changes are made to project objectives, nor are the underlying reasons for these changes ever explained to him. Ernest finds that his isolation limits his ability to grow professionally, and he has trouble contributing to the work of the company because he is unable to describe his company's needs accurately to outside vendors without being so informed himself.

Ernest has asked to have a formal job description and stated performance objectives based on the format suggested by a human resources consultant hired by the company, but he has received no response. Meanwhile, Ernest has been asked to complete the contracts he has negotiated with several outside vendors, and he is told he now reports to an outside consultant who has been hired to help coordinate technical operations, including information systems. This outside consultant tells Ernest not to proceed with these contracts the very day after the CEO tells him to complete them.

Ernest attempts to contribute to the sales and marketing efforts of his company by proposing that the company sponsor an institute at a prestigious university, and he wants to contribute his time and energy to make this project a success. He is told it is a good idea, but the vice president of sales and marketing does not keep his commitment to respond to Ernest's proposal. Ernest sends reminders and continues to develop the idea with the university. He is trying to expand his job responsibilities to include business development, but he knows he needs the support of others in his organization to make a meaningful contribution.

Case Questions

1. What should Ernest do?
2. What are the risks to Ernest?
3. How could Ernest have anticipated these problems before accepting his current position?
4. What should be Ernest's priorities in evaluating an alternative career opportunity? Why?

Short Case 2
Manager Morale at Uptown Hospital

By Sofia Agoritsas

John Robbins, MD, the savvy and scholarly chief executive officer of Uptown Hospital, minimized the screen on his computer just before his monthly department chiefs meeting was about to start. He was concerned about the results of the latest employee satisfaction survey that the vice president of human resources had e-mailed him. The survey results were going to be an important part of the report on "Manager Development at Uptown Hospital" that was being produced by the newly hired consulting group, Coaches Like Us, in response to the board chair's special request.

Robbins stared intensely at the light fixture in his office and wondered what would happen when the chairman of the board saw the report that included these survey results. John knew the chairman was eager to see the consultants' report, especially since a close colleague of the chairman owned the consulting group.

Uptown Hospital

Uptown Hospital, a 500-bed community teaching hospital, is one of two tertiary care centers in the area; its main competitor is University Hospital, which focuses more on its medical school and research. Robbins recently became chief executive officer, having been promoted from his previous position as chief medical officer. He had been asked to fill the CEO role last year on an interim basis after the former CEO left for a new position in a major health system. After a year-long executive search failed to produce any viable external candidates, Robbins was offered the permanent position. For the most part, Uptown Hospital has been a financially sound organization, largely because of its location. People in the area are not interested in driving far to get to the next closest health system, and seem to be satisfied with the care provided at Uptown Hospital. Cost management has not been a major focus of the organization, but this has recently become an area of increased attention as costs for labor and supplies seem to be escalating uncontrollably.

If one was asked to describe the organizational culture at Uptown, that individual would likely say that the place is both comfortable and familial. This is partially attributable to the fact that turnover among Uptown employees has historically been low. On average, about 15 percent of employees leave Uptown annually, compared to a national average of 23 percent. Internal movement within the organization is typically slow, but given the relative stability of the workforce, most of Uptown's managers and even many of the physicians seem to have "grown up" at Uptown. Over the past year, though, multiple department and nurse managers have resigned, and this has been noticed.

Community voluntary physicians have a strong influence on the care provided at Uptown Hospital. They are the core referral source for the organization and these physicians play an integral role in the patient care process. The nursing staff know the voluntary physicians personally, as the patient care areas are open units and the physicians round regularly on their patients.

Recently, many of the major physician practices in the area have become affiliated faculty practices within Uptown Hospital. Now, though, physician faculty members seem to be increasingly at odds with hospital residents and administrative managers because of the different practice patterns and care practices used by the voluntary physicians. This has led to a number of complaints filed by the department chiefs, since this lack of standardization results in considerable variation in care. Staff loyalty has also seemed to sway because of constant confusion about care practices. Further, many of the administrative managers and hospital employees have become frustrated by the seemingly non-cooperative and non-collaborative environment. The staff's willingness to take on new responsibilities usually depends on how the attending physicians are acting, but not everyone is on good behavior anymore.

As a result, the managers are often unable to hold their staff accountable for various job responsibilities.

The Survey Results Are In

Robbins was struck by the survey results on several dimensions. First, he wondered how the people in his organization could not know about the key strategic initiatives of Uptown Hospital. It was not as if the executive team was hiding its activities, and the modernization of the patient care building had been an area of focus day in and day out for the past year. However, he was more surprised that on average the managers stated they were unhappy in the organization.

According to the survey results, the chief complaints of the managers included the following:

1. The goals of the organization are not well defined.
2. Staff are reluctant to take on new responsibilities.
3. There is limited use of a team approach to patient care.
4. The overwhelming number of non-cooperative employees makes it difficult to hold the staff accountable.
5. Managers feel the majority of their staff perform at an average to below average level.

Robbins thought about how these results reflected the perspectives of the different managers throughout the hospital. He could name them all. Most had been at Uptown for more than 15 years. He reflected on the brief instances he had run across these individuals and knew that he usually got to see them all at his quarterly management meetings. In contrast, he was able to foster a more personal relationship with each of Uptown's department chiefs.

Robbins swiveled around in his black leather executive chair and realized he needed to take responsibility for this situation at the hospital. He plastered a welcoming smile on his face as the department chiefs entered his office. He knew he needed to become the hero who would save the day, but he wasn't sure how to begin.

Case Questions

1. What should the CEO do after receiving this survey?
2. How could morale have declined so quickly at Uptown?
3. What constraints would you face in implementing your recommendations to the CEO?
4. What are ways to overcome these constraints?

Short Case 3
A Sure Thing

David A. Kaplan and Anthony R. Kovner

Doug Williams received his master's degree in health management from Kings University in 1997. Since then he has enjoyed a successful healthcare career, having worked at some of the city's most prestigious academic medical centers. Williams even spent some time as a healthcare consultant, traveling across the country performing financial turnarounds at multiple medical centers. Williams was always considered to be somewhat of a risk-taker and was willing to give up stability if it meant moving to the next level in his career. The following is a case study based on a real-life situation that happened to Williams.

****

Williams had left consulting and had landed a position as divisional administrator of cardiology at St. Lucy's University Hospital. The division was the largest within the Department of Medicine, and University Hospital was working to make cardiovascular medicine its leading service line. Williams reported to the division chief, Dr. Fishman, as well as to the Department of Medicine administrator, Linda Carter.

Williams worked tirelessly helping Fishman, a relatively inexperienced division chief, to develop a strategic framework for building the division. This included increasing the number of faculty, increasing the clinical practice volume and associated revenues, building a robust research arm, and improving the reputation of the training program.

After nearly two years achieving tangible results across all of these areas, Williams felt it was reasonable to request a salary increase and/or promotion within the organization. Williams first approached Fishman and had the following conversation:

Williams: Dr. Fishman, I have really enjoyed working with you over the past couple of years and I feel that together we have accomplished a great deal, wouldn't you agree?

Fishman: I absolutely agree, and I can't thank you enough for all your efforts in helping me to achieve my vision of making this one of the top programs in the nation.

Williams: Well, after all my efforts, I was hoping that you might be able to help me. I really would like to be considered for a salary increase. I feel that I have earned this and, in all honesty, with everything going on at home, I really could use it.

Fishman: Have you talked to Linda about this?

Williams: I have, but she sent me to discuss this with you.

Fishman: Okay. I agree that you deserve an increase, especially given all your hard work. Let me look into this and get back to you shortly.

Williams: Thanks so much. I really appreciate your help.

* * * * * *

Nearly two months went by without any mention by either Carter or Dr. Fishman of an increase. In the meantime, Williams, who lived outside the city, was approached about becoming vice president of hospital operations at State Hospital. State Hospital was a government-sponsored academic hospital within minutes of his house. However, the state institution was known to be a political land mine, and many people who worked there spoke about their negative experiences. In addition, several people who had worked there had had their careers shattered by controversy.

These legendary stories did not deter Williams from exploring the new opportunity. In fact, with every interview Williams became more and more enthralled with the notion of working at State Hospital. To think that at the age of 30 he could be a vice president of hospital operations overseeing 10 hospital departments. What a dream come true. On top of it all they were offering a salary 30 percent higher than his current salary and the place was located within minutes of his house. His father always told him that any job had three components—money, location, and the role itself. He would say that if you found a job that had two of these aspects, it would be a wonderful opportunity; amazingly, this job had all three.

A couple of days after his final interview Williams received a call from the chief operating officer (COO) of State Hospital, Alex Roberts, who offered him the position. Without blinking, Williams accepted the position, and was set to start his new job in two weeks.

Williams was so excited that he even called his professor from his health management program to tell him the good news. His professor, who was also aware of State Hospital's reputation, warned Williams to reconsider his decision, but it was too late. Williams had already accepted.

* * * * * *

Later that week, Williams went to talk with Fishman about his decision:

Williams: Dr. Fishman, I again want to thank you for the opportunity to help you rebuild this division. I have had the time of my life working with you and the members of this team. That being said, I have decided to accept an offer to become a vice president at State Hospital starting in a couple of weeks.

Fishman: Wow. I wasn't expecting this, but I suppose that a person with your skills is bound to move up the ranks quickly. Congratulations. I don't suppose there is any way to convince you to stay?

Williams: No. This new job just has too much going for it. I would be hard pressed not to take on the new and challenging role.

Fishman: Well, I want to wish you the best of luck. Please keep me informed about your future success.

* * * * * *

A few weeks later, Williams started in his new role at State Hospital. The first year for Williams read like a textbook. He connected with all of his managers, evaluated the operations of his services, and worked hands-on with his managers to make operational improvements. In addition, he worked closely with his boss, COO Alex Roberts, and the CEO, Bob Swanson, to further grow and build his service lines. Williams didn't understand what all the fuss was about working at this organization. As far as he could tell, this new life was perfect. That was until he received the news....

* * * * * *

Williams was in his regular 8:00 a.m. meeting with the other vice presidents reviewing the weekly agenda items. Roberts strolled into the meeting and made the announcement that he had decided to take a new position as COO at UCLA Medical Center in California. Williams felt his heart fall into the pit of his stomach. Williams knew that Roberts had been the individual primarily responsible for recruiting him, and, in fact, had made the decision that he would pull several service lines away from one of the other long-standing vice presidents for Williams to manage. The transition of Roberts away from State Hospital could have major implications for Williams.

To make the matter even worse, within a week of the COO's announcement, the CEO, Swanson, decided that he, too, would be leaving to become the CEO at Boulder University Hospital in Colorado. If anyone could have helped Williams without Roberts to intercede, it was sure to be Swanson. Swanson's announcement was disastrous, as Williams would surely be exposed now.

* * * * * *

Williams was in a quandary with both of his supporters and mentors gone. It soon became evident that the long-standing vice president was going to get her services back at any cost. She tormented Williams by sabotaging his programs, and even recruited some of his managers to aid her in her efforts. Williams, who was inexperienced with these types of politics, was no match for this vice president and she eventually won her services back. Williams saw his dream job start to unravel and quickly realized that he made a mistake in coming to work at State Hospital. Williams ultimately resigned his position, knowing he could not win at this game.

******

Following this experience, you will be happy to know that Williams eventually found a successful position as a department administrator for another academic medical center in the city. He is happy in his position and has learned that while the grass always appears greener on the other side, it isn't. As for Williams's father's saying that a job has three components—money, location, and the role itself, if you find a job that has all three, it is probably too good to be true. In Williams's case, it certainly was.

Case Questions

1. Should Williams have pushed harder to get an increase and/or promotion at St. Lucy's University Hospital?
2. Should Williams have done anything differently before accepting the position at State Hospital?
3. What could Williams have done differently once faced with the change in leadership at State Hospital?
4. Once faced with adversity, what should Williams have done to possibly preserve his position at State Hospital?
5. Do you think Williams made the right decision in accepting the new position at State Hospital? In leaving his position at State Hospital?

Short Case 4
The First Day

Ann Scheck McAlearney

Susan was both thrilled and terrified. Tomorrow was her first day as a manager. Having recently completed her master of health administration degree at a prestigious local university, a thorough job search had resulted in her being hired as the new manager of patient accounts at University Health System. She had had numerous interviews with various directors and other managers in the health system, as well as a lunch interview/meeting with six people who would report to her, but those interviews seemed very far away.

Susan wanted to make a good impression and get off to a positive start, yet she wasn't sure what to do first. She had learned the importance of listening in management, but she also knew she was the boss. Further, her own boss, the director of patient care services, had emphasized the importance of getting her employees to improve productivity at any cost. Susan had heard that while her new direct reports were nice to one's face, they had a tendency to complain and scapegoat, and this had led to the sudden departure of the previous manager of patient accounts. She was particularly nervous about being younger than all of her new employees. To quell her fears, Susan decided to list what she wanted to accomplish in her first days and weeks on the job.

Case Questions

1. As a friend of Susan's considering a similar position, what would you recommend that she put on the list?
2. How would you suggest that she prioritize her goals?

Short Case 5
Mid-Career Change

By Jacob Victory

With a toothy smile on his face, Josh Webber, a young executive in his early 30s, was ready. He walked confidently into his boss's office for his formal performance evaluation after working for five years as the "right hand" of the major healthcare system's president and CEO. Before Webber was even able to sit down, the CEO surprised him by stating, "I think it is time for you to move into operations." Webber was flattered. After 11 years of staff positions in healthcare management, Webber was being promoted to director of operations for a large ancillary service department within the billion-dollar community-based healthcare system. Taking the operational reins of a $100 million business within the 150-year-old health system would be a welcome change.

Though mild-mannered and soft-spoken, Webber had an unquenchable desire to achieve. He had been an English literature major in college, and had then worked full time in two consecutive hospital management residencies while completing his graduate degree in healthcare finance and management at one of the nation's preeminent programs in health administration. After graduation, his primary work experiences over the next decade had been in corporate strategic planning for community-based and academic hospital systems. He had held different positions, including planning associate and acting director of planning, but he had not had a formal management role. Webber had accumulated a broad variety of experiences including staffing executive managers, boards, physicians, and external consultants, and working on market analyses, program development projects, grant writing initiatives, and long-term strategic planning efforts. His strengths were in business analysis, writing, and presenting complex concepts in simple terms. Webber's key function had typically been to support important hospital stakeholders in efforts to implement their visions and business strategies.

Webber's next position was serving as aide-de-camp to the CEO of a major home healthcare organization. In this role he assisted the CEO in developing and monitoring the corporation's strategic objectives and business and clinical outcome targets, writing and researching the CEO's myriad presentations, and serving as chief liaison to the CEO's 20-member executive staff and the organization's board of trustees. While Webber had no staff directly reporting to him, he kept plenty busy. He regularly spent long hours ensuring that the deliverables produced by the executive office were timely and complete. Because Webber dealt with different personalities—all with varying agendas—and because he was under immense pressure to meet deadlines, he utilized every ounce of political savvy and deferential humor he could muster to get his work done. Executive management valued Webber as a skillful diplomat who used a calm, determined demeanor when "working with" senior staff. Webber secretly relished the perks of the president's office as his phone calls were immediately returned and many sought his advice given the tremendous political capital he yielded. Publicly, however, he modestly described his role as helping management complete their projects. At this point in his career, Webber was chiefly responsible for maintaining the management structure and working behind the scenes to ensure that the CEO's own initiatives ran like clockwork.

The New Job

Webber knew that to rise within the industry he needed operational experience. Thus, Webber's promotion to director of operations for one of the organization's ancillary departments had been a welcome opportunity for him to run a major, profitable product line within the organization. More important, he was now an independent decision maker with deliverables of his own. In his new position Webber reported to the program's new administrator (a clinician), and he had seven clinical directors reporting directly to him. Ultimately Webber was responsible for program operations and the productivity of two dozen management and administrative staff—most of whom had been with the organization for 15 years or more—and hundreds of clinicians.

After 60 days on the job, however, Webber observed the following challenges:

1. Executive administration's mandated programmatic growth and profit targets were going to be difficult to meet. The program was currently 15 percent below growth targets.
2. There were few business or quality metrics in place to permit adequate monitoring of the business.
3. No overall management accountability was readily apparent within the program.
4. All of the clinical directors resisted change.
5. Webber's new position was still largely undefined with no formal job description.
6. Comments from members of the program's long-standing management team implied that Webber didn't have "enough gray hairs" for the job he now held.

Clearly, Webber was not in the president's office anymore.

Case Questions

1. How does Webber's new role differ from positions he has previously held?
2. Did Webber do the right thing in accepting the promotion?
3. What should Webber's management priorities be?
4. What skill sets will Webber need to use to implement these priorities?
5. When should Webber look for his next job? What would you recommend he look for in his next job?

PART

II

CONTROL

You may regard as a Utopian dream my hope to see all our hospitals devoting a reasonable portion of their funds to tracing the results of the treatment of their patients and analyzing these results with a view to improving them. You may prefer to ponder over the voluminous discussions now appearing in our journals and in the lay press about the pros and cons for state medicine and who is to pay the cost of medical care. I read these discussions, but they seem to be futile, until our hospitals begin to trace their results.
—*E. A. Codman, 1935*

I envision a system in which we promise those who depend on us total access to the help they need, in the form they need, when they need it. Our system will promise freedom from the tyranny of individual visits with overburdened professionals as the only way to find a healing relationship; will promise excellence as the standard, valuing such excellence over ill-considered autonomy; will promise safety; and will be capable of nourishing interactions in which information is central, quality is individually defined, control resides with patients, and trust blooms in an open environment.
—*Donald Berwick,* Escape Fire: Lessons for the Future of Healthcare, *2002*

COMMENTARY

Hospital cafeteria manager to counter staff before the start of the work day: Give our customers what they want from our daily menu and kitchen selections.

First customer to counter staff: I want a hot dog with mustard and relish. (Counter staff hands out a hot dog with mustard.)

Customer: There is no relish on my hot dog.

Staff: Sorry. (Takes back the hot dog and adds relish.)

Customer: Thanks. (Proceeds down the cafeteria line to the cashier at the end.)

This simple example raises a lot of the concepts related to control in healthcare or in any other organization. Let us set this example into the context of a hospital's mission, vision, and values.

The *mission* of the hospital in this case is to provide the finest care by skilled and pleasant staff. The *vision* is that care will always meet best-practice standards and be timely, error free, appropriate, and provided at a reasonable cost. The key *values* are that patients come first and employee satisfaction is valued.

The cafeteria fits into these goals by providing hospital workers a meal they want at a reasonable price. The hospital leadership is pleased that staff brag about working at the hospital, including the good food in the cafeteria. The cafeteria manager sets rules for appropriate work for the counter staff, leaving it up to them to match food to customer requests. There are clear limits to what the staff can do. The price of one hot dog does not buy two. Chocolate sauce is not offered for your hot dog. These rules are not burdensome because the customers are socialized to know the first rule and don't ever ask for chocolate sauce on their hot dogs.

From an organizational point of view, this example is similar to the nursing supervisor saying to the staff nurse: "These are your patients. With your good skills and education I am confident you can care for them. Call me if you need help."

Management in healthcare means creating the space and support systems that allow skilled people to meet the needs of the people they serve. If the relish jar is empty, the best counter staff cannot meet their customers' wishes. If the procedure kit is not in the examining room ready to use, the patient may not get a Pap smear test.

In our cafeteria example, an *error* was made and because of the customer's rapid *feedback*, it was corrected. If the quality is measured as the end result of this transaction (a hot dog with mustard and relish), the quality score was perfect, the transaction succeeded, and the customer was satisfied. The error was recognized—"Sorry"—and corrected: "Thanks."

Using a more accurate measure of quality, this transaction did not get a perfect score. Ideally, the error should not have occurred. There is a *cost of poor quality* here in the fraction of a minute used by staff, this customer, and other customers backed up in line, while the error was corrected.

This quality problem was observed in time and corrected by the customer. Patients are usually unable to provide such corrective feedback to caregivers. Professional caregivers—not the patient—are expected to define appropriate care. Therefore, caregivers carry a greater burden and responsibility for avoiding errors.

Human beings are bound to make mistakes and errors will occur. The goal of error reduction is to create systems that stop errors. For example, a self-serve condiment station can be placed beyond the cashier so customers can help themselves. This requires a system for regularly replenishing the supply. This kind of system redesign is sometimes called *reengineering* the process.

Did this employee make a mistake due to lack of *motivation*? The vast majority of workers want to do a good job and not make mistakes. In this example, most likely the employee simply forgot. It may do more harm to criticize this employee for negligence and more good to create a system that makes it easier to avoid errors.

The genius of the McDonald's franchise is a system designed to produce the identical package of French fries in thousands of locations using relatively unskilled employees. Such a system works with farmers to produce the right kind of potato, creates a standardized package, and uses a special metal scoop for filling the package. By such attention to the details of its system design, McDonald's can convince millions of people that they make the best French fries, which gives them a great market advantage. Healthcare has a long way to go to create such systems to reduce error.

Standardization and Variation

A hundred years ago, the hot dog might have been handmade and no two were exactly alike. Shopping then was a more complicated process: "I want the fifth hot dog from the left; it looks bigger." Now that hot dogs are standardized and identical, there should be no reason to choose one over another. Although variation is still possible—how well cooked, how hot, how much relish, what kind of mustard—we do not expect this kind of customer-driven variation in a hospital cafeteria line. Hospital care is a combination of standardized activities (hernia surgery) with variation (left or right side). Best-practice standards combined with appropriate variation are required for good quality of care.

Standardization Can Be Cheaper and Variation Expensive

Back to our cafeteria: What about the attractiveness of the plate and napkin? What about the interpersonal relationship between the server and the customer? Does the server smile? Here, quality is in the mind of the customer.

Quality in healthcare is not defined by the customer alone. The hospital nutritionist might say the hot dogs have too much cholesterol and it would be healthier to replace them with meatless "veggie" dogs, and that the employees should set an example of healthy eating. This changes the definition of quality from customer preference to expert knowledge about nutrition and health. A distinctive feature of healthcare is that professional quality criteria are used. Healthcare organizations must sometimes balance patient satisfaction and adherence to expert definitions of quality.

A System of Control

Healthcare delivery where professional judgment, cost, and the patient's perceptions all matter have led to the concepts of the "value compass" and "balanced scorecard." Outcomes are measured in terms of patient satisfaction, cost of care, physical functioning (e.g., less pain, the ability to climb stairs), and physiological measures such as blood pressure and cholesterol levels (issues the patient may be unaware of, but that are key indicators for a future healthy life).

A system of control comprises five elements:

1. *Goals and objectives* (in our example, this is meeting customer needs).
2. *Information* used to measure performance.
3. *Evaluation of performance in relation to goals and objectives.* Did the customer get what she wanted?
4. *Expectations.* Two levels of expectation were described in our cafeteria example. Did the customer eventually get what she wanted? Is this good enough? Or do we have a higher expectation of getting it right the first time? In this case, this transaction fell short.
5. *Incentives.* These can be based on an internalized desire to do a good job or on external rewards. The desire to make the customer happy and the desire to please the supervisor in hopes of a merit raise ideally go together without a conflict. The manager is delighted when good care is

given. Problems start where there is a disconnect between satisfying the customer or the manager.

Goals and Objectives

Mission, vision, values, goals, and objectives are widely used concepts (see Table II.1). Our mission may be to meet the needs of our customers; our vision is to be the best; the values we live by are our religious beliefs; our goal is to survive this year; and our objective is to break even.

A goal is a broadly stated intention or direction—to improve the quality, for example, by lowering the infection rate. Organizational goals are determined by the preferences of individuals with power. Organizations are collectives of people and things brought together to achieve a common purpose. Individuals with similar goals create the organization. Goals are important because they provide organizational focus. They provide a long-term framework for dealing with conflict, and they encourage commitment from those who work in the organization. Goals are implemented by individuals working together on budgets, allocation of functions, and the authority structure.

The individual wants housing and food and health and entertainment. This person decides he can do this best by working for pay as a nurse in a clinic. Nursing can be both a means (paycheck) and an end in itself (the satisfaction of helping people in a friendly work environment). The clinic's goal of good quality and reasonable cost assumes that this nurse continues to have an enjoyable job and a paycheck. It is the role of the manager to make this happen.

TABLE II.1
Organizational
Directions

Concept	Definition	Example	Requirement
Mission	Reason for existing	To meet the primary healthcare needs in our town	System maintenance
Vision	What we hope to do	People will move to our town because our care is so good	Adaptive capability
Values	The philosophy that guides behavior	Mutual respect for both caregivers and care receivers	Values integration
Goals	An intention or direction	To open a new clinic this year	Goal attainment
Objectives	A measurable intention	The new clinic will see 200 patients a week by the end of the year	

Organizations may have objectives to measure production, sales, profit, and quality. Unit or organizational objectives can be determined by reading formal official goal statements or by observing what is happening in an organization. These observations may reveal shifts in resources or decision-making power among units or individuals, what types of individuals are leaving or being recruited to the organization, and what the organization is not doing and which population it is not serving. Many large corporations expend a lot of effort in goal specification.

What happens if healthcare organizations do not specify objectives? Organizations may lack focus in their programs and may be less likely to abandon products and services that are neither effective nor efficient. The powerful and their short-term interests will tend to be favored over the weak and the long-term; there will be less adaptation to the environment; and there will be a greater tendency to retain the status quo.

Healthcare managers should determine their organization's operative objectives. Official goals may not always provide reliable guidelines for managerial behavior. When those in power go against what a manager sees as the long-range interests of an organization, the manager should be careful, speaking out only if he or she is willing to pay the price and is certain about the facts.

Information

Healthcare managers must obtain information for key product lines about volume of services, the quality of care, service and production efficiency, market share, system maintenance, and the health status of the population served. They may use the following measures to assess performance: cost per case, cost per visit, cost per day, profit, fixed and variable costs, market share, capital expenditures as a percent of sales, days of receivables and payables, top admitting physicians and their characteristics, staff turnover and overtime, sick time, and disability and fringe benefits costs. In addition, healthcare information systems are being expanded to include revenue by service line, budgeting and variance reporting, and clinical performance review. Computerized medical records are linked to cost and revenue data, concurrent review for quality of care, and final-product cost accounting for groups of similar patients at alternative levels of demand. Risk management relies on incident reports of untoward events, which are then aggregated and analyzed.

With the continuing investment in electronic medical records, required performance reporting, and standardized patient satisfaction surveys, healthcare is entering an era of information overload. Instead of the previous lack of quality of care data, now there is more information than management can cope with. What measures should take priority? What are the key quality characteristics?

Performance Evaluation

One of the problems with control systems is that they may measure the wrong thing. They may also measure the right thing inaccurately. These issues are particularly relevant for outcomes-of-care measurement. The easiest response to information we do not like is to say the data are wrong. There is no information accurate enough to be accepted in a hostile, fearful environment. One of the important aspects of quality improvement (QI) is to create a climate "free from fear," where data can be accepted for what they are despite their inaccuracies and still be used to make improvements.

Increasingly, healthcare managers have access to performance data comparing their organizations to other similar ones. In the past, a nursing home board of directors may have simply believed that its care was outstanding without question, but now comparative data allow the board to see how the nursing home stacks up. The first step is to measure its care; for example, the frequency of bed sores or the percent of patients under physical restraint. The next step is to compare measures. Why are 15 percent of our patients under restraint while the statewide average is 8 percent? The third step is to make this information public on accessible websites. This is being done by third-party payers such as Medicaid for nursing homes. Concurrent with these steps is a change from denial (our patients are sicker) and fear to a desire to improve. Managers can visit another similar nursing home with a very low restraint rate to learn how to improve their own situation. This requires collecting performance data over time to track improvements. This process of systematic comparison to best-practice organizations is called "benchmarking."

Expectations

It is well documented that medication errors occur frequently in hospitals. The wrong medicine, the wrong dose, and the wrong time are all parts of this problem. Although no clinic wants medication errors, there are different ways to respond to this problem. What is the level of expectation for good performance? It could be "zero tolerance for error." It could be that "we will make yearly improvements to continuously reduce out error rate." It could be "Everyone has this problem and we are no different" or "We have the best nurses and physicians so I am sure our error rates are lower than anyone else's." One's performance expectations make a difference. Six Sigma is one method for reducing unwanted events.

Incentive Systems

How does the manager transform the individual worker's desire for a paycheck into a pursuit of organizational goals so that both are achieved exactly together? Incentives are stimuli to affect performance. Adoption of incentives is usually based on the answers to the following questions: Does the incentive contribute to the desired results? Is the incentive acceptable to those workers whose behavior managers wish to affect? Could implementation of the incentives produce other dysfunctional consequences (e.g., rewards for cutting costs might lead inadvertently to reduced quality of care)?

Organizations use both positive and negative incentives. Incentives can be monetary or not. One of the underlying ideas of QI is that monetary incentives are often disruptive. The assumption is that people want to do a good job and that faulty systems, not the intentions or abilities of the employees, prevent that from happening. How can the admissions clerk rapidly process an admission when the computer has crashed? How can the dietary department provide hot food at the bedside when the patient is waiting in the x-ray department? QI calls for management to lead the effort in improving these systems, whereas rewarding individuals monetarily may create rivalry rather than teamwork.

To improve care requires "just in time" data about key quality characteristics and an observer who has the expertise to understand this information, whose job it is to improve care, and who is given the power to do so. For example, say the goal is to reduce the burden of asthma for kids. This is measured by the number of school days missed in the area due to asthma. A just-in-time information system would show how many children missed school yesterday (not last year or even last month). There is an asthma expert who has the assignment to reduce this rate and is given the power to do something about it. This would likely be an effective system, but there are too few examples of such management approaches in healthcare.

THE READINGS

How do we know we are meeting the needs of the people we serve? Healthcare organizations have many stakeholders, including patients and future patients, family, government, payers, insurers, employers, labor unions, professionals, and accreditation agencies. They all have an interest in the quality and safety of the care given and its cost. This interest translates into requests for information. With multiple stakeholders this can become a substantial burden. Patrice Spath in the reading lays out the consequences of this societal popularity.

Taming the Measurement Monster

Patrice L. Spath
From *Frontiers of Health Services Management* 23 (4): 3–14

Summary

The healthcare performance measurement landscape continues to evolve. Despite questions about the value of performance data, healthcare organizations are being challenged to meet the data demands of a growing number of mandatory and voluntary measurement projects. Standardization of measure specifications and definitions is months (if not years) away. For healthcare organizations, the measurement "monster" may seem impossible to tame. Although the measurement capabilities of healthcare organizations are being stretched, there are some solutions. First, senior executives must be actively involved in promoting a meaningful measurement system that is compatible with the organization's quality goals and meets regulatory, purchaser, and accreditation requirements. Next, efficiency improvements in the way of system-wide collaboration and expanded information technology support can help reduce the administrative burdens. There is no denying that the focus on measurement has advanced the quality of patient care. Healthcare organizations must create the systems necessary to sustain these gains and move forward toward ever better patient care.

Perhaps it has become a cliché, all this talk about change as a constant in the healthcare industry and the need to stay ahead of the curve. But clichés develop for a reason—usually because they have a ring of truth. In the case of performance measurement, and particularly publicly available performance data, the pace-of-change platitudes are meaningful. Performance measurement was relatively static until the 1990s. For the most part, healthcare organizations used to have considerable latitude in selecting performance indicators and establishing quality standards. All that began to change in the 1980s, and the rate of change has rapidly accelerated in recent years.

It seems that hardly a month goes by without some new voluntary or mandatory initiative aimed at evaluating another aspect of the quality or safety of healthcare services. Like kids in a candy store, everyone—purchasers, regulators, accrediting bodies, researchers, and clinicians—wants more and more data with seemingly little regard to the provider's financial burden of capturing that information. According to one study, a hospital can spend up to $100,000 annually to collect, report, and analyze data for just three of the Joint Commission's Core Measure sets (heart attack, heart failure, and pneumonia) (Anderson and Sinclair 2006). Even when the data can be gathered from existing information systems, the cost of linking different data sets, cleaning the data, doing the calculations, and writing the reports is still quite high. Although the burden of data collection is one of the considerations the Institute of Medicine (2001) uses to select measures for the National Healthcare Report Card and one of the attributes of the Joint Commission's Core Measures (Joint Commission, no date), increasingly external groups seem to place little weight on this criterion when endorsing measures.

Most would agree that having a publicly available, standardized set of healthcare performance measures would be a good thing. Yet there is still little consensus on what that measurement set should look like. If the maxim "what gets measured, gets done" is true, then measures that make the approved list should encourage practices that result in improved patient outcomes. Yet after hospitals spent several years (and several thousands of dollars) collecting data that evaluate the process of care for patients with acute myocardial infarction, heart failure, and pneumonia, researchers recently reported that the measures are not clearly linked to reductions in patient mortality (Fonarow et al. 2007; Werner and Bradlow 2006).

Does this mean performance measurement and public reporting of results data should be abandoned? Definitely not. The value of such reporting goes well beyond its intended use to help consumers make wise healthcare choices. In the past few years more providers are placing a higher priority on quality and patient safety. By knowing how other organizations perform on various measures, senior executives and clinicians are becoming aware of long-standing improvement opportunities. Teamwork among caregivers who seek to improve performance rates has greatly improved. Sharing of best practices and collaboration between healthcare organizations is unprecedented. The performance measures we have now are not perfect (and probably never will be) but the mere threat of transparency has had a positive impact on the quality culture of healthcare organizations. The near mandatory nature of some performance measurement systems has stimulated active involvement in quality and safety improvement initiatives, even by organizations that have not engaged in such activities in the past. Although healthcare transparency and the requisite measurement activities are onerous for providers, most would agree that the resulting quality improvements are good for healthcare consumers.

For all of the apparent flaws in measurement data, the marketplace is not delaying performance measurement initiatives in hopes that better evaluation tools will come along (Gosfield 2005). Healthcare organizations are increasingly expected to provide clinical performance information to purchasers, accrediting bodies, and the public. It is estimated that hospitals now have more than 300 external reporting requirements—and very little private or public funding to help defray the administrative burden. Many healthcare facilities are scrambling to meet current reporting requirements and are seeking new or upgraded information technology (IT) solutions in anticipation of even more reporting requirements in the future (Pham, Coughlan, and O'Malley 2006). Within the limits of organizational resources, senior executives are being challenged to find ways to tame this "measurement monster" without jeopardizing quality, market share, and financial viability.

To strategically plan for the effect of performance measurement and publicly reported data on their organizations, administrative leaders must first understand the measurement evolution and driving forces. Next, leaders must be personally involved in identifying appropriate measures to gauge individual and organizational practices and supporting efforts to develop and sustain organizational capacity for continual performance improvement.

How We Got Here

The notion of using performance data for comparative purposes can probably be traced back to the population-based studies of utilization conducted by Wennberg and Gittelsohn in the late 1960s. These studies, called small area analyses, revealed enormous variations in the use of surgical procedures among different hospital service areas within individual states (Wennberg and Gittelsohn 1973). The seemingly unexplained practice variations sparked the interest of purchasers and health policy analysts, but the findings were largely discounted or ignored by the provider community. At the same time, healthcare expenditures were growing at an increasing rate. Seeking opportunities to hold these costs in check, payers and regulators began in earnest to promote comparative measurement initiatives, many of which included public disclosure of the results.

Once it became apparent that the Pandora's box of healthcare data could in fact be opened, voluntary and mandatory performance measurement projects began springing up at local, state, and national levels. For the sake of brevity, only the national initiatives that influenced the measurement evolution are described in the following section.

Initial Measurement Efforts

In 1986 the Centers for Medicare & Medicaid Services (CMS)—then known as the Health Care Financing Administration—calculated raw death rates for Medicare patients at all hospitals and allowed this information to be made public (U.S. Department of Health and Human Services 1987). Instead of embracing the results as an opportunity to investigate the cause of variations, some healthcare leaders and clinicians cried "foul" and attacked the validity of the methodology used to calculate actual versus expected mortality rates. Not to be dissuaded, CMS developed a more statistically sophisticated model that not only examined in-hospital deaths but also any death that occurred within 30 days of admission. These hospital-specific mortality data were publicly reported by CMS for another few years, although consumer and provider interest in the data seemed to quickly subside after the initial release.

Plans are now underway by CMS to revive the use of mortality data for hospital comparison purposes. Soon the CMS Hospital Compare web site (http://www.hospitalcompare.hhs.gov/) will include provider-specific mortality rates for conditions such as heart attack and heart failure.

The Joint Commission's attempts to gather performance data for comparative purposes met with similar misgivings by the healthcare community. In 1987 the Joint Commission began plans to require accredited facilities to collect and report clinical indicator data that could be used for performance comparison purposes. The indicators the Joint Commission suggested as part of its "Agenda for Change" initiative would be used to measure care processes, clinical events, complications, and other outcomes. The intended purpose of sharing comparative data, according to the Joint Commission, was to help surveyed organizations continuously assess where they stand and where they need to improve relative to comparable organizations (Couch 1989). After testing five sets of indicators at more than 450 volunteer hospitals from 1987 to 1993, the complexities of measuring hospital performance became increasingly apparent. Differences in patient populations, data collection methods, and definitions distracted from the goal of collecting valid comparative data for quality improvement.

Although many of the challenges identified during the initial testing of the measures remained unanswered, the Joint Commission did not abandon its original goal of comparing performance at surveyed organizations. In 1995 the Joint Commission embarked on its ORYX initiative, which eventually led to the development of standardized Core Measure sets and mandatory reporting of measurement data.

Focus on Processes of Care

At the same time researchers were experimenting with various methodologies for risk-adjusting patient outcome data, the measurement focus began to shift from patient outcomes to healthcare processes. Purchasers were already familiar with the process measures found in the Health Plan Employer Data and Information Set (HEDIS), a core set of performance measures for managed care organizations. Many of the HEDIS process measures were based on guidelines first published by the U.S. Clinical Preventive Services Task Force in 1989 (U.S. CPSTF, 1989).

It seemed reasonable to assume that process measures could also be used to determine whether individual practitioners and organizations were providing appropriate patient care. But before this issue could be satisfactorily addressed the medical community needed to establish more nationally recognized definitions of best practice based on scientific evidence and expert opinion. To jump-start the effort, in 1991 the Agency for Healthcare Research and Quality—then known as the Agency for Health Care Policy and Research—published an organized, rigorous, and explicit methodology for guideline development and began sponsoring clinical practice guideline development task groups. Within a few years, medical, nursing, and allied health professional groups took up the challenge of developing practice guidelines, and the federally sponsored task groups were phased out. Even before guidelines were translated into performance measures, organizations began using them to improve the quality of patient care (Grimshaw and Russell 1993; Makulovich 1995).

Once rigorously developed clinical practice guidelines became available, conformance to the recommendations could be measured for populations of patients, and the average rate of conformance could be compared among practitioners and organizations. However, guideline recommendations are not created equal. For measurement purposes purchasers and accrediting bodies focused on evaluating those recommendations derived from strong evidence—meaning that failure to perform such actions appears to reduce the likelihood that optimal patient outcomes will occur.

Consumer Ratings of Quality

An initial purpose of comparative outcome and process measurement data was to help consumers make informed healthcare choices. Yet numerous studies suggest that the performance rates purchasers and even the healthcare industry view as being important are not necessarily evaluating what consumers view as significant (Pelling and Spath 1999). According to Crawford and Sena (1999), some of the most common factors considered to be important by healthcare consumers include

- interpersonal aspects of care;
- communication or information giving;
- timeliness of services;
- access and availability of services; and
- physical environment.

Publicly reported measures of health plan performance have included enrollee satisfaction indicators since the early 1990s, and for several years providers have gathered some type of patient satisfaction data for internal evaluation purposes. Measures of consumer satisfaction with healthcare services have now been incorporated into the Medicare and Medicaid performance evaluation requirements with the intention of making comparative reports available to the public.

Measurement Evolution Implications

What providers face today is an ever-changing kaleidoscope of performance measures that may be used to evaluate resource use, patient outcomes, compliance with important processes, and consumer satisfaction. The politics of measure development and varying priorities among developers caused the efforts to be siloed; there was little coordination among the competing interested parties. The result is that providers are being pulled in many different directions to meet the disparate and sometimes conflicting requirements of accrediting, quality, and purchasing groups (Denham 2005). Recently, national organizations began harmonizing efforts to standardize, as much as possible, measure specifications and definitions. This work could take several years, and in the meantime, providers must contend with reporting data to dozens of different national, state, and local entities that may require slightly different measures. This represents an incredible duplication of efforts, which, from the providers' perspective, translates into waste and inefficiencies (Kusterbeck 2006).

Despite the challenges, the staying power of efforts to measure healthcare performance is clearly evident. When providers and clinicians questioned the validity of outcome measures, more sophisticated severity-adjustment methodologies were created. When there was a scarcity of evidence-based patient care recommendations, development of clinical practice guidelines was encouraged and eventually embraced by the medical community. When consumers voiced the importance of measuring interpersonal quality and amenities, these dimensions of performance were incorporated into health-care report cards. And when providers balked at gathering and reporting additional data to external groups, financial reimbursement and accreditation decisions were linked to participation in the measurement systems. It's clear that the measurement monster can't be stopped, but there are ways for senior leaders to tame its pervasive influence.

Taking Control

All healthcare organizations are, and must be, interested in developing and deploying effective performance measurement systems. It is only through such systems that organizations can see how they are progressing, what isn't working, and what still needs improving. The goal for senior leaders should be to create a meaningful and efficient performance measurement system that complements the quality mission of the organization and meets the expectations of purchasers, accrediting bodies, and consumers.

Meaningful Measurement System

To be meaningful, an organization's performance measurement activities must provide intelligent information for decision makers, not just compile data. Ideally, measures should flow from strategic goals and objectives developed by the board of trustees and senior leaders (Spath 2005). This ideal is being compromised by the growing number of measures that organizations must track to satisfy data requests from external groups. Healthcare organizations often discover that the measures requested by purchasers, regulators, and accrediting bodies differ somewhat from internally established performance management priorities. Thus, senior executives are faced with a decision: Should we modify our strategic quality goals and performance measures to more closely align with the priorities established by external groups? Or should we continue to strive toward achieving our improvement priorities *plus* work to improve the aspects of care that external groups are measuring?

This question is easier to answer when the measurement data are not made public. Transparency and the fear of being labeled a "low performer" are causing some organizations to shift attention and resources away from what trustees and senior leaders might view as more important clinical or service topics (Pham, Coughlan, and O'Malley 2006). Once comparative performance data are presented to the public, there is strong evidence that hospitals are more likely to initiate improvement efforts in those areas affected by the measures (Hibbard, Stockard, and Tusler 2003).

This is not to suggest that national priorities such as reducing surgical wound infections or improving the care provided to patients who suffer a heart attack are not good things to do, but healthcare organizations often have local problems that deserve just as much attention as national priorities. It would be unfortunate for patients if an organization did not attempt to resolve a significant quality concern just because the issue is not an improvement priority for external groups.

Pay-for-performance initiatives will most likely place further pressure on organizations to link public reporting of measurement results and internally set improvement priorities. Whether purchasers and accrediting bodies should be wielding such power—the power to influence the quality goals of individual healthcare facilities—is a subject that merits further consideration by senior executives.

Stay informed

To effectively integrate externally defined measures with the organization's measurement priorities, senior executives must be kept apprised of what external groups are currently measuring and what they might add or subtract in the future. The quality department should be responsible for maintaining an up-to-date list of externally defined measures. Resources for these measures are listed in Box II.1. Ideally, the list should be updated at least quarterly, although

---

BOX II.1
Resources for Healthcare Performance Measures

- Centers for Disease Control and Prevention: www.cdc.gov
- Commission on Accreditation of Rehabilitation Facilities: www.carf.org
- Institute for Healthcare Improvement: www.ihi.org
- The Joint Commission: www.jointcommission.org
- National Association of Children's Hospitals and Related Institutions: www.childrenshospitals.net
- National Association of Health Data Organizations: www.nahdo.org
- National Committee for Quality Assurance: www.ncqa.org
- National Quality Forum: www.qualityforum.org
- National Quality Measures Clearinghouse: www.qualitymeasures.ahrq.gov
- *The Guide to Quality Measures: A Compendium* published by CMS: www.cms.hhs.gov/MedicaidSCHIPQualPrac/Downloads/pmfinalaugust06.pdf
- AQA Alliance: www.aqaalliance.org
- The Leapfrog Group: www.leapfroggroup.org

some organizations, such as Sisters of Mercy Health System in St. Louis, Missouri, choose to make weekly updates (Anderson and Sinclair 2006).

Just because an external group endorses measurement of a particular aspect of healthcare performance, it does not mean organizations should automatically start gathering data for those measures. Data collection, reporting, and analysis are costly, and measurement resources are limited. Try to save your resources for measures that appropriately focus the organization's attention on the right priorities.

Choose wisely

Senior executives, with input from medical staff leadership, should periodically review the existing measures and the newest additions to the list to determine which are currently relevant to the organization's strategic goals and patient populations. For each measure, a set of questions needs to be answered using your best judgment whenever the answers are not readily available. The questions are listed in Box II.2.

How many performance measures are sufficient to meet externally imposed requirements and support your organization's quality objectives?

BOX II.2
Questions for Evaluating Performance Measures

- Is reporting of the data currently mandatory?
- Is it likely that reporting of the data will soon become mandatory?
- Are we financially rewarded for reporting the data?
- Are we financially rewarded for good performance in this measure?
- Is it likely that reporting of the data and/or good performance in this measure will be financially rewarded in the future?
- Is our performance in this measure currently reported publicly?
- Is it it likely that our performance in this measure will soon be reported publicly?
- Does this measure evaluate an aspect of care that represents a strategic objective for our organization?
- Does this measure evaluate an aspect of care that represents an improvement opportunity in our organization?
- Would we benefit from knowing the performance rates at other organizations for this measure?
- Is it likely that affected caregivers will be supportive of initiatives aimed at improving performance in this measure?
- What resources will it take both in time and money to collect, report, and analyze the measurement results?

There is no simple answer; the decision is influenced by many factors. A rule of thumb is found in the 2007 Baldrige Healthcare Criteria for Performance Excellence (National Institute of Standards and Technology 2007):

> An effective healthcare service and administrative management system depends on the measurement and analysis of performance. Such measurements should derive from healthcare service needs and strategy, and they should provide critical data and information about key processes, outputs, and results.

Efficient Measurement System

Cost is a major consideration in maintaining a meaningful performance measurement system. Based on a survey of its customers, CareScience found that it takes 50 to 90 hours per month to collect data for just three of the Joint Commission Core Measure sets (heart attack, heart failure, and pneumonia) and another 23 hours per month to analyze the data (Anderson and Sinclair 2006). Often organizations must add fulltime-equivalent employees to keep up with the growing demand for detailed clinical information that can only be obtained through a review of patient records. Even in organizations with an electronic medical record staff may need to access separate data systems (electronic or paper based) to get complete information (Pham, Coughlan, and O'Malley 2006). In addition, it may be necessary to dedicate additional staff time to documentation enhancement activities to ensure that needed information is recorded in patient records.

The resources necessary to support a meaningful performance measurement system can sometimes seem endless. These resources include the following (Spath and Stewart 2002):

- Facility-specific capital costs
- Data collection costs for
    - recruiting/training data collectors/record reviewers;
    - sampling/screening/selecting cases for review;
    - retrieving records or database;
    - abstracting records and/or downloading data;
    - implementing data quality control and supervision measures;
    - providing clerical and administrative support; and
    - performing data entry.
- Data processing and analysis costs
- Costs related to support staff and professional time devoted to interpreting data, providing feedback, and using the findings for improvement activities

With the potential for continuing cost increases associated with performance measurement activities, the need for efficient data collection and analysis is paramount. Following are some steps senior leaders can take to maximize the capabilities of the organization's performance measurement system.

Encourage systemwide solutions

Efficiencies can be realized if physicians and staff document needed information as part of routine patient care. For example, at one hospital the bedside nurse and physician complete a checklist after inserting a central venous catheter. This checklist primarily serves as a point-of-care reminder of best-practice guidelines for this intervention. Once completed, the checklist is sent to the quality department where it is used to gather data for measuring compliance with the guidelines. Without the checklist, the quality staff would need to search through patient records to look for evidence of guideline compliance. Using the checklist as a data source is much more efficient.

Even if patient care staffing has been cut to the bare minimum, there are often opportunities for point-of-service data collection. Tapping into these opportunities can relieve some of the pressure on an already overburdened quality department. A multidisciplinary approach is needed to achieve systemwide performance measurement solutions. As new measures are introduced, the departments affected by the measures should jointly develop a plan for gathering the data. Some organizations have established a performance data management committee with members from key clinical areas, as well as representatives from the IT and health information management departments. In addition to creating data collection plans for new performance measures, the group maintains an inventory of existing data sources; resolves issues surrounding data integrity; and oversees process improvement on data collection/entry, interrater reliability, and data definitions. This last issue—data reliability (accuracy and completeness)—is the focal point of increased scrutiny by CMS, the Joint Commission, and other external groups (U.S. GAO 2006).

Expand IT support

Many of the inefficiencies in performance measurement systems can be traced to inadequacies of the organization's existing IT system (Pham, Coughlan, and O'Malley 2006). Some healthcare facilities still rely solely on paper records, while others have a patchwork of IT systems that are poorly linked. Even those few organizations with advanced integrated systems find it challenging to create data warehouses with flexible reporting capabilities that can keep up with ever-changing performance measurement requirements.

Given the large costs associated with IT, organizations must begin planning now for short- and long-term solutions. It may be necessary to

- modify existing information systems to include data elements required for particular performance measures;

- write programs to calculate performance measures based on data elements included in the existing information systems; and
- upgrade existing information systems to enable efficient downloading and transmittal of data to a central location for analysis and reporting.

When selecting new IT systems, the potential for gathering reliable performance measurement data should be one of the considerations. Ideally, the technology chosen to support patient care and administrative functions will also support realization of the organization's performance measurement goals.

Prevent measurement creep

Efficiencies gained through systemwide solutions and better IT support can quickly slip away if senior leaders do not actively manage the organization's measurement system. Requests for new measure sets can come from a variety of sources. Some health plans want to create a unique measurement database. Regulators or accrediting bodies often seek volunteers for measure validation projects or other performance-related experiments. National or state medical professional associations actively solicit members to become involved in evaluating topics of professional importance. Physicians and staff within your organization may have areas of special interest for which measurement data are requested.

Although the additional information gained from new measure sets may ultimately prove worthwhile, senior leaders must save the organization's limited resources for high-priority measurement activities. Even if the data appear easy to gather and report, the quality department staff can be quickly overwhelmed by multiple requests for unique data elements.

Use the measure evaluation questions found in Box II.2 to determine whether new measure sets should be added to your performance measurement system. If you have a performance data management committee, use this group to evaluate requests and endorse new measurement sets. If no such committee exists, the responsibility should be given to the quality council or other group with senior executive and quality department representation. Rather than turn down requests for performance data, senior executives can often work with the requesting group to suggest comparable measures already in use by the organization.

Conclusion

Strategies for measuring healthcare performance are in constant flux, and newly introduced financial incentives have upped the ante. For providers to survive and flourish in this era of expanded performance measurement, administrative leaders must deal with a host of strategic, technical, and resource issues. The problem healthcare organizations face is the ever-evolving nature of performance measurement. The solution is for senior leaders to actively support an ever-evolving structure that can tame the measurement monster. This will only be achieved by creating a meaningful and efficient measurement system that has sufficient flexibility to meet current and future requirements.

Of course, the results are the real test of your measurement system's value. It's not just about gathering data or looking good in publicly available comparative reports. It's not about gaining financial rewards when your organization's performance exceeds some externally defined threshold. The real value of your measurement system is knowing where improvements are needed in your organization and acting on that information.

References

Anderson, K. M., and S. Sinclair. 2006. "Easing the Burden of Quality Measures Reports." *H&HN Online*. [Online article; retrieved 1/23/07.] http://www.hospitalconnect.com/hhnmag/jsp/hhnonline.jsp.

Couch, J. B. 1989. "The Joint Commission on Accreditation of Healthcare Organizations." In *Providing Quality Care: The Challenge to Clinicians*, edited by N. Goldfield and D. B. Nash, 201–22. Philadelphia, PA: American College of Physicians.

Crawford, J. M., and J. F. Sena. 1999. "Gathering Satisfaction Data to Share with the Public." In *Provider Report Cards: A Guide for Promoting Healthcare Quality to the Public*, edited by P. L. Spath, 97–117. Chicago: Health Forum/American Hospital Association.

Denham, C. R. 2005. "The Quality Choir: From Warm-up to Harmony." *Journal of Patient Safety* 1 (3): 170–7.

Fonarow, G. C., W. T. Abraham, N. M. Albert, et al. 2007. "Association Between Performance Measures and Clinical Outcomes for Patients Hospitalized with Heart Failure." *JAMA*. 297 (1): 61–70.

Gosfield, A. 2005. "The Performance Measures Ball: Too Many Tunes, Too Many Dancers?" In *Health Law Handbook* by A. Gosfield, 227–84. Eagan, MN: West.

Grimshaw, J. M., and I. T. Russell. 1993. "Effect of Clinical Guidelines on Medical Practice: A Systematic Review of Rigorous Evaluations." *Lancet* 342 (8883): 1317–22.

Hibbard, J. H., J. Stockard, and M. Tusler. 2003. "Does Publicizing Hospital Performance Stimulate Quality Improvement Efforts?" *Health Affairs* 22 (2): 84–94.

Institute of Medicine, Committee on the National Quality Report on Healthcare Delivery, eds. M. P. Hurtado, E. K. Swift, and J. M. Corrigan. 2001. *Envisioning the National Healthcare Quality Report*. Washington, DC: National Academies Press.

Joint Commission on Accreditation of Healthcare Organizations. No date. "Attributes of Core Performance Measures and Associated Evaluation Criteria." [Online information; retrieved 1/2/2007.] http://www.jointcommission.org /NR/rdonlyres/7DF24897-A700-4013-A0BD-154881FB2321/0/ AttributesofCorePerformanceMeasuresandAssociatedEvaluationCriteria.pdf.

Kusterbeck, S. 2006. "More Alignment of Measures on Horizons—But Not Soon Enough for Many QPs." *Hospital Peer Review* 32 (1): 1–4.

Makulovich, G. 1995. "Users of AHCPR-Supported Guidelines Report Improvements in Quality of Care." *Research Activities* 183 (2): 13–14, 17.

National Institute of Standards and Technology (NIST). 2007. *Malcolm Baldrige Criteria for Healthcare Performance Excellence*, 4, Gaithersburg, MD: NIST.

Pelling, M. H., and P. L. Spath. 1999. "Determining What Consumers Want to Know About Providers." In *Provider Report Cards: A Guide for Promoting Healthcare Quality to the Public*, edited by P.L. Spath, 3–19. Chicago: Health Forum/ American Hospital Association.

Pham, H. H., J. Coughlan, and A. S. O'Malley. 2006. "The Impact of Quality-Reporting Programs on Hospital Operations." *Health Affairs (Millwood)* 25 (5): 1412–22.

Spath, P. L. 2005. *Leading Your Healthcare Organization to Excellence*. Chicago: Health Administration Press.

Spath, P. L., and A. Stewart. 2002. *From Quality to Excellence: Using Comparative Data to Improve Healthcare Performance*, 9, Forest Grove, OR: Brown-Spath & Associates.

U.S. Clinical Preventive Services Task Force. 1989. *Guide to Clinical Preventive Services*. Chicago: Health Administration Press.

U.S. Department of Health and Human Services, Healthcare Financing Administration. 1987. *Medicare Hospital Mortality Information, 1986*. Washington, DC: U.S. Government Printing Office.

U.S. Government Accountability Office (GAO). 2006. "Hospital Quality Data: CMS Needs More Rigorous Methods to Ensure Reliability of Publicly Released Data." Washington, DC: GAO.

Wennberg, J. E., and A. Gittelsohn. 1973. "Small Area Variations in Healthcare Delivery." *Science* 182 (117): 1102–8.

Werner, R. M., and E. T. Bradlow. 2006. "Relationship Between Medicare's Hospital Compare Performance Measures and Mortality Rates." *JAMA* 296 (22): 2694–702.

Discussion Questions

1. How would you advise the CEO of a 75-bed hospital to respond to these demands for information?
2. How could this required information be used to improve care?
3. Check out one of the websites listed in Box II.1 of the Spath reading (or other similar websites). Find examples of information being requested.

How difficult do you think it would be for a healthcare organization to comply with these requests?

4. Suppose your neighbor came to you and said "I have just been diagnosed with X condition (for example, diabetes, multiple sclerosis, or the need for heart surgery). Can you help me find a high quality provider for my condition?" Pick a condition and go to the web and see what you can find out about good care.

Required Supplementary Readings

Berwick, D. M. 2005. "My Right Knee," *Annals of Internal Medicine* 142 (2): 121–25.

Bradley, E. H., E. S. Holmoe, J. A. Mattera, S. A. Roumanis, M. J. Radford, and H. M. Krumholz. 2003. "The Roles of Senior Management in Quality Improvement Efforts: What Are the Key Components?" *Journal of Healthcare Management* 48 (1): 15–28.

Jha, A. K., J. B. Perlin, K. W. Kizer, and R. A. Dudley. 2003. "Effect of the Transformation of the Veterans Affairs Healthcare System on the Quality of Care." *New England Journal of Medicine* 348 (22): 2218–27.

Rindler, M. E. 2007. "Extraordinary Success at Northeast Georgia Medical Center." In *Strategic Cost Reduction*. Chicago: Health Administration Press.

Discussion Questions for the Required Supplementary Readings

1. For any specific healthcare organization, what are the most important things for the information system to measure?
2. Errors are frequent in healthcare. They often have serious consequences. What would you recommend to reduce medical errors?
3. What is the role of senior management in promoting quality improvement?
4. What are the barriers to cost containment in healthcare organizations, and how can these be overcome?

Recommended Supplementary Readings

Batalden, P., and P. Stoltz. 1993. "Performance Improvement in Healthcare Organizations: A Framework for the Continued Improvement of Health Care." *The Joint Commission Journal of Quality Improvement* 19 (10): 424–52.

Berwick, D. M. 1995. "The Toxicity of Pay for Performance." *Quality Management in Health Care* 9 (1): 27–33.

Black, J. 2008. *Toyota Way to Health Care Excellence*. Chicago: Health Administration Press.

Bradley, E. H., E. S. Holmoe, J. A. Mattera, S. A. Roumanis, M. J. Radford, and H. M. Krumholz. 2003. "The Roles of Senior Management in Quality Improvement Efforts: What Are the Key Components?" *Journal of Healthcare Management* 48 (1): 15–28.

Eisenberg, J. M. 1996. *Doctors' Decisions and the Cost of Medical Care*. Chicago: Health Administration Press.

Gawande, A. 2004. "The Bell Curve." *The New Yorker*, December 6, 82–91.

Griffith, J. R., and K. R. White. 2007. *The Well-Managed Healthcare Organization*, 6th edition. Chicago: Health Administration Press.

Hebert, C., and D. Neuhauser. 2004. "Improving Hypertension Care with Patient Generated Run Charts: Physician, Patient and Management Perspectives." *Quality Management in Health Care* 13 (3): 174–77.

Institute of Medicine. 2001. *Crossing the Quality Chasm*. Washington, DC: National Academies Press.

Lewis, L. E. 1996. "Improving Productivity: The Ongoing Experience of an Academic Department of Medicine." *Academic Medicine* 71 (4): 317–28.

Longo, D. R., J. A. Hewett, B. Ge, and S. Schubert. 2007. "Hospital Patient Safety: Characteristics of Best-Performing Hospitals." *Journal of Healthcare Management* 52 (3).

McDonagh, K. J. 2006. "Hospital Governing Boards: A Study of Their Effectiveness in Relation to Organizational Performance." *Journal of Healthcare Management* 51 (6).

McGlynn, E. A., S. M. Asch, J. Adams, J. Keesey, J. Hicks, A. DeCristofaro, and E. Kerr. 2003. "The Quality of Health Care Delivered to Adults in the United States." *New England Journal of Medicine* 348 (26): 2635–83.

McLaughlin, D., and J. Hays. 2008. *Health Care Operations Management*. Chicago: Health Administration Press.

Pointer, D. D., and E. Orlikoff. 2002. *Getting to Great: Principles of Health Care Organization Governance*. San Francisco: Jossey-Bass.

Rundall, T. G., P. F. Martelli, L. Arroyo, R. McCurdy, I. Graetz, E. B. Neuwirth, P. Curtis, J. Schmittdiel, M. Gibson, and J. Hsu. 2007. "The Informed Decisions Tool-Box: Tools for Knowledge Transfer and Performance Improvement." *Journal of Healthcare Management* 52 (5).

Smaltz, D. 2008. *Information Systems in Health Care*, 7th edition. Chicago: Health Administration Press.

Umbdenstock, R. J., and W. M. Hageman. 1990. "The Five Critical Areas for Effective Governance of Non-Profit Hospitals." *Hospital and Health Services Administration* 35 (4): 481–92.

Watts, B., R. Lawrence, D. Litaker, D. C. Aron, and D. Neuhauser. 2008. "Quality of Care by a Hypertension Expert: A Cautionary Tale for Pay-for-Performance Approaches." *Quality Management in Health Care* 17 (1): 35–46.

Yap, C., E. Siu, G. R. Baker, and A. D. Brown. 2005. "A Comparison of System-wide and Hospital-Specific Performance Tools." *Journal of Healthcare Management* 50 (4).

Zelman, W. N., D. Blazer, J. M. Gower, P. O. Bumgarner, and L. M. Cancilla. 1999. "Issues for Academic Health Centers to Consider Before Implementing a Balanced Scorecard Effort." *Academic Medicine* 74 (12): 1269–77.

******

In addition to the above readings, these three journals about quality and safety are worth following:

The Joint Commission Journal on Quality and Patient Safety, www.jointcommission.org (At this site also check out the Codman Award videos for interesting examples of excellence in care improvements.)

Quality and Safety in Health Care, www.qshc.bmj.com

Quality Management in Health Care, www.qmhcjournal.com

THE CASES

Peter Drucker (1973) commented, "the basic problem of service institutions is not high cost, but lack of effectiveness." In those days all hospitals believed they provided the best care with the best nurses and doctors, and patients believed these claims in the absence of any information to the contrary. However, three recent trends with glacial-like power have changed this perception. First is the development and acceptance of evidence-based medicine. How do we know the care we give is beneficial? The Cochrane Collaborative has now registered over half a million randomized clinical trials that demonstrate treatment effectiveness or the lack of it. Now that there is much more evidence-based agreement about what works, it is easy to create clinical guidelines for best practice care and ask that they be followed.

The quality and safety movement is the second major force for change. The quality improvement movement encourages the use of best practices for all patients, and disparity research focuses on who and what groups do not get such good care.

The third and most important force in the long run is the steady, relentless growth of computer capacity combined with the declining cost of computing power. While the first health management applications were for insurance billing and finance, the new wave emerging is related to clinical information.

The three case studies that follow reflect the process of adoption. Case D by McAlearney describes the introduction of an electronic medical record system. Case E by Kovner shows a management information system for staffing and cost control that compares actual and budgeted performance. Case F by Struk and Neuhauser shows a home care agency overwhelmed with comparative clinical performance data of many sorts. It shows we are moving from Drucker's absence of data to information overload.

The six short cases consider parallel issues. These include the introduction of quality improvement programs (Cases 6 and 7), new computing capacity (Case 11), priority setting (Case 8), analysis of existing budget information (Case 10), and recognition of good performance through pay for performance (Case 9).

Reference

Drucker, P. 1973. "Managing the Public Service Institution." *The Public Interest* 33: 43–60.

Case D
An Information Technology
Implementation Challenge

Ann Scheck McAlearney

Introduction

Geneva Health System is a large academic medical center based in Longwood, a mid-size metropolitan city in the Southwest. Geneva Health System is associated with the state university, and includes three hospitals, a medical clinic facility, a medical research complex, and affiliated primary and specialty group practices spread throughout the region. Geneva University Hospital is the main hospital campus with 500 inpatient beds and equipment and facilities that are considered state of the art. Geneva Health System is well known for its cancer and rehabilitation service lines, and has recently expanded its cardiac service line in an attempt to keep up with the increasing demand.

Despite strong clinical services lines and an excellent reputation, Geneva Health System has been reluctant to adopt new clinical information technologies (IT) such as computerized provider order entry (CPOE) systems or a more comprehensive electronic health record (EHR) system. Instead, Geneva Health System's services are mainly supported by paper-based processes, and a strong team in the medical records department that has been able to expand with the health system's growth.

Changing Health System Leadership

Dr. Dan Johnson has just been appointed CEO of Geneva Health System, and has come to the Longwood area after serving five years in his previous position as CEO of a 200-bed community hospital. Johnson's predecessor, Jeffrey Ash, had retired after serving 20 years as Geneva Health System's CEO. While the announcement of a new CEO was not unexpected, this change in leadership has left the organization unsettled, and staff and affiliated physicians are anxious about the new changes Johnson may bring to Geneva Health System.

Assessing the Situation

Johnson is a definite fan of EHR and electronic medical record (EMR) systems, and is enthusiastic about the potential for incorporating an EMR system with CPOE capabilities into Geneva Health System. In particular, he is aware of the opportunities to use an EMR system to improve Geneva's ability to provide care according to evidence-based guidelines, and to capitalize on patient safety improvements that are possible with an EMR system. Johnson knows that his daughter, Ellen, uses a handheld computer, or personal digital assistant (PDA), to help her keep track of her patients, check medications, and access important clinical information in her internal medicine practice, and he has seen PDAs in the pockets of many of the Geneva physicians as well.

Yet Johnson is aware of the likely resistance he will face in his efforts to introduce an EMR system throughout Geneva. He has followed some of the IT implementation literature, and knows that common barriers to implementation, such as physician resistance to changes in workflow and a reluctance to use practice guidelines or "cookbook medicine," may create challenges at Geneva. He also predicts resistance from the strong and capable medical records department. Given that successful EMR implementations are associated with a reduced need for space and personnel in medical records, it is unlikely that such changes will be warmly received.

Johnson schedules a meeting with Barb Northrop, director of information services, because he suspects Northrop might have some ideas about how to proceed.

Meeting with the Information Systems Department

Once Johnson scheduled his meeting with Northrop, excitement grew in the IS department. Northrop and her department had been enthusiastically following all of the changes in EMR systems, but had met with resistance when they suggested that Geneva consider adopting a new system. The previous CEO had been decidedly "old school" and had little interest in leading the charge to put Geneva on the EMR map. Instead, Ash chose to placate the established physicians and the director of medical records, Amy Chapman. Even though he was aware that the newer physicians were all carrying PDAs and iPhones, he had no interest in rocking the proverbial boat at Geneva.

Northrop knew this was her opportunity to make the case for a system-wide EMR introduction at Geneva. She had full confidence in her IS team's ability to carry out this initiative. Northrop had the group compile the information they had collected from different vendors about the various systems and capabilities, and summarize everything in an "issue brief" document that would be easy to skim. She also had her summer resident, Austin Mitchell, collect some of the key articles from the research literature that highlighted the potential and the pitfalls of such a system-wide implementation.

Northrop's meeting with Johnson went even better than she had hoped. Armed with the evidence, Northrop laid out the various issues, pro and con, for a system-wide implementation of an EMR, and then explained the different vendor options that might be appropriate for Geneva. Already convinced that this was a good idea, Johnson gave Northrop the green light to develop a formal proposal for presentation to the Geneva board, and directed her to Chase Aukland, Geneva's CFO, to make sure the cost proposal IS developed would be appropriate for Geneva.

A Hallway Conversation

Johnson left the meeting with Northrop smiling, but his smile faded when he was stopped in the corridor by Amy Chapman, who was leaving the Medical Records Department.

Johnson: Hi, Ms. Chapman. How is everything going in Medical Records?

Chapman: Not well, Dr. Johnson. I heard a rumor that you were considering bringing an electronic medical record system to Geneva, and that makes me very concerned.

Johnson: Well, Ms. Chapman, nothing has been decided yet, but there is a strong push nationwide to introduce EMR systems in all hospitals and we don't want to be left behind.

Chapman: I understand that, Dr. Johnson, but I just don't think we want to do any of this too quickly. Mr. Ash had been very consistent in his message that Geneva had no reason to be an "early adopter" of such systems. As he repeatedly said, "Let all those other health systems make the mistakes first. Then we can learn from their mistakes and make our own decision. And, in the meantime, we can keep doing well what we already do well."

Johnson: I appreciate that perspective, Ms. Chapman, but I have to admit, I am a bit more likely to push the envelope than Mr. Ash. I believe an EMR system would be a great boost for Geneva, helping us to track everything electronically, and potentially helping us to reduce medical errors in the process.

Chapman: But don't we already have the ability to track everything? I'm just not sure what's wrong with paper. Our medical records team is very capable and responsive. I certainly haven't heard any complaints about our ability to access patient records.

Johnson: That's true, Ms. Chapman, but I don't think that we're looking far enough ahead. As other hospitals and health systems go digital, we're going to be left behind. I truly believe we do not have a choice in this situation. It is not a matter of "whether," but a question of "when." I think it would be in the best interests of Geneva to get this going on the sooner side so that we can take advantage of the capabilities of an electronic medical record system as soon as possible.

Chapman: Well, Dr. Johnson, I disagree. I tend to believe "If it ain't broke, don't fix it." And the Medical Records Department "ain't broke."

Johnson: I understand your concerns, Ms. Chapman. Thanks for sharing them with me. Would you be interested in participating in a task force charged with investigating this opportunity?

Chapman. I'm not sure I think this is much of an opportunity. But since you're asking, I guess I'll need to participate.

Johnson: Thanks so much, Ms. Chapman. I appreciate your time.

As Johnson headed back to his office, he was once more reminded that none of this was going to be easy. Even though Northrop and her IS department seemed fully capable and on board with the idea, there were plenty of others throughout the health system who might not share their enthusiasm. He was especially concerned about resistance from the physicians. While he was a physician himself, that did little to improve his credibility when he was making a case "from the dark side" of administration. He decided to seek out Dr. Jody Smith, the chair of internal medicine, to begin to gauge some of the sentiments from the physicians. He headed to her office to see if he could catch her for a moment.

A Physician's Perspective

Johnson (knocking as he enters Dr. Smith's office): Hi, Jody. How's everything going?

Smith: Dan. Just the person I wanted to see. I heard a rumor that you were considering an EMR for Geneva and I wanted to make sure that it was just a rumor.

Johnson: Well, Jody, the rumor is actually true. I just met with Barb Northrop, the head of IS, to get her and her team to begin to develop some estimates and plans for what an EMR adoption would mean for Geneva.

Smith: But Dan! Have you been following the latest research? Despite what the vendors claim, every place that puts one of these systems in reports that it actually takes the docs *more* time to do what they used to do on paper. Even after having the system in place for awhile, the docs are still spending more time doing record-keeping than before—and that time is time that they used to have to care for patients! Also, when they put in a system somewhere in Pittsburgh, the EMR system was actually associated with an *increase* in the number of medical errors!

Johnson: I have followed that research, Jody, but I think there's a bigger picture to consider here. While it's true that EMR systems do require the physicians to spend more time entering data and so forth, there's also evidence that with an EMR it is actually the right people who are entering the data—not some non-clinical person trying to decipher a physician's notes about what was done, or trying to figure out if a visit was long or short. Also, evidence is beginning to build that when EMR systems are coupled with decision support logic such as order sets within CPOE systems, this type of system can actually save time. Instead of going through multiple screens to find all the meds and tests that need to be ordered, the physician can just click on the asthma order set, for instance, and review the options there.

Smith: But what about patient-centered care? Who says that every patient is alike? For heavens sake, what if your patient needs something different? How long does it take to find that when everything is based on a standardized order set? And how about the resident physicians? Maybe they will stop thinking about making patient-specific clinical judgments and just click the standard order set for everyone! Have you really thought this through?

Johnson: I know there are issues, Jody, but I truly believe the future of medicine is in electronic records. I'm guessing you've been following what's going on at the national level, and there are policy-type folks involved making a strong push toward expansion of EMRs into outpatient settings as well. Policymakers are concerned that hospitals and physicians have been too slow to adopt these systems, which they believe will improve both patient safety and the quality of care delivered, and they are beginning to propose incentive systems to encourage adoption. As I just mentioned to Amy Chapman, the director of medical records, I don't think this is a question of "whether" any more—it's just a question of "when." Geneva is a terrific health system that should be at the forefront of medical and technological advances, not waiting to see what everyone else does.

Smith: I'll bet Ms. Chapman was thrilled with the prospect of losing control of her medical records area. I think I understand your desire to help Geneva, but I don't think you've been here long enough to appreciate how great we already are. Mr. Ash repeatedly emphasized that we didn't need to be early adopters and that we could "let others make the mistakes first" and I think that makes a lot of sense. Our docs are content with paper, we have a functional and responsive medical records department, and I'm not sure I sense any burning need to be the "most wired" or anything. This isn't Boston, after all. A lot of us chose to practice here because we could do what we do best—provide excellent clinical care—without the distractions of a push to be number one in the world or something like that. I'm just not sure you can make a major change like putting in an EMR and keep everyone happy like they've been for so long here.

Johnson: I realize I haven't been here at Geneva very long, but I've been working very hard to get a sense of this place before I propose any major changes. I also realize that introducing an EMR system to a place that is completely paper-based is no easy task. At this point I know there is still considerable work to be done to better understand both Geneva and the opportunities and risks associated with implementing an EMR. However, I strongly believe the future of medicine will require the electronic capabilities associated with an EMR system, and I am not willing to "watch and wait" much longer. I'd like to make an EMR system implementation a major goal for the coming year, and I'd appreciate it if you would consider being on a task force to make this happen. What do you think?

Smith: I think this is crazy. I agree with Mr. Ash. We should wait and see what happens at other hospitals and health systems and learn from their mistakes. There is no reason to stick our necks out on the "cutting edge" of EMR system implementation. And by the way, I'm not alone in my beliefs. Lots of other physicians agree. What we do here works just fine, and the people who work here are happy doing things the way they are done now. As for your task force, I don't have the time to participate in more silly administrative meetings. I need to use my time to help ensure that the clinical care we deliver here is as good as it can be. And that requires me to use my time seeing patients and overseeing our physicians in training who are learning to be better physicians.

Johnson: Well, I'm sorry you won't be able to participate more in this initiative, but I respect your time and your priorities. Thanks so much for sharing your thoughts.

Johnson left Smith's office with his mind reeling. Was this really a shared sentiment among Geneva's physicians? Were they truly content with paper-based records and letting other hospitals pass them by with electronic capabilities? Regardless, Johnson knew he was right about the future. He knew Geneva needed to get on the EMR bandwagon, and the sooner the better. However, he now knew the implementation challenge was even greater than he had anticipated. Not only were the members of the medical records department threatened, but apparently physicians weren't all that interested in changing their practice patterns either. His only allies appeared to be among Northrop's IS team.

Considering the Resistance

Johnson recognized that in addition to uncovering some attitudes toward EMRs, he had learned quite a bit about Geneva's organizational culture during these exploratory conversations about EMR adoption. It appeared that the predominant culture was comfortable clinging to the status quo, and that few individuals were open to considering the possibility of change. He had felt strong resistance from Chapman and Smith, and knew that resistance to change was a major hurdle he would have to overcome if there was any hope that an EMR implementation process could succeed.

Yet Johnson sensed that this resistance was not merely resistance to change, but resistance to change that would result in a loss of control for the individuals involved. As he reflected upon his conversations with Chapman and Smith, he thought about some of the unspoken messages they had sent. Champman and her group felt threatened by the loss of control they would have over the medical records process. With electronic systems in place, they would no longer have a major role to play in health systems operations, and their jobs might even be at stake.

Smith's comments suggested that the physicians were uninterested in changing their practice patterns because they would lose some of their control as well. The introduction of standardized order sets and other decision support tools could truly change the way physicians practice medicine, thus leading to less discretion for individual providers with respect to viable treatment options. As both Smith and Johnson knew, with electronic medical records, there would be a searchable digital trail, which could be used to monitor those providers' practice patterns. While Smith mentioned her fear that newer physicians would come to rely too much on decision support systems and stop thinking for themselves, there was also an unspoken fear that if a physician did not do what the order set had defined as the "right things," they might face problems.

Learning More

Johnson knew of several IT implementation failures that had occurred over the past several years, with the most notorious at Cedars Sinai in Los Angeles.

There, he had learned, the hospital had rolled out a CPOE system across both the inpatient and outpatient settings and the process was deemed an utter failure. Physicians revolted and the hospital had to retreat, going back to paper-based processes while they decided what to do. On the other hand, he had also heard anecdotal stories about implementation successes, such as an incremental implementation that had been taking place at Nationwide Children's Hospital in Columbus, Ohio. While the Children's physicians were all hospital-employed and thus had little ability to "just say no," as the physicians at Cedars had, the process at Children's had been carefully planned and seemed to be proceeding according to schedule—without alienating the entire provider population.

Johnson had to plan his next steps carefully. He knew doctors valued evidence, and he had to build a good case for moving forward with an EMR implementation. He suspected there might be value in learning more about implementation successes and failures, but he also guessed there was other information out there he was not aware of. Johnson decided to recruit Northrop's summer resident to help him expand his search for evidence and help build the case for EMR adoption.

Case Questions

1. What types of information should Austin Mitchell collect to build the overall evidence case for an EMR system implementation? Where should he look to find this evidence?
2. What would you suggest that Dr. Johnson say to physicians who are concerned that an EMR will limit their ability to practice patient-centered medicine and provide individualized care to each individual patient? What evidence could you seek to support your argument?
3. How would adoption of an EMR affect organizational control systems at Geneva? How would it affect individuals?
4. What could be learned from speaking with hospitals and health systems about their experiences with EMR implementation? With whom would you like to speak at these organizations?
5. Beyond the director of medical records, who should be on the task force to consider the EMR alternatives and issues?
6. What would be critical success factors associated with implementation of an EMR at Geneva? What steps would you recommend to maximize the likelihood of success?

Case E
Improving Financial Performance in the Orthopedic Unit

Anthony R. Kovner

Dinah Ward is the patient care director (PCD) of the orthopedic service line at South Division, a 1,000-bed teaching hospital in a large eastern city. She has been in the position three years, and worked previously at another teaching hospital. The unit has 36 beds, and is primarily orthopedic, although it includes ear, nose, throat and plastic and oral surgery patients. Ward's first master's degree was in education and she has an MBA from a local college's Saturday executive program.

South Division is one of four hospitals in the University Health System (UHS). Ward is one of nine PCDs in the medical/surgical service line that is headed by Clara Stone. (There are two other divisions of nursing and 18 other PCDs at the South Division.) Stone reports to Rose Costello, who is the director of nursing operations at South Division. Costello is responsible for developing and monitoring the nursing budget; monitoring operations of departmental staffing, payroll, and financial performance; and overseeing the information system initiatives.

Costello estimates PCD level of performance in the finance areas as follows: 60 percent of the PCDs are great; 20 percent are satisfactory; and 20 percent need improvement. She identifies the causes of the problem as both PCD and department of nursing problems:

1. PCDs have a knowledge deficit in calculating what their staffing needs are. Some PCDs lack experience because they are new. Some PCDs lack aptitude because they were good nurses, but appear to be weak as managers, especially when it comes to the numbers/finance side.
2. The hospital administration doesn't supply PCDs with resources to do these calculations.
3. There is a lag in the timing of when financial reports are distributed. The reports are distributed three weeks after the last day of the previous month, which causes problems. For example, PCDs are required to justify what happened during the first week in July during the last week of August.
4. The hospital administration gives PCDs little opportunity to successfully influence the budget. PCDs feel they consistently are required to justify their variances, often similar variances over successive time periods, but have not been able to successfully do so with the available information.

(For the Monthly Departmental Variance Report, see Figures II.1 and II.2.)

Costello's recommendations are as follows: (1) PCDs should collaborate more intensively with other managers in developing the budget for their unit. Then they will take more ownership of the process. (2) Reports should be distributed in a more timely manner from finance, which should be possible because of improved IT investments and systems. (3) More education should be provided for PCDs on how to manage and monitor their budgets.

What Ward finds most challenging about financial performance is that "we are required to run the unit with a significant lack of necessary data, such as information about acuity, patient needs, and other units' needs. Also, the current structures don't allow for staffing efficiency, and I don't always feel as if we have the discretion to make those decisions." Ward has raised the issue with nursing leaders who are working to achieve institution-wide goals, such as increased patient satisfaction scores. Ward comments, "I would be able to raise patient satisfaction scores if I had appropriate staffing to address these initiatives." Patients may need more care because of acuity, regardless of the budget. To address the boundary concerns between nursing and finance, South Division created the position of director of nursing operations, which had formerly been a position within the UHS Finance Department but now reports directly to nursing leadership. This position was created to coordinate dollars and FTEs (full-time equivalents) based on acuity in the units, in collaboration with finance. Prior to this position being created, plans were developed solely by finance.

Ward says there are no real financial problems in her unit, unlike other units where the nurses in charge lack MBAs or other formal training in financial management. Ward thinks that master's programs in nursing "don't teach you financial management, how to influence the budget process, or how to lead a team in maintaining a financially successful unit. Those kinds of nurse leaders don't take ownership, lack accountability, and are passive managers."

With regard to financial performance, Ward gets the expense reports every month for staffing and supplies, allowing her to compare actual operating expenses to budget. FTEs are budgeted according to midnight census counts, but the census often changes from midnight to 7:00 a.m. so the budget doesn't account for variations in acuity. Ward and her nursing colleagues find it difficult to explain the impact of acuity on staffing and expenses without the appropriate data. They are asked to justify this case consistently, but find no way of reasonably doing so. Ward feels that incentives for a managed budget are not strong enough to compete for her attention given other priorities for the unit.

Also impacting the financial performance of her unit, Ward reduced average LOS (length of stay) for the unit from 6.0 to 4.1 days. In addition,

FIGURE II.1

Monthly Departmental Variance Report

UNIVERSITY HEALTH SYSTEM

Fiscal Year: 2006

Month Ending on

May 31st

ACCT DESCRIPTION	AU	May, Current				May, YTD			
		ACTUAL	BUDGETED	$ VARIANCE	% VAR	ACTUAL	BUDGETED	$ VARIANCE	% VAR
Salaries & Wages									
Gross Salaries & Wages									
0500 PAYROLL-GENL									
0510 OTHER PAYROLL-O.T.									
2300 REGISTERED NURSES									
2310 R.N.-O.T.									
2320 R.N.-HOLIDAY O.T.									
2330 ELECTIVE B/O-SNA									
2340 HOLIDAY B/O-SNA									
2350 SICK B/O-SNA									
4400 1199 PAYROLL-GENL									
4410 1199 OVERTIME									
4420 1199 HOLIDAY O.T.									
4050 AGENCY FEES									
Non-salary & Wage Expenses									

Monthly Departmental Variance Report

UNIVERSITY HEALTH SYSTEM

Fiscal Year: 2006

Month Ending on

May 31st

ACCT DESCRIPTION	AU	May, Current				May, YTD			
		ACTUAL	BUDGETED	$ VARIANCE	% VAR	ACTUAL	BUDGETED	$ VARIANCE	% VAR
Med/Surg Supplies									
7200 CHEMICALS & STAINS									
7250 NEEDLES & SYRINGES									
7300 OXYGEN & MED GASES									
7350 I.V. SOLUTIONS									
7370 GLOVES-MED/SURG									
7380 OTHER MED SUPPLIES									
7400 IRRIG SOLUTN/ACCESS									
7450 LAB & DIAG SUPPLIES									
7500 RESPIR & ANESTH SUPP									
7550 DRESSINGS & BANDAGES									
7560 SKIN APPLIC. SUPPLY									
8000 UROLOGY SUPPLIES									
8050 DIALYSIS FLUID/ACCESS									
8130 OSTOMY SUPPLIES									
8160 CUSTOM SURG PROC PAC									

(continued)

FIGURE II.2

FIGURE II.2
(*continued*)

Monthly Departmental Variance Report

UNIVERSITY HEALTH SYSTEM

Fiscal Year: 2006

Month Ending on

May 31st

ACCT DESCRIPTION	AU	May, Current				May, YTD			
		ACTUAL	BUDGETED	$ VARIANCE	% VAR	ACTUAL	BUDGETED	$ VARIANCE	% VAR
Med/Surg Supplies									
8200 SUTURE-NON-U.S. SURG									
8240 SUTURE-U.S. SURGICAL									
8300 SURGICAL INSTRUMENTS									
8310 DISPOSAL INSTUMENTS									
8320 SURGICAL DRAPES									
8480 IMPLANTS-ALL OTHER									
8680 OTHER O.R. SUPPLIES									
8690 OTHER SURG SUPPLIES									
8700 OTH MED/SURG SUPPLY									
Total Med/Surg Supplies									
Blood Products									
8520 BLOOD PRODUCTS									
8620 BLOOD PROCESS SUPP									
Total Blood Products									

she looked into best practices at a competitor teaching hospital. These included pre- and post-operative education, developing a good interdisciplinary team, obtaining good commitment from the staff, providing early physical therapy for the patients, monitoring patient pain, and eliminating bedpans. Ward developed discharge planning protocols for patients that are initiated before patients are admitted, and she implemented clinical pathways. Each patient is told what to expect concerning the day and time of discharge and this is posted in the patients' rooms.

Staffing on the unit includes a unit-based nurse practitioner, two dedicated nurse social workers, and one case manager (who is shared with another unit). As a result of the extra efforts Ward has made to reduce LOS, the nursing hours per discharge have dropped significantly, but the hours per patient day (HPPD) have risen. For example, it used to be 4 HPPD × 6 LOS = 24 hours per discharge; now it is 5 HPPD × 4.1 hours = 20.5 hours per discharge. From Ward's perspective she has reduced nursing hours by 3.5 hours, which is a 15 percent reduction in nursing cost per patient. Yet the finance department is upset that Ward is using 5 HPPD when they say the standard for a med/surg unit is 4. They ignore the savings per discharge and give her a poor performance rating for being over budget on a patient day basis. Ward feels she is being given an incentive to revert to the old approach, which costs the hospital more per patient discharged but gives her a better performance rating. She wishes Costello would address this issue with finance so incentives would align what is in the best interests of the hospital with how her work as a manager is evaluated. (For the Patient Days and ADC Census reports, see Figures II.3, II.4, and II.5).

Ryan Connor is the director of nurse credentialing and operations for UHS, supervising 87 patient care directors at the four hospitals. Although he has no direct responsibility for management of units, he has responsibility for budget and financial performance related to hospital initiatives, such as lowering overtime and the use of agency nurses over four campuses. Connor reviews the upcoming budget requests, and makes sure that nursing care hours are captured correctly.

Connor agrees with Ward about the challenges of untimely reports and lack of familiarity with how the budget is developed. Connor states that PCDs need to manage financially the following: FTEs relative to budget, overtime, traveler/agency usage and regular staffing, vacancies, and average daily census. He says PCDs should be asking themselves: "Are you where you should be with respect to staffing and patient load? Do you have the most efficient mix of resources? And what do you do if you're not where you should be?"

Connor frames the problem as follows: PCDs aren't fluent with the budget process and financial management. They must evaluate performance,

FIGURE II.3
Patient Days Spreadsheet

UNIVERSITY HEALTH SYSTEM HOSPITAL
PATIENT DAYS AND ADC - 2006
SOURCE: CENSUS REPORT

NOTE: THIS REPORT REFLECTS THE MIDNIGHT ADC FOR CENSUS DRIVEN INPATIENT UNITS ONLY.
ADC FOR OTHER UNITS WHERE BUDGETED STAFFING IS NOT CENSUS DRIVEN IS NOT INCLUDED.

Acct Unit	Nursing Unit	Staffed Beds	Description	YTD PATIENT DAYS	YTD ACTUAL ADC	Jan-06 PATIENT DAYS	Jan-06 ACTUAL ADC	Feb-06 PATIENT DAYS	Feb-06 ACTUAL ADC	Mar-06 PATIENT DAYS	Mar-06 ACTUAL ADC	Apr-06 PATIENT DAYS	Apr-06 ACTUAL ADC	May-06 PATIENT DAYS	May-06 ACTUAL ADC
105156	S5HS (Temp to S4HS)		MED ICU												
105157	S5HS		CARDIAC ICU												
105158	S6GN		MEDICINE												
105159	S6GS		MEDICINE												
105160	S5GN		CARDIAC (@ 100%)												
105161	S5GS		CARDIAC												
105162	S6HS		SURG ONCOLOGY												
105163	S7GS		MEDICINE												
105164	S7HN		CHEST / STEPDOWN												
105165	S7HS		SURG / RENAL												
105166	S8GN		REHAB												
105167	S7GN		ORTHOPEDICS												
105168	S8HN		NEUROSURGERY												
105169	S8HN - EU *		EXPRESS UNIT - EU												
105170	S8HS		NEUROLOGY												
105171	S9GN (E6X)		PSYCH												
105172	S9GS		AIDS UNIT												
105173	S9HS/N		MCKEEN SURGERY												
TOTAL SOUTH DIVISION															
GRAND TOTAL															

*S8HN-EU is a mid year new unit. Days for Jan through April are not included in the ADC calculation for YTD ADC.

FIGURE II.4
Year-to-Date Average Daily Census

UNIVERSITY HEALTH SYSTEM HOSPITAL
UHS CAMPUS
YTD AVERAGE DAILY CENSUS - 2006
SOURCE: CENSUS REPORT AND BUDGET

NOTE: THIS REPORT REFLECTS THE MIDNIGHT ADC FOR CENSUS DRIVEN INPATIENT UNITS ONLY.
ADC FOR OTHER UNITS WHERE BUDGETED STAFFING IS NOT CENSUS DRIVEN IS NOT INCLUDED.

Acct Unit	Nursing Unit	Staffed Beds	Description	#### Actual ADC	Jan-06 Budget ADC	Feb-06 Actual ADC	Feb-06 Budget ADC	#### Actual ADC	Mar-06 Budget ADC	#### Actual ADC	Apr-06 Budget ADC	#### Actual ADC	May-06 Budget ADC	YTD Patient Days	YTD Actual ADC	YTD Budget ADC	YTD ADC VAR	Budget Nursing Care Hours	Expected FTE Var at Actual Census	Med/Surg Nursing ADC Variance	Med/Surg Expected FTE Var at Actual Census	Crit Care Nursing ADC Variance	Crit Care Expected FTE Var at Actual Census	VCH Nursing ADC Variance	VCH Expected FTE Var at Actual Census
105151	S5HS (was S4HN)		CARDIOTHOR ICU																						
105152	S4HS		SURG ICU																						
105153	S8GS (was S4HS)		NEURO ICU																						
105154	S6HN		ONCOLOGY																						
105155	S5HN		SURG STEPDOWN																						
105156	S5HS (Temp to S4HS)		MED ICU																						
105157	S5HS		CARDIAC ICU																						
105158	S6GN		MEDICINE																						
105159	S6GS		MEDICINE																						
105160	S5GN		CARDIAC (@ 100%)																						
105161	S5GS		CARDIAC																						
105162	S6HS		SURG ONCOLOGY																						
105163	S7GS		MEDICINE (was Surg)																						
105164	S7HN		CHEST / STEPDOWN																						
105165	S7HS		SURG / RENAL																						
105166	S8GN		REHAB																						
105167	S7GN		ORTHOPEDICS																						
105168	S8HN		NEUROSURGERY																						
105169	S8HN - EAU *		NEUROSURG-EAU																						
105170	S8HS		NEUROLOGY																						
105171	S9GN (E6X)		PSYCH																						
105172	S9GS		AIDS UNIT																						
105173	S9HS/S		MCKEEN SURGERY																						
TOTAL SOUTH DIVISION																									
GRAND TOTAL																									

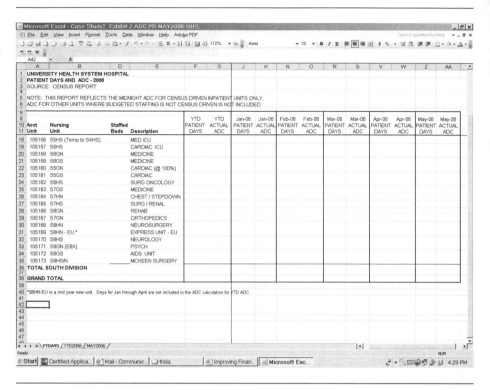

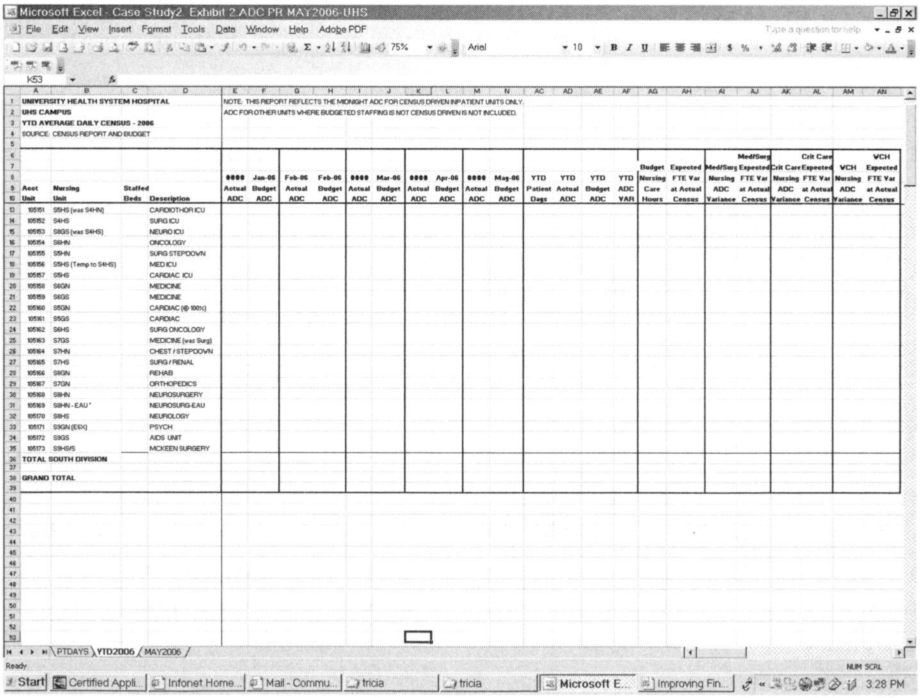

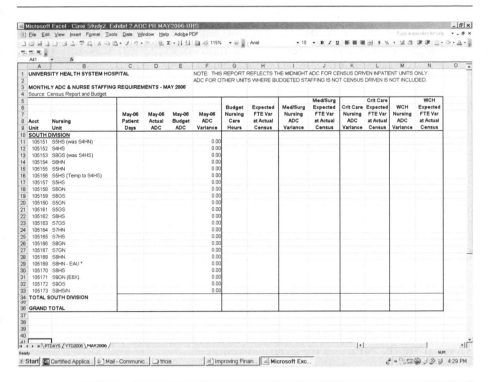

FIGURE II.5

Monthly
ADC and
Nurse Staffing
Requirements

staff to their census, access the appropriate data available to them, and communicate with staff about how the unit is performing in financial metrics. Connor feels PCDs struggle to manage this way because of competing priorities, including spending a lot of their time responding to regulatory agencies. What PCDs could do better, Connor suggests, is "explore alternative skill mixes, improve advanced planning for fluctuations in staffing, and enforce attendance policies effectively with all staff."

On October 1, 2006, Ward, Costello, and Connor had lunch in the South Division cafeteria to discuss the financial responsibilities of the patient care directors. A summary of their discussion follows:

Connor: I think the main opportunities to improve financial performance at the level of the patient care units lie in increasing patient volume (the number of admissions) and in continuing to decrease the length of stay. If this is so, I wonder where exactly the patient care directors figure into all of this.

Ward: Well, I know in my case I've been doing just that. I have a great rapport with the orthopedic surgeons who know they will always be able to admit a patient to my unit when they want that patient admitted. We've been lowering patient stays in the unit for two years now, and we expect to continue to manage innovatively to hold and increase the gains. But, Ryan, I do think PCDs figure into all of this significantly, and it is critical for us to manage finances and anticipate demand. My issue is that we don't have the necessary data to effectively manage.

Costello: It's really important to properly orient PCDs to the financial process. And I agree with you, Dinah, I'd like to see more PCD involvement in the budget process, and some factor built into that process to deal with acuity—something that's rough and ready, even if it's not that complicated. Of course, the whole thing should be automated soon.

Case Questions

1. What are the most important things that the patient care directors can do to improve unit financial performance?
2. What are the priorities for Dinah Ward?
3. What are the priorities for Rose Costello?
4. What are the priorities for Ryan Connor?
5. What would you advise Phil Leewerth, COO of South Division, to do to help Dinah, Rose, and Ryan respond to these challenges?

Case F
Evidence-Based Quality Management in a Home Health Organization

Cynthia Struk and Duncan Neuhauser

Introduction

The Visiting Nurse Association Health Care Partners of Ohio (VNAHPO) is a not-for-profit, community-based agency that provides home health services, hospice care, private duty nursing, and home-based physician care. The organization, founded in 1902, consists of six corporations (Figure II.6). It is a leading community healthcare organization in Ohio, recognized for innovation, quality improvement, and community service. It is also one of the largest, annually providing more than 500,000 units of service to

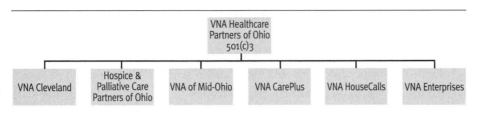

FIGURE II.6
Organization Chart of VNA of Ohio

Used with permission of the Visiting Nurse Association Health Care Partners of Ohio

more than 12,000 families in the region. Home health is the organization's largest service, in terms of volume of services and revenues (approximately $30 million per year).

Home care is part of the continuum of healthcare services and has become a diverse and dynamic service industry. More than 20,000 providers deliver home care services to some 7.6 million individuals with acute illnesses, long-term healthcare needs, permanent disabilities, or terminal illnesses. National expenditures for home health care totaled $47.5 billion in 2005. Medicare remains the single largest payer for home care services.

Home health and hospice care are regulated by both state and federal agencies, such as the Centers for Medicare and Medicaid Services (CMS), state health departments, and agencies that oversee services for special populations, such as people receiving mental health services. In addition, many agencies participate in voluntary accreditation by organizations that use professional peer review to assess quality and safety standards, such as the Joint Commission, the Accreditation Commission for Health Care, Inc., and the Commission on Accreditation of Rehabilitation Facilities. Agencies also must meet various safety regulations, information access and privacy rules, legal requirements, and ethical practice standards.

All of these provider and professional oversight groups have different data collection and reporting requirements. The healthcare sector's concerns about quality and costs have prompted additional data collection, and the availability of electronic information systems has made data collection and storage easier. VNAHPO, like virtually every other home health organization, finds itself potentially awash in data, but, as is so often pointed out, there's a big difference between data and actionable information. Thus, earlier in this decade, the organization was challenged "to sort out the wheat from the chaff," and create a data collection and monitoring approach that would truly contribute to quality improvement and the bottom line.

Home Health Services and Quality

VNAHPO has a quality improvement program that is directed by the vice president of performance improvement and research. This program provides an ongoing, systematic, planned mechanism for objectively monitoring customer satisfaction, the quality and appropriateness of patient care, utilization of services, efficiency of agency operations and business practices, and risk management. It enables problem identification and resolution and has two major goals: (1) to monitor the processes and outcomes of services and (2) to comply with quality improvement program requirements established by regulatory and accrediting bodies.

A professional advisory committee includes both internal employees and external members who also serve on subsidiary boards for home health, private duty, hospice, and physician services. Committee members' duties include approving and monitoring the annual quality improvement (QI) plan, and serving as expert resources. The executive and management staff ensure the development, implementation, monitoring, and evaluation of QI activities, and help staff at all levels carry out their roles in quality improvement.

Over the past several years, quality monitoring in home health care organizations has become much more complex. An increasing volume of data is generated and required by regulatory agencies. Quality measurement has become a key driver in home care as public and private insurers and regulatory bodies have begun to use it to assess the effectiveness of healthcare delivery among providers, to control expenses, and, ultimately, to improve healthcare outcomes. Consumers have become more aware of quality initiatives, too, through the educational efforts of their healthcare providers, insurers, and consumer advocacy groups, and by educating themselves as they seek information related to care and treatment.

Two national quality initiatives have had a tremendous effect on home health and, more recently, hospice services. CMS is currently piloting several quality initiatives that link performance and reimbursement. These initiatives are directly linked to the Medicare Modernization Act of 2003, which created a set of measures to evaluate the clinical care provided by home care agencies. The Home Health Quality Initiative is based on data from the Outcome and Assessment Information Set (OASIS), a survey completed by patients at admission, every 60 days, and at discharge. OASIS measures data are aggregated by provider, monitored over time, and publicly available on http://www.medicare.gov/HHCompare/Home. They permit comparison and benchmarking among home care providers nationally and locally on measures such as improvement in pain or medication management (Figure II.7).

FIGURE II.7

OASIS
Outcome
Data from
Home Health
Compare

Percentage of patients who get better at taking their medicines correctly (by mouth)

This information comes from the Home Health Outcome and Assessment Information Set (OASIS) during the time period October 2005–September 2006.

Why is this information important?
For medicines to work properly, they need to be taken correctly. Taking too much or too little medicine can keep it from helping you feel better and, in some cases, can make you sicker, make you confused (which could affect your safety), or even cause death. Home health staff can help teach you ways to organize your medicines and take them properly. Getting better at taking your medicines correctly means the home health agency is doing a good job teaching you how to take your medicines.

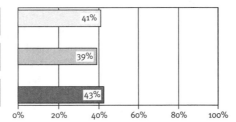

Percentage of patients who get better at taking their medicine correctly (by mouth)

This is the average for all the home health agencies in the United States — 41%

This is the average for all home health agencies in the State of Ohio — 39%

VISITING NURSE ASSOCIATION OF CLEVELAND — 43%

Used with permission of the Visiting Nurse Association Health Care Partners of Ohio

In another recent initiative, CMS redefined the Conditions of Participation for hospice providers by instituting a more comprehensive quality assessment and performance improvement program. This program enables hospices to take tailored, proactive steps to ensure quality and focuses on the results of care. A core list of measures is published by the National Hospice and Palliative Care Organization, and each hospice can select the measures that are most critical to its own performance. Table II.2 lists the core categories with examples of the measures. The new program is intended to ensure high-quality care for this particularly vulnerable patient population.

Evidence-Based Management for Quality Improvement

In the past, VNAHPO had available some anecdotal information related to the quality of care but little quantitative data. In the absence of any contrary information, the agency believed the care provided was excellent and that the staff was outstanding. Meanwhile, national quality initiatives were maturing, and the agency faced increasing requirements to evaluate many aspects of its performance. It became difficult to prioritize and manage all of the clinical, financial, risk, and other types of data that the agency needed to evaluate the effectiveness of the healthcare it was providing.

TABLE II.2

Quality
Assessment and
Performance
Improvement
(QAPI) for
Hospice

Core Categories	Examples of Measures
Family- and patient-centered care	• Avoid unwanted hospitalizations • Emotional support prior to death
Ethical behavior and patient rights	• Percent of patients responding to survey as not having been treated with respect
Clinical excellence and safety	• Comfort within 24 hours of admission • Evening and weekend staff responsiveness
Inclusion and access Workforce excellence	• Percent admissions by ethnicity/race • Overall patient satisfaction • Willingness to recommend
Standards Compliance with laws and regulations	• Deficiencies from last survey • Medical director approval • Percent of medical record review requests
Stewardship and accountability	• Average length of stay • Contributions per patient served
Performance measurement	• Comparison to national benchmarks by submitting data to National Hospice and Palliative Care Organization

Thinking About the Problem

Early in 2006, the Professional Advisory Committee, with the support of the VNAHPO board, recommended creation of a better model for quality monitoring that would enable consistent presentation, communication, and monitoring of quality measures across the organization. The challenge was considerable, since the many stakeholders presented different views and had varying levels of understanding about which data should be tracked for corporate purposes and which were necessary for regulatory or corporate compliance.

Step 1. Formulating the Question

The vice president of performance improvement and research, Cynthia Struk, was put in charge of the project and decided to use the techniques of evidence-based management to address the board's question, which she interpreted as: *How can we better marshal and utilize data to meet a diverse—and growing—set of management needs?*

Step 2. Using the Internet to Acquire Evidence-Based Performance Indicators

As Struk began to address the board's question, she first examined the vast and accessible Web-based information available on quality improvement. She utilized various Internet quality improvement sites to help ensure that her approach would be consistent with national quality efforts and aligned with evidence-based management. The following sites were particularly helpful in defining indicators, framing the approach, and ensuring that the measures she ultimately selected would be consistent with industry approaches to quality management:

Joint Commission. This website, www.jointcommission.org/Performance Measurement/, features information related to quality improvement, but most helpful for this project were the descriptions of core performance measure attributes and the criteria used to select them. For example, the site managers recommended that measures:

- Target improvement in the health of populations, based on protecting and improving health or addressing important areas of healthcare;
- Be specific and precisely defined, with respect to standardized data sources, sampling procedures, algorithms for calculation, and risk adjustment, if applicable;
- Be reliable and capable of being consistently measured over time, and reproducible when applied across settings;
- Be valid—that is, based on evidence that they actually measure what they purport to measure;
- Be interpreted, understood, and presented in a useful way to stakeholders;
- Help in the organization's accreditation process or in decision making about quality improvement efforts; and
- Be available in the public domain.

Institute for Healthcare Improvement (IHI). IHI, www.ihi.org, focuses on the need to define the aims of quality improvement initiatives and supports the use of Plan-Do-Study-Act (PDSA) cycles as the means to achieve them. Its concept of Whole System Measures encourages creation of a set of strategic performance measures that can give leaders information about important processes and outcomes over time, provide comparative metrics for benchmarking across organizations, and inform strategic quality improvement planning. The Whole System Measures are aligned with the Institute of Medicine's six dimensions of quality: safety, effectiveness, patient-centeredness, timeliness, efficiency, and equitability. Struk found these approaches supported models already in use within her organization. She had been using PDSA cycles for several years in performance improvement efforts, and the Whole System Measures approach appeared compatible with VNAHPO's multi-corporate structure.

Medicare Quality Improvement Community (MedQIC.) This organization, www.medqic.org, assists quality improvement organizations and providers in finding, using, and sharing quality improvement resources. Its website helped Struk find tools that could be used to share results, identify critical points for control, suggest areas for improvement, and help explain and solve problems. The site's creators supported the use of flow charts, check sheets, Pareto diagrams, cause-and-effect diagrams, and many other charts, again consistent with many of the data analysis approaches already being used within VNAHPO.

Armed with knowledge about some of the measures and tools that could be used for the new quality monitoring model and confident that she was on the right track, Struk moved to the next step.

Step 3. Assessing the Applicability of the Evidence

Struk scheduled meetings with Professional Advisory Committee members and agency leaders. Given the tremendous amount of information she *could* obtain, it was critical that both groups assist in narrowing the scope of the project. She asked them to help define the quality characteristics and performance measures that would best align with the mission, vision, and values of the organization, the demands of external regulators, the needs of the agency's clients, and the agency's imperative to remain financially sound.

She used VNAHPO's major strategic initiatives to frame the discussion at each meeting, and she asked participants questions that would enable her to distill the indicators into key areas:

1. What indicators are most important to you in measuring or reporting on progress in your major strategic initiatives?
2. Do these indicators, for the most part, meet standards of reliability, validity, relevance to stakeholders, utility, ease of collection, availability over time, and so forth?

3. How do you see the indicator being shared or displayed, and how often does it need to be reported?
4. Can the indicator be benchmarked against local or national data?
5. Will the indicator provide information relevant to the mission, vision, and values of the organization?
6. Is this an indicator that could be used across VNAHPO's six corporations?

As Struk's meetings progressed, she recognized that it would be imperative that not only should the indicators be defined similarly across the six corporations, but also that she consider how data could best be presented given the many different venues within the organization to share quality data and the multiple audiences, from staff to the board to external groups, with whom those data would be shared.

Step 4. Defining the Quality Measures

What soon became apparent to Struk was that the set of indicators would need to differ for each of VNAHPO's corporations, but that each set would contain components tied to their strategic objectives and could be categorized similarly. The indicators that were emerging appeared to meet at least 75 percent of the criteria for a "good measure," and they could be categorized into four main groups:

1. *Customer Satisfaction,* which is defined corporately as the experience of the "customer" during the process of service. Several types of customers are involved in this experience, including patients, referral sources, and internal customers—employees.
2. *Clinical Performance*, which focuses on the processes or outcomes of service delivery. This area includes measures related to **corporate compliance** (regulatory requirements and care outcomes) and aligned with several of the external quality initiatives for both home health and hospice, and measures of **service utilization** (concentrating on the processes of care, such as length of stay, trends and patterns of use, gaps in service, referrals, and so forth). Some service utilization measures can be applied organization-wide, such as those related to preventing falls, while some are unique to specific programs, such as those affecting only hospice.
3. *Operational Performance* relates to measures of fiscal viability and operations in three areas: business practices (such as budgetary indicators and financial performance indicators), personnel management (such as recruitment and job performance), and information technology (such as reliability of the IT system, measures to reduce risk, responsiveness to users, and return on investment).

4. ***Risk Management*** focuses on prioritizing events that have the greatest potential impact on the organization, either because they are highly likely or potentially very costly. Measures include patient concerns and incidents (e.g., falls, medication errors, quality-of-care concerns), risk prevention (e.g., fire drill evacuation time, employee safety), business vulnerability (e.g., lapses in data security), and patients' rights (e.g., informed consent).

The measures developed for each corporation were tested, compared with organizational strategic objectives, categorized in one of the four preceding categories, and matched with regulatory or other external standards to provide a validity check for the entire process. Table II.3 illustrates the application of this process to one of the corporations, VNA of Cleveland.

Step 5. Aligning the Quality Measures with Quality Improvement

With the tested measures in hand, Struk took several more steps to make sure that each corporation would be able to use its set of measures and indicators effectively. She did this by:

- creating reference documents supporting each measure set;
- defining data sources for each measure;
- selecting the best methods for monitoring the indicators; and
- determining the most effective way to display the data.

Identifying primary data sources helped ensure that the measures were evidence-based and would generate consistent, reliable, valid data that could be easily assessed and comparable over time (Table II.4). The agency also has access to many external data sets, including the OASIS data set, which is aggregated by the state of Ohio and includes comparisons to state and national benchmarks. Similarly, Medicare and Medicaid often provide comparison data useful for benchmarking.

With the performance measures selected and the data sources defined, Struk found it relatively easy to determine the quality improvement thresholds and recommended thresholds for measurement based on internal or external (regulatory) requirements (Table II.5).

Step 6. Final Results

At the end of this process, Struk developed a summary description of each set of QI indicators that listed each individual indicator and described its purpose, its data source, the established threshold/benchmark if applicable, and the frequency of monitoring required. This summary document was made available to the Professional Advisory Committee, organization management,

TABLE II.3
Examples
of Strategic
Measures
and Quality
Measures for
Home Health

Strategic Measure	Quality Category	Quality Measure/Goal	Alignment with Regulatory Compliance
Program growth in key strategic areas, including mental health, heart failure, and rehabilitation services	Clinical Performance	Re-hospitalization of heart failure patients at or below national benchmark	OASIS indicator for re-hospitalization
	Human Resources	Retention of physical and occupational therapists above the national rate for home health agencies	No
	Clinical Performance	Improvement in medication management	OASIS indicator for improvement in medication management
Customer satisfaction at national benchmark	Customer satisfaction	Overall written customer satisfaction at national benchmark	No, but it is being evaluated in the CMS pay-for-performance model
Improve cash flow	Operational Performance Business Practice	Decrease the mean number of days for submission of a Requested Anticipated Payment (RAP) for a home health episode	No
Evaluate the satisfaction of internal customers for IT support	Operational Performance Information Technology	Internal customer service satisfaction trends	No

and the entity that made the request for this research—the corporation's board. Table II.6 presents an excerpt of the summary report created for VNA of Cleveland (VNAC).

As this summary document was being developed, Struk further considered the most effective and feasible way to share the data. While each corporation limited the measures it used to the most important subset, it still became onerous to display and share all these data each quarter. To help with this issue, Struk identified key indicators for each entity in the corporation that could be pulled into a quick snapshot to show status on a quarterly basis. This very high-level summary then ties the data to strategic initiatives in order to inform decision making about and monitoring of the organization's most important work (Figure II.8).

TABLE II.4
Data Sources

Data Source	Public (Yes/No)	Comparable to Other Home Health Data	Required (economic consequence)	Web-site	Reporting Delay
OASIS	Yes	Yes	Yes	Yes	Agency data immediate; state and national data about 4-month delay
Hospice QAPI	No	Yes with Hospice	No, but required by CMS for licensure as a hospice provider	No	Yes, about a 4-month delay to have data aggregated against other providers
Patient satisfaction	No	Yes	Being considered under CMS pay-for-performance models	No	Monthly
Fiscal measures • Cost report • Internal for budget and cash flow	Some required for cost report submission	Yes	Yes	No	Agency data immediate; cost report data are from 2003/2004
Risk management	No	Some, depending on the data	Some indicators required for reporting to accrediting bodies (e.g., sentinel events)	No	Agency data immediate; comparative data 3-month delay
Licensing/ accreditation measures	No	No	Yes, required by government, state, or specialty organizations	No	Quarterly
Clinical data • Processes of care	No	Yes, depending on the data	No	No	Real-time

Compliance Level	Threshold	Criteria
High	95% or greater or against external benchmark, if available	• Required by licensing, accrediting bodies, and/or Conditions of Participation • Critical to staff safety • Critical to patient outcome or safety • Client/patient satisfaction with services • Process indicators controlled by regulations (e.g., OASIS submission time frames)
Medium	90% or greater or against external benchmark, if available	• Not controlled by regulation, but critical to clinical or business practice (e.g., billing cycle times, paperwork submission) • Coordination/communication indicators
Low	85% or greater or against external benchmark, if available	• Indicators not controlled by regulation and less critical to clinical or business practice (e.g., supervisor performance evaluation submission)

TABLE II.5
Performance Thresholds

CQI Activity	Purpose	Source	Threshold	Frequency
Satisfaction Outcomes				
Written Satisfaction	To monitor and evaluate client satisfaction corporately for VNAC based on key drivers of care	OCS compiles the data based on discharges sampled within the quarterly time frame	Changes quarterly based on national benchmarks compiled by OCS for home health agencies (Goal: at or above national threshold)	Quarterly

TABLE II.6
Excerpt of Continuous Quality Improvement Activities for Home Health

(continued)

TABLE II.6
(*continued*)

CQI Activity	Purpose	Source	Threshold	Frequency
Satisfaction Outcomes				
Telephone Satisfaction Survey	To monitor and evaluate client satisfaction focusing on critical elements of service delivery	Internal random audit of patients who have been receiving care for 6 weeks	90% overall satisfaction	Reported quarterly
"Concern for Quality"	Mechanism for reporting concerns by patients, physicians, and staff. May be related to care delivery issues, agency operations, or business practices	Completed Concern for Quality Form	Qualitative analysis for trends	Analyzed corporately at least annually
Clinical Performance				
OBQI Re-hospitalization	To analyze and trend the results of state CMS re-hospitalization data, comparing them to state and national benchmarks	OASIS data submitted to the state for CMS patients exclude OB and hospice patients. Data are retrievable from state database with statistically significant re-hospitalization outcomes	Comparison to local and national benchmarks for state reports, based on aggregate sample for time frame	Quarterly

VNAHPO, like all healthcare organizations, is entering an era of quality data overload due to the steady spread of accessible electronic information and increasing emphasis on performance by external payers and regulatory bodies concerned about both quality of care and reimbursement. As a result, organizations must maintain a clear focus on what information is truly important for the people they serve (consumer mindfulness); develop a greater

FIGURE II.8

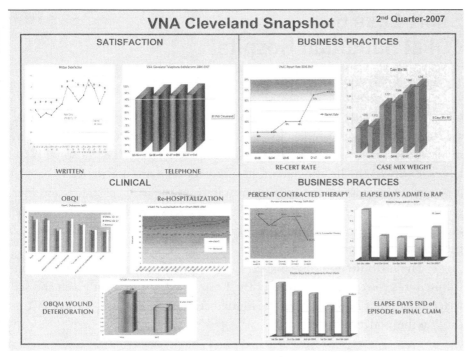

Used with permission of the Visiting Nurse Association Health Care Partners of Ohio

understanding of data accuracy and interpretation (statistical mindfulness and clinical meaningfulness); and exercise greater selectivity in picking measures that can effectively signal where more attention must be paid or improvements made (organizational transformation). Healthcare organizations today need the *right* information, in order to validate that their healthcare activities and practices produce optimum value and are safe and appropriate and, when they are not, to enable prompt and effective correction.

Case Questions

1. Construct a summary report for the quality management advisory board of VNAHPO. Sometimes such reports are called dashboards.
2. What is the value added by the evidence-based process that Struk pursued?
3. Select one of the indicators and develop a target for performance; specify the process you went through to select this target.
4. What can VNAHPO do differently or better as a result of using the dashboard?
5. Specify a process for changing the items used in the dashboard.

Short Case 6
CQI at Suburban Hospital

Larry K. McReynolds

Clara Maass Health System is composed of a 475-bed community hospital, a 120-bed long-term care facility, a 10-bed subacute care unit, and a visiting nurse agency. It is located in north Newark, New Jersey. The hospital is the largest entity of the health system, having been in existence for 125 years. It is a community-based non-teaching hospital and the medical staff is an older, conservative group, wary of change. The employees typically pride themselves on being part of their local hospital, but have recently become disturbed by the changes occurring.

The introduction of managed care into the local marketplace has contributed to growing unease among the hospital administration given the service changes that must occur in the immediate future. Some of the key factors causing this concern include:

1. The county in which Clara Maass is located has 14 other hospitals, making the county over-bedded by 200 percent.
2. The competitive environment is enabling managed care companies to force hospitals to accept reimbursement rates below their costs.
3. The hospital's average length of stay and average cost per discharge are significantly higher than those of other hospitals in the area.
4. Many of the physicians at Clara Maass are close to retirement and see little reason to change their ways of practicing medicine at this stage of the game.
5. Employee morale is low as a result of cost-cutting, two recent layoffs, and no raises for two consecutive years.

In an attempt to help bring about some of the needed changes in the organization, administration decided to implement a CQI program. The hospital CQI program had been approved by the board of trustees and had now been in place for almost two years.

The CQI program was implemented through required CQI training for managers, all employees, and as many physicians as possible. Initially, quality action teams (QATs) were chartered to examine operational and clinical issues. Operational QATs were chartered by the steering committee to address processes and procedures that were high-volume, problem-prone, costly, or likely to have an adverse effect on the patient. Elements predictive of patient satisfaction were also used to determine if a QAT should be chartered.

The patient services department selected the CareMap format for addressing physician and complex patient care issues. CareMaps are multidisciplinary tools that help establish care protocols and delineate expectations about factors such as clinical outcomes and length of stay based on the patient's case type. CareMaps were developed using the primary nurse model, placing the nurse as the responsible party for keeping the patient on the specific CareMap.

To facilitate integration of CQI principles among all employees, managers attend an ongoing workshop. This monthly meeting is designed to provide a non-threatening forum for managers to examine their department processes and outcomes, and to determine the degree of the department's success in meeting customer needs. Ideas from the workshops and suggestions from the QATs and CareMaps process are approved by the steering committee and implemented by the team.

Case Questions

1. Employees have the feeling that eliminating "wasted work" and improving processes is a fancy way of eliminating more jobs. Identify strategies to overcome this impression.
2. Managers feel this is the management philosophy of the week. Identify and describe effective means to overcome this barrier.
3. Physicians see CareMaps as cookbook medicine imposed upon them by the nursing department. Describe ways to get them to buy into CareMaps.
4. Identify organizational strategies that the hospital should adopt to make the institution more viable in the marketplace.

Short Case 7
ED at Queens Hospital Center

Anthony R. Kovner

Currently 83 percent of patients at the Queens Hospital Center Emergency Department (ED) are treated and released. They wait six to eight hours for treatment. The goals are to decrease waiting time and the number of number of people who leave without being treated and to improve care and patient satisfaction.

Current Procedure

Step 1. Patient seen by triage nurse.
Step 2. Patient sent to registration.
Step 3. Patient waits to be seen by physician.
Step 4. Patient sent for any necessary lab or x-ray.
Step 5. Patient waits for test results to be reviewed by MD.
Step 6. Patient treated, discharged, or admitted.

Case Question

1. What do you suggest to improve the process? What do you suggest to reduce errors by the triage nurse?

Short Case 8
Sparks Medical Center and the Board of Trustees

Anthony R. Kovner

Sam Phillips, chairman of Sparks Medical Center's board of trustees, wondered why hospital board meetings were so different from those at his spice company, Phillips' Flavors, Inc. The hospital board discussed the reports of various committees, reviewed accreditation and licensing reports, and listened to reports and recommendations about state regulations and reimbursement. At Phillips' Flavors, Inc., the board discussed the future of business, what the competition was doing, and strategies to increase market share and profit margins.

Clara Burns, CEO of Sparks Medical Center, made the following recommendations to Phillips regarding more effective board meetings:

1. Board discussion should focus on the organization's mission.
2. Objectives and strategies should be established.
3. A startegy to plan and measure board performance should be developed.

Sam realized that it would be difficult to address these issues given the board structure and organization, which led to excessive amounts of meeting time spent on routine committee and management reports. The current process resulted in a full agenda and little time to deal with issues critical to the future of the medical center.

Case Questions

1. What do you recommend that Sam do now?
2. Identify constraints and opportunities that Sam will face when implementing your recommendations.

Short Case 9
Pay for Performance: Hypertension

Brook Watts and Duncan Neuhauser

Chris Hebert, MD, is in charge of coordinating ambulatory hypertension care at the Cleveland Clinic. Hebert is highly respected by his colleagues there, and the Cleveland Clinic is proud of its excellent reputation for cardiovascular care. Hebert is a general internist who has specialized in treating patients who have difficulty controlling their blood pressure. His colleagues refer such patients to him. One innovation he has introduced is to give patients graph paper so that they can record sequentially their own blood pressure measures every day at home. Patients bring in their graphs to discuss the reasons why there may have been variation and what they can do to improve.

In his clinical leadership role, Hebert has been asked by a large national insurer to give advice about pay for performance (P4P) for excellent hypertension care. Three different P4P measures are being proposed. The insurer wants to know which one is the best measure of quality. It wants to know if these measures can be "gamed." The three proposed measures are:

1. Pay a bonus if the patient's end state (end of year or most recent measure) blood pressure is low (<140/90).
2. Pay a bonus if the patient's blood pressure has improved after a year of care. There also must be recorded changes in prescribed medicines (titration) to show active physician involvement in care management.
3. Process measures only are used to measure performance. There must be documentation in the electronic medical record of screening diagnosis, follow-up care, and patient education about lifestyle changes.

Like all general internists, Hebert knows that a patient's blood pressure can vary due to the disease, but it can vary for other reasons. This list of reasons includes measurement error, stress, relaxation, eating salty food, "white coat hypertension" (a worried patient's blood pressure goes up just by entering the doctor's office), which medicines are prescribed in what doses, whether the patient actually takes the medicine, and even time of day (e.g., blood pressure can be low after a good night of sleep).

Considering these P4P measures, Hebert decided to pull up the record of one of his current patients, Mr. Norton. When Mr. Norton had first come to see Hebert, his blood pressure was high, 170/90. Mr. Norton had six office visits and there were nine medication changes. Discussions about stopping smoking were not recorded in the record, but Hebert knew they had occurred. Mr. Norton's most recent blood pressure was 150/80. According to the proposed measures, Hebert found that he would not qualify for a bonus based on measures 1 and 3, but he would for measure 2.

Hebert next pulled out Mr. Smith's chart. Mr. Smith's blood pressure remained consistently high over time, despite Hebert's close work with Mr. Smith, including multiple calls to the patient's home. In the case of Mr. Smith, Hebert would get a bonus according to measure 3, but not according to measures 1 or 2. With this closer review of cases, Hebert began to realize that because he was seen as an excellent physician, he tended to get referrals of really difficult cases. Under the proposed P4P system, Hebert's colleagues—who kept the patients they could manage well—would get their bonuses, but Hebert might not. Hebert then considered how performance using these proposed measures could be gamed.

Case Questions

1. What kind of P4P measure, if any, should Hebert recommend for hypertension care? Why?
2. Do you think it would make a difference in blood pressure control if the patient were paying out of pocket?
3. Do you think Hebert's opinion would be different if this were his whole medical group's incentive plan rather than a fee-for-service payment by an insurer?

Short Case 10
Financial Reporting to the Board

Anthony R. Kovner

Act I

At the December board meeting for Christian Health System, board member Sam Brown received the following 2008 Operating Budget Highlights from Larry Dolan, chief financial officer:

HOSPITAL 2008 OPERATING BUDGET HIGHLIGHTS

- The surplus for 2008 is projected to be approximately $640,000.

VOLUME

- The budget is based on 28,000 inpatient discharges, or 76 discharges per day. This rate is 1.4 discharges a day higher than the hospital's projections for 2007 (74.4).
- The closing of Clark Hospital and the recruitment of new physicians are expected to produce the projected growth in discharges.
- Other hospital outpatient services (emergency, ambulatory surgery) are conservatively budgeted to continue at current volumes.

REVENUE

- Total revenue is budgeted to increase by 5.7%:
  - Net patient service revenue is projected to increase by 7.6%.
  - Other revenue is budgeted to decrease by 17.8%, mostly due to the loss of one-time items such as donations, and a projected decrease in investment income.
  - The reduction in investment income is a product of an anticipated decline in cash and investment balances due to amounts owed to Eastern State, pension payments, and capital purchases.
- New rates were included in the budget for Medicare, Medicaid and other payers:
  - New Medicare rates included an inpatient increase of 1.5%. In the 2008 rate there is a decrease in the city wage index.
  - Medicaid rates have been budgeted at the preliminary January 2008 issued rates, which includes an adjusted trend factor of 1.88%.

o New negotiated rates for managed care are included in the revenue model by payer. The following are some examples of these increased rates:

- Blue Cross +6%
- Aetna +4%
- Plan 1 +10%
- Plan 2 +6%
- United Medicaid +15% and Commercial +3%
- Plan 3 +5%

• Case-mix indexes for Medicare (1.43), Medicaid (1.38), and Plan 4 non-maternity (1.22) are budgeted at the actual levels through October 2007.

EXPENSES

• Total expenses are budgeted at 5.8% above projections of 2007 spending.
• This reflects the following:
  o The expansion of the available medical/surgical acute care beds by 16, with 8 beds as of January 1, 2008 and another 8 beds as of February 29, 2008, for a total increase of 16 beds.
  o The following contractual increases:
    - RN union: 3%, as of January 1, 2008.
    - Technical and professional union: 3% as of January 1, 2008, and 3% as of December 1, 2008.
    - Security guards union: 3% as of January 1, 2008.
    - A 3% salary increase for non-union staff as of April 1, 2008.
  o Supplies and other expenses were increased for inflation at a rate of 3%.
• Other noteworthy expense changes included in the budget:
  o Benefits: An 11.8% increase from projected 2007 to 2008 as a function of the increased cost of union benefits and increases to non-union healthcare benefits.
  o Physician contracted services: the 11.9% reflects both changes in salaries and increased coverage (e.g., labor and delivery, 24/7 coverage).
  o Bad debt: A decrease of 10.4% from projected 2007 to 2008 as a continuation of the "Stockamp Effect" and increases in charity care.

Act II

The day after the board meeting, Brown sent the following e-mail to Dolan:

To: Larry Dolan
From: Sam Brown

Re: Financial Reporting to the Board

1. The purpose of this memo is to improve the quality of financial reporting to the board so that the board can add more value to hospital performance.
2. This is not the first time I have expressed these concerns to you. I become especially frustrated around budget time. The board spends way too little time examining the budget.
3. I do not feel sufficiently informed about the choices that underlie financial performance despite 17 years of service on the board, including several years on the Executive Committee as chair of the Performance Committee and as vice chair of our Medicaid managed care plan.
4. I would like to see a plan and a commitment from you to do better.

Questions that Came to Mind from Reading Your Distributed Materials and from Listening to Your Presentation

- You made no report on last year's results in relation to what you had forecast when last year's budget was presented.
- There was no summary of nor explanation of variance in the financials presented.
- What are the assumptions on which next year's budget is based? For example, what are the specifics regarding the impact on admissions of Clark Hospital's closing?
- How can we increase revenues?
- What are we doing to decrease re-hospitalizations?
- What investments should we be considering to improve quality of care?
- How do our expenses compare with benchmark hospitals?
- Why can't we make greater improvements in our lengths of stay, and what would be the impact of such improvements on our operating financials?
- What is the relationship between our financials and our strategic plan?
- What is our community service budget? How do we spend these funds currently? How could we spend them better?
- You don't seem to be getting much help from the board with these matters. Is there a problem with leadership of the Finance Committee?
- What are our options with respect to controlling the increase in health benefits each year?
- Where is the discussion about how Christian will meet its capital needs in the future?

Act III

Two days after his e-mail, Brown received the following e-mail reply from Dolan:

> Thanks for your thoughtful questions. Most of these issues are discussed in great detail by the Finance Committee. I think if you read some of the minutes from those meetings you could get a better sense of the issues that are discussed.
>
> Regarding capital, as we have said at the past several board meetings, we are in the process of refinancing our housing complex. This effort will allow us to continue to operate the housing and allow us to continue providing existing subsidies to tenants, while at the same time draw significant funds from the refinancing. We are currently estimating approximately $30 million. In addition to this we continue to explore with the state options for moving funds from our Medicaid managed care plan to Christian Health System. And as I mentioned last night, we are obtaining $5 million in TELP financing and $2.1 million in state ERDA financing. Additionally, we were able to come to final endorsement with HUD much faster than any facility in the region on our $87 million borrowing. So all in all, while the capital picture is not great, primarily due to the funding needed for our pension plan, I think we are doing better than most hospitals in the city that serve high proportions of Medicaid and uninsured patients.
>
> I also think the finance staff works very closely with the program side of the house in trying to figure out new ways to fund productive, high-quality programs. Two examples of that were discussed last night: our relationship with University Hospital and our collaboration with the family health center on rehabilitation services. Our budget process is a "bottom-up" process, with detailed discussion at the cost center level, building up to cost groups, and then up to facility-wide discussion. In those discussions we review old programs for viability and quality, and consider new proposals that will enhance our strategic direction. It should also be noted that over the past four years we have met our budget targets, and enhanced quality of care throughout the facility, while working in a fiscally restrained environment that has experienced reductions in both Medicaid and Medicare reimbursements that encompass approximately 75 percent of our patients.
>
> I will continue to work with the Finance Committee and the board to make our financial presentations more meaningful.

Case Questions

1. What are the strengths and weaknesses of board member Brown's e-mail about health system financial reporting?
2. What are the strengths and weaknesses of Dolan's e-mail response to Brown's e-mail?
3. How would you have responded to Brown's e-mail?
4. Why didn't Dolan respond as you have recommended?

Short Case 11
A Purchasing Decision

Abhi Kasinadhuni and Ann Scheck McAlearney

Bill Richardson, the director of information systems (IS) for a large academic medical center, must make a final decision about whether or not to purchase personal digital assistants (also known as PDAs or handheld computers) for hospital-based physicians. During the past couple months he and his team have been meeting with representatives of various PDA software companies pitching their products to the medical center. It seems that it is now possible to put just about anything on a PDA. They have been shown everything from basic reference table software to very specialized decision support systems. However, they have learned that not all PDA hardware options are compatible with the various software applications. They have also realized that as technology is constantly improving, Richardson and his team will need to seriously consider the options provided by lower-end PDAs compared to the higher-end models. Richardson's true preference is to purchase higher-end models, viewing the larger investment as a form of insurance against some level of technical advance, but this option would swallow much of his current budget allocation.

As Richardson reflects upon the numerous discussions he has had with the members of his IS team, though, he recognizes that there are other considerations beyond budget. For one, the medical center has a system that can allow doctors to synchronize medical records from the server to the individual PDA device, thus providing portability and efficient handling of patient data. However, this functionality also poses a potential threat to patient privacy according to the HIPAA bylaws. If the PDA was lost or stolen, sensitive information could be accessed by unauthorized individuals. Further, he is aware that not everyone likes PDAs. Some co-workers have complained that

PDAs are difficult to use because of things like tiny buttons, the small screen, and limited battery life. Finally, Richardson has heard that expenses associated with demands to support PDAs often exceed the cost of the devices themselves. In a colleague's hospital he heard how the successful distribution of PDAs was well received initially, but device users later swamped the IS department with calls to help them fix problems they encountered.

Richardson suspects that putting PDAs in the hands of all physicians could be helpful, but he's just not sure how such an investment will play out. Given the relatively low price of PDAs, Richardson has the authority to make a decision about the investment on his own, and plans to make his recommendation to the executive team by the end of the week.

Case Questions

1. What are the advantages and disadvantages of purchasing high-end versus lower-end PDA devices for the medical center physicians?
2. What might be the implications of a decision about purchasing PDA devices for physicians at this medical center?
3. What are the limitations of the current decision-making process about a PDA investment?
4. What decision-making process would you propose for IS investment decisions at this medical center? Should others be involved? Who? How much?

ORGANIZATIONAL DESIGN

To understand how the Professional Bureaucracy functions in its operating core, it is helpful to think of it as a repertoire of standard programs—in effect, the set of skills the professionals stand ready to use—which are applied to predetermined situations, called contingencies, [which are] also standardized.

—*Henry Mintzberg*

COMMENTARY

Understanding Organizations

Organizations are people and things combined to achieve an agreed upon goal in a changing and resource-scarce environment. Organizations have socially defined boundaries. They have a structure, a process, and outcomes. Understanding these concepts and how they relate to each other is at the core of organization theory.

Each of these basic concepts can be subdivided. *People* include workers, professionals, managers, and trustees. *Things* include long-term assets and short-term supplies. *Combination* includes dividing people and equipment into departments and a hierarchy aligned to the process of work and goals. *Resource scarcity* implies that achieving the goals of improved health must be constrained by the people and things available. The *organization's environment* can be described legally (laws governing behavior), economically (competition or monopoly), socially (how people define their work), and historically (our hospital is located where it is because that's where the donor gave us the land 100 years ago). *Goal achievement* can be estimated by measuring outcomes (patient census, mortality rates, vaccinations given). For-profit, not-for-profit, and government ownership of healthcare organizations relate to legal definitions and different goals: For example, long-run shareholder value maximization may be the goal of a for-profit organization. Organizations create different internal cultures. A faith-based organization may have a different vision and values than a for-profit organization, even though both may achieve their ends through the provision of high-quality care.

"I am a nurse working in the intensive care unit of Memorial Hospital." This simple statement describes an organization, its boundaries and goals, the work being done there, the technology in use, and a point in time. Another way to describe an organization is to explain its scarcities. The statement "We do what we can do best and let others do what they do best" is one way of understanding the "make or buy" managerial decisions that define the organization's boundary. "Our hospital needs computers and a food service, but we buy the former and contract out the latter because others can make and do these things better than we can."

Organizations must transform individual goals (my paycheck, my job satisfaction, my desire to help) into a unified overall good or mission. Everyone who is a member of the organization is there because it fulfills his or her personal goals. Keeping the balance of all these personal incentives favorable over time and through changing circumstances in a way that achieves the organizational goals is central to the role of management.

Understanding Organization Design

Organization design describes the way elements of an organization are arranged to meet the organization's goals. These elements include and affect the people and things that are combined in an organization. Mintzberg (1979, 1983) has suggested five basic types of organizational design or structure: simple, machine bureaucracy, professional bureaucracy, divisionalized firm, and "adhocracy" (Mintzberg's term for a mutually adjusting structure). These basic types represent different ways to organize work, and some ways work better than others. However, strictly causal relationships between technology and organizational design, or between environment and design, have not yet been proven.

The basic parts of Mintzberg's organizations are the strategic apex or top managers, middle management, the technological structure (such as planners and industrial engineers), support staff (such as personnel and security), and the operating core (or workers). Each of the five types of organizational design has a different configuration of these five parts. For example, the simple organization (e.g., a doctor's office) has managers, support staff, and an operating core, but little or no technological structure or middle management.

Visually, organization design may be depicted in an organizational chart showing relationships among these basic parts of organizations. Thus a good organization chart will illustrate linkages between and among top managers, middle management, the technological structure, support staff, and the operating core. Case G and Short Case 15 provide examples of organization charts, but they can be considerably more complex.

The key means of organizational coordination vary according to the type of organization, and include approaches such as direct supervision, work standardization, standardization of professional skills, standardization of outputs, or mutual adjustment (Mintzberg 1983). In a simple organization, direct supervision is the key means of coordination. In a machine bureaucracy, such as a large outpatient department for the poor, work standardization is the key means of coordination. In a professional bureaucracy, such as a community hospital, standardization of professional skills is a key means of coordinating the work. In a divisionalized firm, such as a multi-hospital corporation, the key means of coordination is the standardization of outputs, such as profits or market share. Finally, in an adhocracy, work is coordinated as the clinicians adjust on the spot to working with one another.

Work is sometimes organized according to the available physical facilities and may be influenced by an organization's history and the initial design of its founders. For example, most doctors still are not employees of hospitals because most physicians have been traditionally independent professionals.

According to Mintzberg (1979, 1983), work in the operating core can be organized in one of three ways: by process or occupation (e.g., all nurses report to the director of nursing, all physicians to their department chiefs); by purpose or division, cutting across occupational specialties (e.g., all nurses and physicians report to the local clinical leadership, which may be surgery, women's health, or emergency services); or by both process and purpose, in a matrix organization. Under this matrix method of organization, all nurses report to the clinical leadership of the division for some activities and to the director of nursing for others. Matrix organization solves certain coordination problems by process and by purpose but adds another layer to management, thereby increasing coordination costs. Managers must decide when to use which form of organization and whether the benefits, if any, outweigh the costs.

Organization Design and Healthcare Delivery

Today, many hospitals are being seen as just part of larger systems of care. Some health systems are organized to provide a "continuum of care" including primary care, secondary care in community hospitals, tertiary care, home care, and long-term care all in a single market area. Such integrated delivery systems bring increased managerial challenges in planning organization and performance measurement. Twenty-five years ago, a large city may have had 40 independent hospitals. Now these hospitals have either closed or merged into a few large competing networks. These systems are diversifying through vertical integration. At the same time, industry is going in the opposite direction. Business conglomerates with many subsidiaries and product lines are dropping those that are not performing well and sticking to "core competencies." Will healthcare follow this lead? Will these large integrated systems be dissolved back into their component parts?

Declining hospital occupancy rates resulting from shorter lengths of stay and fewer admissions combined with the high fixed costs of hospitals have fueled the competitive frenzy of the last decades. This competition has led to many new organizational forms, and these changes are far from over. In addition, this competition has compelled closer attention to the wishes of the public and a growing emphasis on market understanding and patient satisfaction.

One new organizational form that has seen tremendous recent growth is the retail health clinic, such as the convenient care clinics described in the reading (Lin 2008). Different ownership and operating models for these clinics have emerged, including clinics associated with a hospital or health system, those owned or operated by a drugstore retailer, and those independently financed and operated (Laws and Scott 2008). Yet this new care delivery option has raised issues around access to care for consumers, the quality of care provided by physician extenders such as nurse practitioners and physician assistants who staff the clinics, and business entities' motivations for opening and operating the clinics. While this organizational form is still new to most markets, its rapid expansion across the United States has sparked interest and controversy in both the business and policy arenas (Laws and Scott 2008; Mehrotra et al. 2008; Paulus, Davis, and Steele 2008; Pollert, Dobberstein, and Wiisanen 2008; Fenn 2008; Newbold and O'Neil 2008).

Variation and Innovation in Organizational Design

Organizational variation is unending, both across the United States and around the globe. Some hospital-centered systems—such as the Hospital Corporation of America, the Voluntary Hospitals of America, or the Veterans Administration—cross healthcare markets. Health maintenance organizations (HMOs) combine the insurance function and provision of care under capitation, which is a reversal of the economic incentives of fee-for-service. Once, one could describe Kaiser-Permanente and say "That is what HMOs are or expect to be." No longer. For example, point-of-service (POS) plans, which give enrollees a choice of care and payment levels, have become increasingly popular. Under this model, if patients use the core physicians and hospitals, they do not make copayments; if the larger preferred provider list is used, they do. The patient can go out of the network and pay even larger copayments. However, allowing patients more choice of providers than they would have in an HMO makes it more difficult to control quality and costs in such POS plans.

Other variations in organizational design are emerging as a result of the information revolution in healthcare. When information about patients is available electronically on a timely basis, providers may be able to make decisions about patient care alternatives without needing to be present. For instance, radiologists are now able to read films and make recommendations remotely. Surgeons can perform surgery remotely using computer-based technologies. Telemedicine is extending the reach of providers into remote and rural areas. Such technological innovations are encouraging healthcare organizations to consider new approaches to delivering healthcare services that can reduce costs and improve the quality of care provided.

Process innovations are also important, as seen in the spread of techniques such as the Toyota Production System (TPS) or Lean production processes (Chalice 2007; Grunden 2008; Printezis and Gopalakrishnan 2007), and quality improvement methods such as Six Sigma (Trusko et al. 2007). In addition, there has been increasing emphasis on opportunities to apply best practices to healthcare organizations, whether such practices are found in healthcare or outside the industry. For instance, Fred Lee's exploration of what hospitals would do differently if they were run by Disney (Lee 2004) emphasizes the importance of culture in improving the quality of service. Berry and Seltman similarly present the findings from their extensive research into the Mayo Clinic, highlighting the fundamental roles of organizational culture and shared values in delivering high-quality care (Berry and Seltman 2008).

External organizations and foundations are promoting these efforts by helping healthcare organizations learn improvement techniques, many of which require design changes. The Boston-based Institute for Healthcare Improvement (IHI) has made important strides in addressing quality improvement issues, such as the need to reduce the number of medical errors in its 5 Million Lives Campaign (www.ihi.org/ihi). Through its website and educational programs, IHI helps hospitals improve patient safety. Similarly, recent projects funded by the Robert Wood Johnson Foundation have emphasized the need to address organizational design and quality-of-care issues, such as the Urgent Matters program, which focused on the need to improve flow in hospital emergency departments to reduce overcrowding (www .urgentmatters.org/), and the Expecting Success program, which explored ways of improving the quality of cardiovascular care provided in inpatient and community settings (www.expectingsuccess.org/).

Innovations in organizational design are producing improvements in care quality and reductions in healthcare costs. Within the United States, the Intermountain Healthcare system has successfully used TPS methods to reduce waste and improve efficiency while increasing the quality of the products they deliver (Jimmerson, Weber, and Sobek 2005). Similarly, results reported for Virginia Mason Medical Center of Seattle have sparked interest in both the healthcare and business communities (Spear 2005). Geisinger Health System's recent success has involved addressing issues such as clinical leadership, electronic health information systems implementation, and alignment of financial incentives to foster organizational innovation (Paulus, Davis, and Steele 2008). Organizational innovations overseas have produced startling results in the area of cardiac care, demonstrated by two hospitals in India that have been able to perform open heart surgery for 10 percent of what such surgeries cost in the United States (Richman et al. 2008).

Yet healthcare in the United States remains extremely expensive and of variable quality. Barriers to change include misaligned reimbursement systems, regulatory limits on innovation, and the lack of a financial incentive system for the majority of patients to seek higher value in the care they receive. While the cost of making an international phone call, taking a transcontinental flight, or purchasing stocks are all decreasing in the United States, there is still a need for lower-cost materials, equipment, and sites of care within the healthcare system.

Organization Design and Health

Some cost-cutting measures can be initiated with little change in the way care is organized. For example, using generic drugs and self-administered pregnancy tests and substituting physician extenders such as nurse practitioners and physicians' assistants for physicians save money. The next step is to "reengineer" care—or pursue "disease management" as it has come to be called. Reengineering care is based on answering a question: What is the best care for a defined population and how do we organize to achieve it? For example, how do we keep asthmatics out of the hospital? How do we reduce the loss from work caused by back pain? The Chronic Care Model, developed by Edward Wagner of Group Health Cooperative of Puget Sound (Wagner 1998; Wagner et al. 2001; Bodenheimer, Wagner, and Grumbach 2002), addresses the needs associated with caring for those with chronic diseases by examining the roles of primary care, care coordination, and the ability of patients to care for themselves.

From an organizational perspective, this type of approach calls for improving the organization of care and achieving measured outcomes. Case H describes the potential for use of a disease management program at Superior Medical Group to organize care delivery and improve patient care outcomes. Self-care presents another important opportunity to improve health. Asthma, diabetes, hypertension, and stress can be largely self-managed. Community coaches meeting in church basements with groups of diabetics who are trying to lose weight and exercise may be the future of healthcare focused on wellness in the community.

The Role of Management in Organization Design

Organizations are often described at a moment in time (a photograph). They can also be described as changing over time (a movie). It is easier to describe the organization as a photograph, but the leader's task is to guide the organization over time: to envision a future preferred state and to get the organization from its present condition to that future.

Changes in organizational design, however, can be expensive and difficult to implement. It can be challenging and time-consuming to get individuals and organizations to change. Politics can also create barriers to change when powerful individuals or groups openly or covertly resist a change.

One key task of today's senior health executives is to determine which organization design will best fit tomorrow's environment and how their organizations can get there ahead of others. This is indeed leading in uncertain times with great rewards for the visionary who understands the environment well enough to predict correctly.

References

Berry, L. L., and K. D. Seltman. 2008. *Management Lessons from Mayo Clinic: Inside One of the World's Most Admired Service Organizations.* New York: McGraw-Hill.

Bodenheimer T., E. Wagner, and K. Grumbach. 2002. "Improving Primary Care for Patients with Chronic Illness: The Chronic Care Model." *Journal of the American Medical Association* 288: 1775–79.

Chalice, R. 2007. *Improving Healthcare Using Toyota Lean Production Methods: 46 Steps for Improvement,* 2nd ed. New York: ASQ Quality Press.

Fenn, S. 2008. "Integrating CCCs into the Hospital System." *Frontiers of Health Services Management* 24 (3): 33–36.

Grunden, N. 2008. *The Pittsburgh Way to Efficient Healthcare: Improving Patient Care Using Toyota Based Methods.* New York: Productivity Press.

Jimmerson, C., D. Weber, and D. K. Sobek II. 2005. "Reducing Waste and Errors: Piloting Lean Principles at Intermountain Healthcare." *Joint Commission Journal on Quality and Patient Safety* 31 (5): 249–57.

Laws, M., and M. K. Scott. 2008. "The Emergence of Retail-Based Clinics in the United States: Early Observations." *Health Affairs* 27 (5): 1293–98.

Lee, F. 2004. *If Disney Ran Your Hospital: 9 1/2 Things You Would Do Differently.* Bozeman, MT: Second River Healthcare Press.

Lin, D. Q. 2008. "Convenient Care Clinics: Opposition, Opportunity, and the Path to Health System Integration." *Frontiers of Health Services Management* 24 (3): 3–11.

Mehrotra, A., M. C. Wang, J. R. Lave, J. L. Adams, and E. A. McGlynn. 2008. "Retail Clinics, Primary Care Physicians, and Emergency Departments: A Comparison of Patients' Visits." *Health Affairs* 27 (5): 1272–82.

Mintzberg, H. 1983. *Structure in Fives: Designing Effective Organizations.* Engelwood Cliffs, NJ: Prentice Hall.

———. 1979. *The Structuring of Organizations.* Engelwood Cliffs, NJ: Prentice Hall.

Newbold, P., and M. J. O'Neil. 2008. "Small Changes Lead to Large Effects." *Frontiers of Health Services Management* 24 (3): 23–27.

Paulus, R. A., K. Davis, and G. D. Steele. 2008. "Continuous Innovation in Healthcare: Implications of the Geisinger Experience." *Health Affairs* 27 (5): 1235–45.

Pollert, P., D. Dobberstein, and R. Wiisanen. 2008. "Jumping into the Healthcare Retail Market: Our Experience." *Frontiers of Health Services Management* 24 (3): 13–21.

Printezis, A., and M. Gopalakrishnan. 2007. "Can a Production System Reduce Medical Errors in Healthcare?" *Quality Management in Healthcare* 16 (3): 226–38.

Richman, B. D., K. Udayakumar, W. Mitchell, and K. A. Schulman. 2008. "Lessons from India in Organizational Innovation: A Tale of Two Heart Hospitals." *Health Affairs* 27 (5): 1260–70.

Spear, S. 2005. "Fixing Healthcare from the Inside, Today." *Harvard Business Review* 83 (9): 78–91.

Sutherland, J. V., W. J. van den Heuvel, T. Ganous, M. M. Burton, and A. Kumar. 2005. "Towards an Intelligent Hospital Environment: OR of the Future." *Studies in Health Technology and Informatics* 118: 278–312.

Trusko, B. E., C. Pexton, J. Harrington, and P. Gupta. 2007. *Improving Healthcare Quality and Cost with Six Sigma*. New York: FT Press.

Wagner, E. H. 1998. "Chronic Disease Management: What Will It Take to Improve Care for Chronic Illness?" *Efficient Clinical Practice* 1 (1): 2–4.

Wagner E. H, B. T. Austin, C. Davis, M. Hindmarsh, J. Schaefer, and A. Bonomi. 2001. "Improving Chronic Illness Care: Translating Evidence into Action." *Health Affairs* 20 (6): 64–78.

THE READINGS

L in describes how convenient care clinics (CCCs), which have sparked interest and controversy, provide an opportunity to bridge the gap between consumers and healthcare.

Convenient Care Clinics: Opposition, Opportunity, and the Path to Health System Integration

Dean Q. Lin
From *Frontiers of Health Services Management* 24 (3): 3–11,
Spring 2008

Summary

As the terrain of the healthcare system grows increasingly more difficult to navigate for healthcare professionals, health systems, and consumers, the country is forced to seek new ways to align our healthcare needs with our healthcare capacity. In its quest to meet this challenge, the healthcare system—already besieged with rising costs and diminishing reimbursements, rapidly changing demographics, heightened demands for pricing, transparency demands, stringent regulations, and rising consumer expectations—is forced to examine new healthcare business models. One of the new healthcare business models, the convenient care clinic (CCC), has spurred great debate among healthcare professionals. Viewed as a threat that compromises quality by some and a viable business model that delivers much-needed basic healthcare services by others, convenient care clinics continue to multiply at a rapid pace. This article examines traditional healthcare delivery systems and ways that CCCs can begin to bridge the widening gap between healthcare and consumers.

The Advent of Convenient Care Clinics

Convenient care clinics (CCCs) are retail-based medical clinics offering a defined scope of diagnostic and treatment services for common medical ailments, as well as preventive health and wellness. These walk-in clinics are conveniently located in places where people shop, such as grocery stores, drugstores, and general merchandise retailers. They are usually staffed by certified family nurse practitioners or physician assistants, medical professionals who are able to write prescriptions when clinically appropriate.

Many in-store clinics have up-front menu-style pricing prominently displayed to address issues of price transparency. The first CCC opened in 2000, and today there are more than 800 clinics operated by more than 25 companies and health systems nationally (Convenient Care Association 2008).

This is a small but fast-growing segment of the healthcare marketplace. The growth in the number of CCCs is expected to accelerate due to increasing consumer desires for convenience, reliability, accessibility, and affordability, as well as business demands for cost control and quality improvements.

The Citizens' Healthcare Working Group (2006), created through bipartisan legislation and consisting of citizens from all walks of life and the Secretary of Health and Human Services, was charged with exploring the values and aspirations held by the American people regarding the American healthcare system and health reform. The third recommendation of the five-point plan developed after gathering input from thousands of Americans was: foster innovative integrated community health networks.

Participants cited many healthcare delivery system problems, including a lack of primary care providers, difficulty in accessing specialty care, and obstacles in navigating a complicated system. They also emphasized the importance of having access to healthcare in local communities and the need to keep systems simple and easy to navigate. In addition to consumers and businesses, other positive industry drivers include growing retailer interest, health system entrants, insurance industry support, and venture capital funding.

Growing Gaps in the U.S. Healthcare Delivery System

Innovations such as convenient care are driven by necessity. CCCs emerged and proliferated in response to the growth of obstacles that hinder or prevent the delivery of healthcare services to Americans.

The convergence of overcrowded emergency departments (EDs), the growing physician shortage, and escalating insurance costs translate into less access to care for many Americans. An Advance Data report from the Centers for Disease Control and Prevention (CDC) issued in 2006 showed that EDs are under increasing pressure to provide care for more patients, resulting in overcrowding and ambulance diversions. According to the National Center for Health Statistics (NCHS 2008), there were 110.2 million visits to hospital EDs in 2004—an increase of 18 percent over the previous 10 years. In part,

ED overcrowding is attributed to the increasing use of the ED for non-urgent care. A recent report from the National Association of Community Health Centers, Inc., found that at least one-third of all ED visits are "avoidable," meaning non-urgent or ambulatory-care-sensitive and therefore treatable in primary care settings (Choudhry et al. 2007).

Why people have resorted to non-urgent use of the ED is part of a complex, growing problem that reflects financial and insurance issues, physician shortages, and the need for convenience. Longer waiting times for physician appointments are one factor that contributes to the growing reliance on the ED as a patient's usual source of care (USC). A study published in *Academic Emergency Medicine* found that patients are more likely to use the ED for non-urgent visits when they believe their USC is not meeting their needs. About 20 percent of the uninsured say the ED is their USC (Henry J. Kaiser Family Foundation 2006).

CCCs may be part of an overall strategy for hospitals looking to decrease ED use for non-urgent visits. According to a number of industry clinic operators, up to 40 percent of patients who have used a CCC report that, had there not been an in-store clinic, they would have sought treatment at an emergency room.

Shortage Drives CCCs

The growing physician shortage is also an industry driver for CCCs. A growing number of patients report that they cannot schedule a timely appointment with their physician. For patients without a primary care physician, there are fewer physicians accepting new patients. It's also estimated that approximately 35 percent of physicians in the United States are over age 55, and most will likely retire within the next five to ten years, according to a report from the American College of Physicians (2006), "The Impending Collapse of Primary Care and Its Implication for the State of the Nation's Healthcare." The population is aging too, making the physician shortage even more critical. Older people visit a doctor at a much higher rate than younger people. The National Hospital Ambulatory Medical Care Survey reports that people between the ages of 25 and 34 visit a physician 2.2 times per year, while people 65–74 visit a physician six times a year (McCaig and Nawar 2004).

Whatever the predictions, trusted sources concur that the United States is facing a critical physician shortage. Some experts predict that by 2020 or 2025, the shortage could be as high as 200,000, or 20 percent of the needed workforce (Cooper 2004). Although there is inconclusive evidence at this time, logic tells us that the physician shortage may be playing a role in the overcrowding of EDs.

In addition, the demand for preventive services has increased significantly due to proven efficacy and patient requests (Bodenheimer 2006). CCCs may be a good alternative resource for primary physicians who are too time-constrained to provide these services. In fact, CCCs, located where healthy people congregate, may provide a more suitable venue for delivering preventive health services.

Uninsured Use CCCs

The growing number of individuals who are under- and uninsured is creating a financial burden on hospitals, which provide about $34 billion of uncompensated care per year (Institute of Medicine 2003). The Center on Budget and Policy Priorities reports that in 2006, 47 million Americans were without health insurance (DeNavas-Walt, Proctor, and Lee 2006). Rapidly rising health insurance premiums prevent a third of firms in the United States from offering coverage to their employees (Henry J. Kaiser Family Foundation 2006). Even in cases in which insurance is offered, employees cannot always afford their portion of the premium.

The consequences of this lack of insurance may be compromised health, because the uninsured receive less preventive care, are diagnosed at more advanced disease stages, and, once diagnosed, tend to receive less therapeutic care and have higher mortality rates than insured patients (Institute of Medicine 2004). Increasingly, those who are under and uninsured are paying for services up front, before they are rendered (Henry J. Kaiser Family Foundation 2006).With affordable, up-front, menu-style pricing, CCCs can mean the difference between someone receiving or not receiving healthcare.

A Promising Concept

Innovations in medicine have led to increased life expectancy. Drug and treatment protocols have changed illnesses that were once death sentences into manageable chronic conditions. As we begin the twenty-first century, medical technology continues to advance.

Yet in spite of remarkable progress in the medical field, the country continues to struggle with a healthcare delivery system that is inefficient, unwieldy, and often not consumer-friendly. Escalating costs, shifting demographics, and declining reimbursement levels have mired our healthcare system in bureaucracy. While raging debate continues over exactly how to fix or redesign our ailing healthcare system, the number of Americans without access to healthcare continues to rise.

As Albert Einstein said, "In the middle of every difficulty lies opportunity." The same spirit of innovation that continues to drive medical advances has also paved the way for convenient care as an innovation in healthcare delivery.

The concept of CCCs is based on a well-thought-out business model. CCCs epitomize a "disruptive innovation"—a phenomenon identified by Harvard Business School professor Clayton Christensen.

In a 2000 *Harvard Business Review* article, "Will Disruptive Innovations Cure Healthcare?" Christensen, Bohmer, and Kenagy define "disruptive innovations" as powerful innovations that disrupt industries by enabling a larger population of less-skilled people to do things in a more convenient, less expensive setting that historically could be performed only by expensive specialists in centralized, inconvenient locations.

The in-store clinic, however, may be more than a disruptive innovation to the healthcare delivery system. It has the potential to be a catalyst in improving healthcare access and affordability in this country. CCCs should be viewed as a step in the maturation process for health systems that are focused on creating a more consumer-friendly healthcare environment (PricewaterhouseCoopers 2005). They are not the singular solution to the nation's disjointed healthcare delivery system, but rather one step in an incremental improvement in healthcare delivery.

Critics and Their Concerns

CCCs have been met with the same skepticism faced by other innovations. Critics have raised myriad issues, including quality and continuity of care. They are concerned that the healthcare delivery model of the CCC does not support the "medical home" model and that increased use of CCCs will further fragment patient care and threaten the provision of episodic care to patients with special healthcare needs and chronic conditions.

Concerns about CCCs typically center on quality of care and safety. Quality of care and patient safety should be a priority for any healthcare provider, and this is no different for organizations that operate CCCs (see Convenient Care Association standards sidebar).

The narrow scope of services offered at CCCs is based on highly standardized interventions.

Diagnoses are made using protocol-based decision rules, which are grounded in evidence-based medicine and guidelines published by respected healthcare bodies. In addition, studies have shown that, for the scope of services they are licensed to provide, the care provided by nurse practitioners is comparable to care from physicians (Mundinger et al. 2000).

Convenient Care Standards

The CCC industry has taken it upon itself to ensure quality and safety. The Convenient Care Association (CCA 2008), a nonprofit organization for the industry, has developed and issued mandatory standards that ensure timely, accurate treatment from qualified healthcare professionals for patients. They include:

1. All providers will be thoroughly credentialed for license, training, and experience, with rigorous background checks to verify training and licensing.
2. All CCA members are committed to monitoring quality on an ongoing basis, including but not limited to: peer review; collaborating physician review; use of evidence-based guidelines; collecting aggregate data on selected quality and safety outcomes; collecting patient satisfaction data.
3. All CCA members build relationships with traditional healthcare providers and hospitals, and work towards a goal of using EHRs to share patient information and ensure continuity of care.
4. All CCA members are committed to encouraging patients to establish a relationship with a primary care provider, and to making appropriate and careful referrals for follow-up care and for conditions that are outside of the scope of the clinic's services.
5. All CCA members are in compliance with applicable OSHA, CLIA, HIPAA, and ADA standards. All CCA members follow Centers for Disease Control (CDC) guidelines for infection control through hand washing.
6. All CCA members provide health promotion and disease prevention education to patients. All CCA members provide written instructions and educational materials to patients upon leaving the clinic.
7. All CCA members use Electronic Health Records (EHR) to ensure high-quality efficient care. All CCA members are committed to providing all patients with the opportunity to share health information with other providers electronically or in paper format.
8. All CCA members provide an environment conducive to quality patient care and meet standards for infection control and safety.
9. All CCA members will establish emergency response procedures and develop relationships with local emergency response service providers to ensure that patients in need of emergency care can be transported to an appropriate setting as quickly as possible.
10. CCA members empower patients to make informed choices about their health care. Prices for services provided at Convenient Care Clinics are readily available in a visible place outside of the examination room. Providers discuss what impact, if any, the provision of additional services will have on the ultimate cost to the patient.

Another concern is that CCCs do not support the medical home model. CCCs can and do play a role in supporting the medical home model by referring patients to primary care physicians in the local community. According to many CCC operators, up to 30 percent of their patients do not have a primary care physician.

In fact, CCCs have made a substantial effort to develop and maintain a symbiotic relationship with local primary care practitioners. CCCs refer patients who are without a "medical home" to area primary care physicians who are taking new patients.

The relationship can go both ways: Doctors who want to alleviate long waits for appointments can direct patients to clinics for vaccinations and other simple, standard healthcare.

Most clinics use proprietary software systems, electronic health records, and technology to enhance the patient experience and continuity of care within the medical community. CCCs operated by health systems such as Geisinger Health System may have a unique advantage in that they can share the same electronic medical record platform used by other parts of the health system, which allows for interoperability and continuity of care.

That said, the cradle-to-grave model of receiving care from the same primary care physician or care setting is no longer the norm for most Americans.

This reflects new lifestyle trends, such as people working for multiple employers, commuting farther daily, moving frequently, and shopping in multiple venues.

Tension Among Doctors

The tension within the medical community is palpable. Although new discoveries and treatments are embraced, even celebrated, new delivery systems are sometimes viewed as unwelcome competition.

The emergence of CCCs should not be viewed as a threat or a step in the direction of substandard care. Instead, it should be embraced as an opportunity to create a push-pull environment that serves both patients and healthcare professionals.

Integration with Traditional Healthcare Delivery

To date, the discussion and debate on CCCs have been largely focused on independent, venture-backed companies and retail hosts with household names.

While insights can be gained from these companies with regard to consumer marketing and experience, health systems are in an excellent position to ensure quality control, safety, and continuity of care. In fact, a few leading health systems and some physician group practices have embraced CCCs to implement these principles and to leverage this new model of care as a way to further their healthcare mission in the community. As the trend continues with healthcare shifting away from hospitals to outpatient care sites and home settings, the retail setting provides an alternate community platform with a strong value proposition.

As a partner in the continuum of care, CCCs can mitigate congestion in EDs and urgent care facilities and enhance access to affordable healthcare for the under- and uninsured. They can also relieve pressure on physician workloads, especially during evening and weekend hours, which may enhance physician satisfaction.

As convenient access points in busy public areas, CCCs provide an opportunity for brand development and revenue enhancement. Many of the retailers where CCCs are located will record daily transactions of 1,000 to 9,000 per store—and an average transaction may include other family members or friends, which multiplies the actual number of individuals visiting. This level of foot traffic presents a unique opportunity to interact with a large number of people on a daily basis and is likely to generate positive impressions. Many CCCs, including the ones operated by Geisinger Health System, report patient satisfaction in the top decile. Health systems may also expect to generate downstream revenues from the initial convenient care encounter, including ancillary lab work, primary care physician referrals, and hospital admissions.

CCCs may also play a role in prevention and early detection. Immunizations and screening to detect problems early—when they can be treated more effectively—can significantly improve health outcomes and quality of life associated with a variety of medical conditions. In fact, the CDC has recognized that vaccination services at CCCs offer an excellent way to expand adult vaccination during influenza season (CDC 2007). Over time, with scale, CCCs may be able to contribute to public health epidemiology and surveillance.

In the long run, CCCs may be able to support aspects of disease management, which is defined by the Disease Management Association of America (2007) as a "system of coordinated healthcare interventions and communications for populations with conditions in which patient self-care efforts are significant." Medical professionals may educate patients about self-management—which includes behavior modification as well as compliance and monitoring—at the in-store clinic. The retail setting itself may serve as a teaching tool. For example, a packaged offering of in-store nutritional tours and health monitoring services may be provided to patients with heart disease and diabetes.

Today, the current business model is focused on treating minor acute conditions in a convenient location where people shop. The future is bright and opportunities from integration are boundless.

CCCs are here to stay and their role is likely to evolve as health systems adopt this model of care to complement their existing services.

Conclusion

The healthcare crisis in this country is convoluted and there is no simple solution; the challenges are enormous.

Issues such as overcrowded EDs and primary care physicians operating in a reimbursement-driven time crunch cannot be resolved easily or quickly. Questions about quality, safety, and continuity of care are important, and should be asked about every aspect of the healthcare continuum. And we should always be sure, regardless of our role in the delivery of healthcare, that we are providing and maintaining the gold standard of care.

CCCs are not the sole answer to the healthcare crisis. But if they're viewed as an extension of the traditional healthcare model, rather than as a competitor, they are positioned to help alleviate some of the obstacles that prevent people from obtaining healthcare. They also offer options for developing more engaged healthcare consumers and a healthier society overall. CCCs have the potential to become a valuable asset in the healthcare continuum that may just help us work together to build a more comprehensive, consumer-friendly healthcare delivery system.

References

American College of Physicians. 2006. *The Impending Collapse of Primary Care Medicine and Its Implications for the State of the Nation's Health Care.* Report from the American College of Physicians, Philadelphia, PA.

Bodenheimer, R. 2006. "Primary Care—Will It Survive?" *The New England Journal of Medicine* 355 (9): 861–64.

Bohmer, R. 2007. "The Rise of In-Store Clinics—Threat or Opportunity?" *The New England Journal of Medicine*, Perspective 356 (8): 765–68.

CDC. 2007. "Strategies for Increasing Adult Vaccination Rates." Atlanta, GA: Centers for Disease Control.

Christensen, C., R. Bohmer, and J. Kenagy. 2000. "Will Disruptive Innovations Cure Healthcare?" *Harvard Business Review* 78 (5): 102–12.

Choudhry, L., M. Douglass, J. Lewis, C. H. Olson, R. Osterman, and P. Shah. 2007. *The Impact of Community Health Centers & Community-Affiliated Health Plans on Emergency Department Use.* Washington, DC: National Association of Community Health Centers.

Citizens' Healthcare Working Group. 2006. "Final Recommendations." Convenient Care Association. "History of the CCI." http://www.convenientcareassociation .org/abou thcci.htm (accessed January 31, 2008).

Convenient Care Association. 2008. "History of the CCI." www.convenientcare association.org/abouthcci.htm (accessed Jan. 31, 2008).

Cooper, R. 2004. "Weighing the Evidence for Expanding Physician Supply." *Annals of Internal Medicine* 141 (9): 705–14.

DeNavas-Walt, C., C. Proctor and C. Lee. 2006. "Income, Poverty and Health Insurance Coverage in the United States." Washington, DC: U.S Census Bureau.

Disease Management Association of America. 2007. *Enhancing Health Care Quality Through Disease Management and Care Coordination.* Washington, DC.

Henry J. Kaiser Family Foundation. 2006. "The Uninsured: A Primer, Key Facts About Americans Without Health Insurance." Menlo Park, California.

Institute of Medicine. 2003. "Hidden Costs, Values Lost: Uninsurance in America." Congressional Briefing. Board on Healthcare Services, Committee on the Consequences of Uninsurance. Washington D.C.: The National Academies Press.

———. 2004. "Insuring America's Health—Principles and Recommendations." Washington D.C.: The National Academies Press.

McCaig, L., and E. Nawar. 2004. *National Hospital Ambulatory Medical Care Survey: 2004 Emergency Department Summary.* Washington, DC: National Center for Health Statistics, Advance Data from Vital and Health Statistics (372).

Mistry, R., R. Hoffmann, J. Yauck, and D. Brousseau. 2005. "Association Between Parental and Childhood Emergency Department Utilization." *Pediatrics* 115:e 147–151.

Mundinger, M., R. Kane, E. Lenz, A. Totten, W. Tsai, P. Cleary, W. Friedewald, A. Siu, and M. Shelanski. 2000. "Primary Care Outcomes in Patients Treated by Nurse Practitioners or Physicians: A Randomized Trial." *JAMA* 283: 59–68.

National Center for Health Statistics (NCHS). 2008. "Annual Number of Visits to Hospital Emergency Departments: United States, 1992–2005." Accessed online at www.cdc.gov/nchs.

PricewaterhouseCoopers. 2005. *Management Barometer Survey.* New York: PricewaterhouseCoopers.

Discussion Questions

1. How do convenient care clinics (CCCs) threaten existing healthcare organizations? How do they threaten local physicians?
2. As CEO of a health system considering developing a CCC within the system, make a case to the board that the CCC model makes strategic sense.

Required Supplementary Readings

Berenson, R. A., T. Hammons, D. N. Gans, S. Zuckerman, K. Merrell, W. S. Underwood, and A. F. Williams. 2008. "A House Is Not a Home: Keeping

Patients at the Center of Practice Redesign." *Health Affairs* 27 (5): 1219–30.

Herzlinger. R. 2000. "Market-Driven, Focused Healthcare: The Role of Managers." *Frontiers of Health Services Management* 16 (3, Special Issue).

Paulus, R. A., K. Davis, and G. D. Steele. 2008. "Continuous Innovation in Healthcare: Implications of the Geisinger Experience." *Health Affairs* 27 (5): 1235–45.

Questions for the Required Supplementary Readings

1. Berenson and colleagues define and describe the "patient-centered medical home" (PCMH) and its potential to transform primary care. How could this model negatively affect patient care? As administrator of a large multispecialty group practice, what challenges would you anticipate to be associated with introducing the PCMH model to your physicians?
2. You are asked to become the CEO of a 200-bed community hospital, one of three in your part of the city, which is trying to be all things to all people. The board has asked you to focus on "what we do best." Using concepts from Herzlinger's article, what would you tell the board? Given Herzlinger's case for focused factories, what are arguments against this approach?
3. Paulus and associates describe a remarkable effort to improve care delivery and service at Geisinger Health System. What made this a successful effort? How might this approach be applied in other health systems? What would be constraints to applying this approach elsewhere?

Recommended Supplementary Readings

Arndt, M., and B. Bigelow. 2000. "The More Things Change, the More They Stay the Same." *Healthcare Management Review* 25 (1): 65–72.

Bush, R. W. 2007. "Reducing Waste in U.S. Healthcare Systems." *Journal of the American Medical Association* 297 (8): 871–74.

Casalino, L. P., E. A. November, R. A. Berenson, and H. H. Pham. 2008. "Hospital-Physician Relations: Two Tracks and the Decline of the Voluntary Medical Staff Model." *Health Affairs* 27 (5): 1305–14.

Conrad, D. A., and W. L. Dowling. 1990. "Vertical Integration in Health Services: Theory and Managerial Implication." *Healthcare Management Review* 15 (4): 9–22.

Cussell, C. K., J. M. Ludden, and G. M. Moon. 2000. "Perceptions of Barriers to High-Quality Palliative Care in Hospitals." *Health Affairs* 19 (5): 166–72.

Gamm, L., B. Kash, and J. Bolin. 2007. "Organizational Technologies for Transforming Care: Measures and Strategies for Pursuit of IOM Quality Aims." *Journal of Ambulatory Care Management* 30 (4): 291–301.

Gerteis, M., S. Edgman-Levitan, J. Daley, and T. L. Delbanco (eds.). 2002. *Through the Patient's Eyes: Understanding and Promoting Patient-Centered Care*. San Francisco: Jossey-Bass.

Glouberman, S., and H. Mintzberg. 2001a. "Managing the Care of Health and the Cure of Disease—Part I: Differentiation." *Healthcare Management Review* 26 (1): 56–69, discussion 87–89.

———. 2001b. "Managing the Care of Health and the Cure of Disease—Part II: Integration." *Healthcare Management Review* 26 (1): 70–84, discussion 87–89.

Goldsmith, J. 2000. "How Will the Internet Change Our Health System?" *Health Affairs* 19 (1): 148–56.

Hearld, L. R., J. A. Alexander, I. Fraser, and H. J. Jiang. 2008. "How Do Hospital Organizational Structure and Processes Affect Quality of Care?" *Medical Care Research & Review* 65 (3): 259–99.

Jha, A. K., J. B. Perlin, K. Kizer, and R. A. Dudley. 2003. "Effects of the Transformation of the Veterans Affairs Healthcare System on the Quality of Care." *New England Journal of Medicine* 310 (22): 1477–80.

Kilo, C. M. 1999. "Improving Care Through Collaboration." *Pediatrics* 103 (1): 384–92.

Kimberly, J. R., and E. Minvielle. 2003. "Quality as an Organizational Problem." In *Advances in Healthcare Organizational Theory*, edited by S. S. Mick and M. E. Wyttenbach, 205–32. San Francisco: Jossey-Bass.

Lathrop, J. P. 1993. *Restructuring Healthcare: The Patient-Focused Paradigm*. San Francisco: Jossey Bass.

Lawrence, D. 2002. *From Chaos to Care*. Cambridge, MA: Perseus.

Leatt, P., R. Baker, and J. R. Kimberly. 2005. "Organization Design." In *Healthcare Management*, 5th edition, edited by S. M. Shortell and A. D. Kaluzny, 314–55. Albany, NY: Delmar.

McAlearney, A. S. 2004. "Hospitalists and Family Physicians: Understanding Opportunities and Risks." *Journal of Family Practice* 53 (6): 473–81.

Mehrotra, A., M. C. Wang, J. R. Lave, J. L. Adams, and E. A. McGlynn. 2008. "Retail Clinics, Primary Care Physicians, and Emergency Departments: A Comparison of Patients' Visits." *Health Affairs* 27 (5): 1272–82.

Pham, H. H., J. M. Grossman, G. Cohen, and T. Bodenheimer. 2008. "Hospitalists and Care Transitions: The Divorce of Inpatient and Outpatient Care." *Health Affairs* 27 (5): 1315–27.

Robinson, J. C., and L. P. Casalino. 1996. "Vertical Integration and Organizational Networks in Healthcare." *Health Affairs* 15 (1): 7–22.

Rosenberg, C. 1987. *The Care of Strangers*. New York: Basic Books.

Rundall, T. G., S. M. Shortell, M. C. Wang, L. Casalino, T. Bodenheimer, R. R. Gillies, J. A. Schmittdiel, N. Oswald, and J. C. Robinson. 2002. "As Good As It Gets? Chronic Care Management with Nine Leading U.S. Physician Organizations." *British Medical Journal* 325 (26): 958–61.

Schweikhart, S. B., and V. Smith-Daniels. 1996. "Reengineering the Works of Caregivers: Role Definition, Team Structures and Organizational Redesign." *Hospital & Health Services Administration* 41 (1): 19–36.

Scott, R. L., L. Aiken, D. Mechanic, and J. Moravcsik. 1995. "Organizational Aspects of Caring." *Milbank Quarterly* 73 (1): 77–95.

Shortell, S. M., R. R. Gillies, D. A. Anderson, K. M. Erickson, and J. B. Mitchell. 1996. *Remaking Healthcare in America*. San Francisco: Jossey-Bass.

Smith, H. L. 1955. "Two Lines of Authority Are One Too Many." *Modern Hospitals* 84 (3): 59–64.

Villagra, V. G. 2004. "Integrating Disease Management into the Outpatient Delivery System During and After Managed Care?" *Health Affairs* Web Exclusives W4 (May 19): 281–83.

Wachter, R. M., and L. Goldman. 1996. "The Emerging Role of Hospitalists in the American Healthcare System." *New England Journal of Medicine* 335 (7): 514–17.

Wachter, R., and L. Goldman. 2002. "The Hospitalist Movement 5 Years Later." *Journal of the American Medical Association* 287 (4): 487–94.

Woolf, S. H. 2004. "Patient Safety Is Not Enough: Targeting Quality Improvements to Optimize the Health of the Population." *Annals of Internal Medicine* 140: 33–36.

Woolhandler, S., T. Campbell, and D. U. Himmelstein. 2003. "Costs of Healthcare Administration in the United States and Canada Hospitals." *New England Journal of Medicine* 349 (8): 760–75.

Zuckerman, H. S., D. W. Hilberman, R. M. Andersen, L. R. Burns, J. A. Alexander, and P. Torrens. 1998. "Physicians and Organizations: Strange Bedfellows or a Marriage Made in Heaven? *Frontiers of Health Services Management* 14 (3): 3–34.

THE CASES

In healthcare, discussion about organizational design occurs at four levels. The first is at the patient care level. New questions are being asked: How do we organize the best care for asthma or hypertension or back pain? Answering this question requires a definition of "best," data on the population served, a team of staff members working to achieve these goals, and management support. How does our organization answer these questions? What is excellent diabetes care? How would we know we are achieving it? The "Future of Disease Management" case raises some of these issues.

At the next level of aggregation are the issues of the design of the hospital, nursing home, and other care organizations. How do we put the component departments together? Restructuring, reengineering, downsizing, and right-sizing are the jargon terms of the moment. The Wise Medical Center short case highlights some of these concepts. In addition, the case "Improving Organizational Development in Health Services" presents the issues associated with centralization versus decentralization at both the health system and service line levels.

Across the country, hospitals, clinics, and insurers are grouping themselves together as systems of care. In an urban area where 30 separate hospitals once stood, there may now be three or four competing groups of hospitals within both regional and national health systems. The competing entities may be not-for-profit organizations, investor-owned, or a mix of both. This new grouping strategy is the third level of organizational design.

One reason for these changes is the recognition that with managed care and alternative financing arrangements we will need many fewer hospital beds than we now have. The leaders of a single hospital left out of such a system may wonder if it will be one of the hospitals that will disappear. One way these mergers are occurring is through the sale of a not-for-profit hospital to a for-profit group. The sale price plus the not-for-profit hospital's existing endowment is put into a nonprofit foundation. The income from this foundation's endowment is used to achieve the charitable and philanthropic goals of the original not-for-profit hospital. The hospital, now part of the for-profit organization, is run along business lines in a competitive environment.

In the rush to become one of the three or four biggest groups in the area, a health system bases its decisions about organizational design on expediency, comfort level, and speed rather than organizing to provide expeditious, excellent care. The local rush for size is of vital importance in a market oversupplied with hospitals. Any one urban hospital priced too high or of average quality can be ignored by insurance providers negotiating contracts. For such a hospital to exist, it will have to accept whatever price the insurance providers choose to offer, which will not be high. If the system is large enough and includes popular, specialized, and prestigious hospitals, all insurance providers and managed care systems must deal with it. As a result, such a system will not be a "price taker" but a "price giver." It can charge a full price for its services because the insurer or HMO has no choice.

The fourth level of design is at the state- or national-policy level. One notable effort to change the context of healthcare delivery was the Clinton administration's unsuccessful national health plan initiative. However, the current devolution of decision making related to Medicaid from the federal to the state level will also change the context of care. Some states, such as Hawaii, Oregon, and Massachusetts, have provided interesting examples of system reform, while the state of California struggled along similar lines.

It is the interaction of all four of these levels of organization and system design that makes healthcare delivery a most lively arena. The field is creating unprecedented opportunities for creative leadership and the organization of whole new ways of providing better care at lower cost. New business models are being introduced, such as convenient care clinics or retail clinics located in pharmacies and grocery stores, and existing organizations are challenged to respond to competition from these new sources of care.

The coordination of many different professional workers with varying skills, views of the world, perceptions of what needs to be done, and licensing statutes lies at the heart of this new design for health services organizations. Yet the field is never static. Short Case 13 presents a question about whether to include a hospitalist program at Plateau University, describing the potential value of a new physician specialty that has developed and flourished in the past decade.

Work can be organized in many different ways in large health services organizations: by task or purpose, by facility, or by client group served. Short Case 15 describes a situation in which the organization of work can create confusion for the individual employee. Often, several different organizing principles operate in the same organization, sometimes appropriately and sometimes for historical reasons. As Clibbon and Sachs (1969) have pointed out, a laboratory is a place, obstetrics is a health condition, outpatients are people, dietary is a service, intensive care is a need, day care is a category of residential status, radiology is a group of techniques, and rehabilitation is a purpose.

The structure of many healthcare organizations was more appropriate for conditions when the organization was founded than it is for today. Organization structure is determined in part by the nature of the work the organization has to do, its physical facilities, the history of the organization, and the culture of the society and of like institutions. As a result, questions about what structure would truly be best for a particular organization or service remain common. The short case about integrating rehabilitation services (Short Case 14) raises both structural and cultural issues associated with needed changes in organization design.

Reference

Clibbon, S., and M. L. Sachs. 1969. "Healthcare Facilities: An Alternative to Baili-wick Planning in Patient Fostering Spaces." *The New Physician* 18: 462–71.

Case G
Improving Organizational Development in Health Services

By Ann Scheck McAlearney and Rebecca Schmale

Who, What, and Where?

John Shea, CEO and president of Worthington Health System (WHS), needed some time to think. He had been leading WHS for ten years, and was contemplating the legacy he wanted to leave. WHS, based in the Midwest, was comprised of four hospitals, a home health company, and an ambulatory care service line (see Figure III.1 and Table III.1). The system had been formed 12 years ago when two of the local community hospitals decided to combine

		FIGURE III.1
Employees	10,400	Worthington
Physicians	1,800	Health System
Volunteers	2,500	Facts at a
Hospitals	5	Glance
Net patient revenue	$1.2 billion	
Patient days	370,000	
Community benefit	$37 million	
Outpatient visits	1.1 million	
Ave. daily census	960	
Emergency room visits	260,000	
Ambulatory centers	6	
Home health visits	125,000	

TABLE III.1
Worthington
Health System
Facilities

Care Sites	Type	Beds	Employees
Riverview Hospital	Tertiary	800	4,600
Lincoln Hospital	Trauma	600	2,980
Graystone Memorial Hospital	Community	200	685
Mount Rising Hospital	Community	124	512
Fairland Memorial Hospital	Community	95	450
Worthington Home Care	Home health	—	440
Ambulatory care centers (6)	Health centers, urgent care, Outpatient surgery	—	690

FIGURE III.2
Worthington
Health System
Service Area

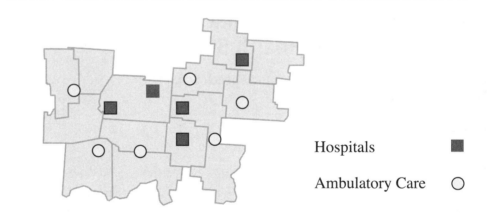

Hospitals ■

Ambulatory Care ○

forces and become a health system. The two freestanding hospitals each served distinct patient populations, with 600-bed Lincoln Hospital located downtown, and 800-bed Riverview Hospital located in a nearby suburb. Rather than take the name of either hospital, the organizing group elected to create a new, neutral name for the health system, and left each individual hospital with its original name. Shea was hired soon after the system's formation so he had personally experienced most of the changes WHS had navigated.

Since the formation of WHS, the rapidly changing healthcare market and shifting patient demographics had presented a series of opportunities for WHS. Shea had successfully managed the acquisition of two other local hospitals for WHS when another local system dissolved, and he had extended the reach of WHS to the adjacent county by forming a strategic alliance with Graystone Memorial Hospital. (See Figure III.2.) Additional market changes led to the formation of Worthington Home Care, and the creation of a network of ambulatory care centers that expanded the reach of WHS. WHS was financially strong, and enjoyed a positive reputation in the area, despite competition from two other health systems and several newly developed specialty hospitals.

Shea's continuing concern was the lack of "system-ness" within the broad WHS system. It had taken quite some time to build community awareness of WHS as a health system, and patients were still primarily loyal to the original flagship hospital, Riverview, rather than to WHS. This loyalty, however, was also evident among employees. The Riverview staff identified with Riverview Hospital, not WHS, and Lincoln Hospital staff exhibited the same silo loyalty. When Shea had arrived at WHS, he was thrilled by the challenge of creating a true system with previously competing entities, but, as he now reflected, he had not succeeded. He wanted his legacy to include a shift in the WHS organizational culture to one of system-focused thinking rather than entity-oriented decision making.

Several functions had been centralized in the last few years to achieve economies of scale and reduce redundancies within the system. The first functions to be centralized under the corporate umbrella were finance and supply chain. Greg Hanson, CFO, was a strong leader, and within one year centralization saved the system over $200 million. There had been some resistance to the centralization but the savings quickly made the centralization decision difficult to dispute.

Given the current financial strength of WHS, Shea realized he had an opportunity to focus on the goal of enhancing system-focused thinking. (See Figure III.3.) Since entity culture seemed to be playing such a major role, Shea knew he must engage his employees to achieve system-ness. He also knew that education, especially leadership development, could play a key role. One of Shea's goals was to advance WHS as a learning organization. This had led to two recent hires in the areas of organizational development and human resources (HR), and both Fiona Sinclair and Blake Snowdon seemed to have

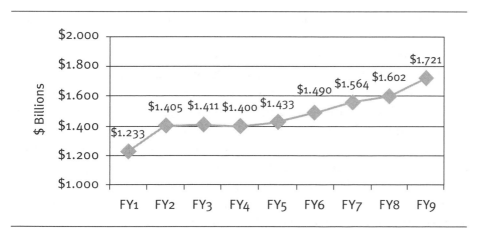

FIGURE III.3

Worthington Health System Total Operating Growth

sensed the non-systemness of WHS quite quickly. Shea decided to schedule a meeting with Sinclair and Snowdon to introduce his ideas.

Behind the Scenes

As system vice president of organizational development, Sinclair had spent the past two months getting to know WHS and its various entities. She had come to WHS from outside the healthcare industry, and had been repeatedly surprised by how "behind" she found the health system. Even basic education and training functions were still delivered at the entity level, and there was no sense of organizational identity at the system level. Yet Sinclair felt there was hope for improvement as signaled by her own recruitment, and the apparent interest of the CEO.

Snowdon, director of human resources, shared Sinclair's perspective about the fragmented nature of WHS, and was also struck by the seeming lack of awareness about the potential for strategic human resources management to help reduce this fragmentation (see Figure III.4). He had come to WHS three months ago from a smaller system based in California, and he now saw how good he had had it. Rather than a fully aligned health system that saw human resources as a strategic capability, Snowdon found WHS to be a collection of individual entities that appeared to compete among themselves for corporate-level attention. Many Riverview staff came across as arrogant because they believed they worked for the "best" hospital in the system. In contrast, Lincoln staff prized themselves on their ability to respond to the needs of the surrounding urban community, despite a largely unfavorable payer mix and staggering use of the emergency department. He hadn't yet characterized the cultures of Mount Rising or Fairland Hospitals, but he felt certain they were as entrenched and individualized as those of Riverview and Lincoln.

Given their similar interests and start dates, Sinclair and Snowdon were in frequent contact. Organizationally, the Department of Human Resources reported to the chief operating officer (COO), and Snowdon was its senior executive. The area of organizational development, however, was new for the organization, and Sinclair had been hired with the charge to create and build the department as she saw fit. She reported directly to CEO John Shea, but knew the strategic importance of close ties to Human Resources if she was going to be able to accomplish anything with respect to organizational development.

In Sinclair's last position she had directed the development of a corporate university in order to centralize training and development for the large organization. Sinclair believed this model held promise for a health system such as WHS, but was aware of the challenges associated with centralizing a previously decentralized and tightly controlled function. Coincidentally,

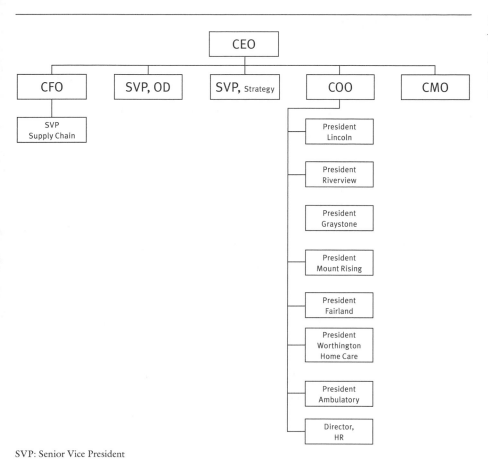

FIGURE III.4
Worthington Health System Organizational Chart

SVP: Senior Vice President

Snowdon's last role as director of human resources for a smaller health system had involved an evaluation of the corporate university model, but that system had rejected it. Instead, Snowdon's previous role had focused on building credibility for human resources as a strategic capability of the health system. The focus was on making targeted investments in strategic human resources capabilities, such as developing hiring managers' abilities to use behavioral interviewing techniques and linking individual performance evaluations to the health system's overall performance through use of a balanced scorecard.

Getting together to prepare for their meeting with Shea, Sinclair and Snowdon discussed their initial assessments of WHS. They agreed that WHS was a disjointed collection of individual entities with little loyalty to the system, but they also agreed that a fragmented culture could change. The key, they felt, would be in centralizing the education and training function for WHS at the corporate level, but they knew this idea would be met with widespread resistance from all entities. They also knew that without the commitment and support of the CEO, a move to centralize any function within WHS would fail.

The First Meeting

Shea decided to meet with Sinclair and Snowdon in Sinclair's office, signaling his willingness to move outside the suite of executive offices to collaborate with others considered experts in their own fields. He had purposely not created an agenda for the meeting, and instead had proposed this as a "conversation" about WHS. Shea opened the meeting with the basic question, "What can we do to make WHS feel like a system?"

Neither Sinclair nor Snowdon was timid, and they had previously agreed to be completely honest and direct with Shea. They described their early observations of WHS and the component entities, and their collective assessment that there was almost nothing that bound WHS as a system other than a common logo and a centralized payroll system. Even though there were several corporate-level functions, such as strategic planning and marketing, it seemed that the individual hospitals often replicated these functions in-house in order to ensure entity-level control. Particularly troublesome, Sinclair and Snowdon reported, was the training and development function. Yet they noted that this also presented a tremendous opportunity to bring WHS together as a system.

While Shea knew WHS suffered from the entity-focused territoriality common to many U.S. healthcare systems, he had been unaware of the magnitude of the problem. He was struck by the financial implications of hospital-based duplication of services. He realized that with respect to the area of education and training alone, duplication of training programs, evaluation processes, tracking systems, and even trainers was costing the system thousands of dollars. However, Shea was also aware that each hospital entity took training and development seriously as an entity-level capability. He knew the hospitals prided themselves on providing continuing education programs for physicians and nurses that were appropriately tailored to the hospital's perceived needs. Any move to centralize what was considered an important organizational competency would be perceived negatively and would likely be resisted. Shea knew that this issue would have to be evaluated thoroughly, and if accepted, introduced carefully.

The Charge

Shea liked the notion of centralizing the training and development function at WHS, and believed this could help him achieve his goal of transforming WHS into a cohesive system and learning organization. Yet he needed to be convinced that this approach could work, and that it would be worth the investment. He felt Sinclair and Snowdon were the appropriate individuals to lead the assessment process, and their newness within the system might help them uncover challenges or concerns less obvious to someone who had worked at WHS for a longer period of time.

Talking this over with Sinclair and Snowdon, Shea outlined what he would need to make his decision. First, he would need a list of the current financial and non-financial costs associated with decentralized training and development. While Shea knew they would not be able to cost out everything, he felt that a list and general estimate of costs could be sufficient for his purposes. Second, Shea wanted options. If, as they suspected, the centralized option was going to prove favorable, he needed to know what this could mean for WHS. Were there alternative models for centralized training and development? If so, which would be appropriate at WHS? What costs would be associated with this type of change? Further, how long would this organizational change take to implement? What would be the "value-add" of a centralized department for the entities? How could programs such as orientation, leadership development, and clinical management training reinforce a new way of thinking beyond the boundaries of each entity?

Shea asked Sinclair and Snowdon to collect the necessary data and prepare to present it to WHS senior leadership at the end of the next quarter. This would give them several months to do their background research, followed by another couple of weeks to refine their assumptions and properly frame the results of their research. Shea also offered to participate in regularly scheduled meetings so that he could remain informed about their ongoing findings and any challenges they encountered. They closed the meeting mutually energized, but Sinclair and Snowdon knew they had to get started right away.

Considering the Options

After Shea left Sinclair's office, Snowdon remained in order to continue the discussion with Sinclair. Their first task was to plan for the work they would have to do in the coming months. In particular, they wanted to determine the scope of the project, and try to get a sense of how to frame the alternatives.

Based on the preliminary conversations they had had with each other and their knowledge of the organizational development and training literature, they were able to outline six separate alternatives that varied based on level of centralization and magnitude of organizational changes required:

1. centralize training and development within the existing Department of Human Resources;
2. centralize training and development within the new Department of Organizational Development;

3. centralize training and development with creation of a new structure, a Corporate University, housed with the new Department of Organizational Development;
4. maintain decentralized delivery of training, but centralize the development function within the existing Department of Human Resources;
5. outsource training and development to a third-party vendor; or
6. maintain status quo with decentralized training and development.

Given these six alternatives, Sinclair and Snowdon's next step was to consider what information they needed to collect to assist Shea in the decision-making process. Their biggest task was to perform an organizational assessment of WHS as a whole with respect to training and development. In particular, they needed to determine what currently was going on in the areas of education, training, and development, including where these activities occurred, who or what department provided them, and how they were delivered. Within education and training, they were curious about factors such as whether any programs were offered online, whether some areas of the organization collaborated with others, and how clinical training and continuing education were delivered. Within development they wanted to know if there was any formal system to track development activities, if employees in any entity or area were required to create professional development plans that could be monitored, and whether developmental programs were tied to annual performance evaluations.

Another important area for their assessment was to identify key stakeholders in the areas of training and development for each health system entity. They knew organizational politics would likely play an important role in either building support or resistance for any initiative that required a change. As a result, they needed to identify important decision makers within each entity, and, ideally, recruit organizational champions who could help them with any change process.

Finally, in order to fully evaluate the different alternatives, they would have to develop some projections about costs associated with current operations (Alternative 6) in comparison with the five other alternatives they had outlined. Shea had recognized that there were likely non-financial costs associated with training and development in addition to financial costs, so they needed to consider these along with the financial and non-financial gains that could be accrued with each alternative.

Building the Case for Change

Shea was known for his ability to make quick decisions and then back his decisions with resource support. However, Sinclair and Snowdon knew they needed not only financial resources, but organizational commitment in order to ensure success for this initiative. They were excited to move forward with their ideas about centralizing the training and development function for WHS, but they knew they needed to build their case carefully.

Case Questions

1. In addition to the several items listed in the case, what other information would need to be collected to fully evaluate the centralization-decentralization decision?
2. What should be included in developing a financial analysis of this decision?
3. What would be the non-financial arguments for or against centralizing training and development at Worthington Health System?
4. With whom should Sinclair and Snowdon speak when considering the impact of each alternative?
5. How might physicians and nurses be affected by the different alternatives?
6. What would be critical success factors associated with the pursuit of a centralization alternative?
7. How could a centralized organizational development department support a culture of system-ness at WHS?

Case H
The Future of Disease Management at Superior Medical Group

Helen Nunberg

Introduction

Five years ago, Superior Medical Group of Paradise County (SMG) entered into a contract with LifeMasters for a disease management program for congestive heart failure. The program achieved improved outcomes, cost savings, and patient satisfaction. SMG's medical director, Dr. Hugh Welly, would like to make a recommendation to the board of directors regarding future chronic disease management. In particular:

- Should SMG develop its own diabetes management program?
- If SMG lacks the resources and competencies to develop its own program, with whom should SMG partner?

Welly, trained as a pediatrician, joined SMG two years ago, after seven years as medical director of Paradise County's Medi-Cal HMO plan. LifeMasters was his first experience with a commercial disease management program. As he prepared for the board meeting, he reflected on the accomplishments and the disappointments of the past year.

Superior Medical Group: History and Development

Prior to the founding of SMG in 1993, the physicians of Paradise County were primarily organized as employees or partners of Northside Medical Clinic, a multispecialty group practice, and as owners of independent solo or small group practices. In addition, there was a small number of physicians in nonprofit community clinics and public county clinics. Sisters of Mercy Hospital acquired the only other hospital in north Paradise County 12 years ago. A second hospital serves the less affluent South County.

The independent physicians organized themselves as SMG, an independent physician association (IPA) soon after Paradise Medical Clinic entered into its first managed care contract. Seven years ago a multi-hospital system acquired Paradise Medical Clinic and began construction of a second hospital in North County. That same year Paradise Sisters Hospital supported the formation of Coast Medical Associates, a primary care group within SMG.

SMG is a private, investor-owned corporation. SMG's current CEO began as the director of contracting in 1994. He is SMG's second CEO. The board of directors makes management decisions based on recommendations from the CEO, the medical director, and board committees. Board members are physicians selected by a formula to balance North and South counties, specialty and primary care, and cognitive and procedural practices (see Figure III.5).

Physician membership in SMG has been consistent at approximately 200, with recent 20 percent overall turnover, 30 percent in primary care. A physician may choose to become a shareholder after participating in the network for two years by buying shares for a nominal fee. There are currently 140 shareholders.

Patient enrollment, currently 36,000, dropped 12 percent in 2001 because of patients shifting from HMO to PPO plans. SMG is legally able to act on behalf of member physicians only with HMOs, not PPOs. The greatest threat to SMG's continued existence as an organization is the possible "end" of managed care.

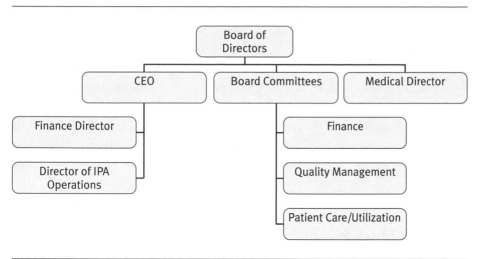

FIGURE III.5
SMG
Organization
Chart

In California, 29 physician groups filed for bankruptcy last year; 56 percent of IPAs have problems with solvency. Explanations include unsustainable reimbursement rates, poor management, poor acquisitions, and lack of reinvestment. Fueled by financial stress, SMG has suffered from internal dissension, especially between the primary and specialist physicians. In June of last year, Sisters Hospital's parent hospital system dissolved its relationship with Coast Medical Associates, bringing instability to SMG's largest primary care group. Sisters Hospital had also supported SMG financially four years ago by installing its intranet system, Elysium.

Despite these difficulties, SMG is now solvent and has strengthened its reserves enough to satisfy regulators. SMG's primary income stream is from capitation, a sum equal to the number of patient members multiplied by the contractual rate. The SMG primary care physicians receive capitated payments while specialists are paid fee-for-service. Additional income sources for SMG include grants from pharmaceutical firms for special programs and a contract to provide credentialing services to Coast Medical Associates.

Welly joined SMG at a time when several specialist groups were threatening to leave unless they received higher reimbursement rates. He identified his role as medical director to be that of "facilitator." He comments, "This person must pay respectful heed to compelling and highly individualized specifics without losing sight of the big picture. The intensified regulatory stringency, escalating consumer activism, and legitimate physician exasperation have made this a delicate balancing act."

Welly's responsibilities as medical director are primarily in the areas of quality and utilization management. His duties include investigating quality deficiencies; reviewing primary care referrals to specialists; reviewing hospital admissions and length of stay; authorizing high-cost procedures; reporting performance measures to HMOs; and supervising SMG's clinical staff and programs, including disease management. He is SMG's third medical director. He believes that quality management and quality improvement are the essence of what a medical group can do that independent physicians can't do, and believes the continued existence of SMG as an organization depends on its ability to bring something new and valuable to the community.

Welly communicates continuously with member physicians via the intranet. SMG does not provide significant education or training for its member physicians and does not get involved in the management of physicians' practices. SMG has not implemented quality incentives for the physicians.

Disease Management: Overview

The last decade has seen a wide range of experimentation in healthcare reform intended to contain costs and promote effectiveness. Disease management (DM) is one key tool managed care organizations have attempted to use to control costs and ensure quality. The goal of a DM program is to offer a continuum of care that uses guidelines and case management protocols to prevent acute care episodes, achieve improved outcomes, and reduce healthcare costs.

Chronic diseases such as diabetes, coronary heart disease, hypertension, asthma/chronic obstructive pulmonary disease, end-stage renal disease, and HIV/AIDS are the most prevalent and most costly of all health problems. Scientific studies have demonstrated that more intensive management of chronic diseases using evidence-based assessments and interventions leads to prevention or delay of complications. Some studies have shown economic benefits as well.

The distinction between efficacy and effectiveness is critical to DM; treatments with proven efficacy in clinical trials do not always perform as well under conditions typical of clinical practice. Clinical guidelines must be implemented to achieve improved outcomes. Intensive management with evidence-based guidelines requires increased resources. Commercial DM vendors promise high-quality, patient-focused care that is effective and reduces cost. DM is one of the fastest-growing investments in healthcare: "a movement" or "bandwagon" or "paradigm shift." Last year DM companies accounted for $600 million in revenue, up from $300 million two years ago and $150 million three years ago.

The Disease Management Purchasing Consortium and Advisory Council's catalogue *DM Vendor Profiles* contains descriptions of 60 independent companies. Health plans and pharmaceutical companies have DM divisions, and physician groups may create their own DM programs. A company or group usually begins with one disease and then expands to multiple disease entities. Vendors primarily contract with at-risk health plans and self-insured employers.

The nonprofit Disease Management Association of America, founded two years ago, defines DM as a system of coordinated healthcare interventions and communications for populations with conditions in which patient self-care efforts are significant. Disease management

- supports the physician/patient relationship and plan of care;
- emphasizes prevention of exacerbations and complications utilizing evidence-based guidelines and patient empowerment strategies; and
- evaluates clinical, humanistic, and economic outcomes on an ongoing basis with the goal of improving overall health.

Disease management components include:

- population identification processes;
- evidence-based practice guidelines;
- collaborative practice models that include physician and support-service providers;
- patient self-management education (may include primary prevention, behavior modification programs, and compliance surveillance);
- process and outcomes measurement, evaluation, and management; and
- routine reporting feedback loop (may include communication with patient, physician, health plan, and ancillary providers) and practice profiling.

A typical DM program requires clinical protocols, a sophisticated information system, a nurse call center, outcomes reporting methodology, claims analysis capabilities, and patient education materials.

American Healthways identifies three key components that must be present and operational to ensure a program's success:

- Clinical expertise, tools, and interventions
- Data and information management systems
- Experienced personnel (management, clinical, financial, and technical)

To implement a program, these three components come together to identify patients and physicians; stratify patients; collect and track data; scan records to determine when a test, exam, or other type of intervention is due; measure and report outcomes; and effectively communicate with patients and physicians.

Physicians' Views of Disease Management Programs

One physician's response to an *American Medical News* interview with Aetna's CEO: "Personally, I can't think of a bigger waste of money than these programs. I receive these assessments from many managed care companies. I have found they provide no further information to me than what I already know after I have spoken with and examined my patient. I am sure that this costs the managed care companies big bucks. This is a waste of healthcare dollars."

A survey of California primary care physicians published in the *Journal of General Internal Medicine* found over half the physicians surveyed were not hostile to DM programs. The crucial element of a favorable program was that it decrease physician workload without decreasing income.

Physicians voice a number of concerns about DM programs:

- Whether outsourced to a corporate vendor or performed within a commercial health plan, the profit motive may be in conflict with meeting medical needs.
- The programs could be made to appear cost-effective by favorable selection, that is, dropping certain populations or diseases because of business considerations.
- Funds dedicated to DM programs could be taken from primary care physicians.
- The DM approach could lead to fragmentation of care if patients with multiple chronic diseases were treated in separate disease-specific programs.
- Primary care physicians who reduce their participation in the care of patients with chronic illness might lose clinical skills, and the physician–patient relationship would be undermined.
- There is a lack of well-designed peer-reviewed studies to support the claims of the DM vendors that their programs improve outcomes and reduce costs.

DM programs could be perceived as a desirable strategy for assisting busy primary care physicians to care for patients who require considerable attention and time. In-house DM programs that assist physicians in doing a better job at Lovelace Clinic, Kaiser-Permanente, University of Pennsylvania, Harvard Vanguard Medical, and the Henry Ford Health System have been well received by the physicians.

Welly is not optimistic about SMG developing its own DM programs. "Physicians lack the organizational expertise to make DM programs work. They also don't trust each other with things like this. It's very odd—they'd rather deal with an outsider, and rather still simply get paid more and let things stay as they are."

Physician organizations say compensation for DM is a tricky area that needs to be addressed. The 2,000-physician multispecialty Brown and Toland Medical Group in San Francisco scaled back its DM programs because insurers failed to compensate the group. The group's DM programs reduced overall costs by shifting care from the hospital to the physician's office. "Neither health plans nor employers rewarded us financially for these programs. As we managed these populations effectively and efficiently and hospital costs went down, there was more pressure to reduce the payments coming in to us," Welly says.

Superior Medical Group's Experience with Disease Management

Congestive Heart Failure (CHF)

SMG entered a contract with LifeMasters four years ago to provide a DM program for patients with Stage 3 and 4 heart failure. The program opened three years ago as a clinical trial; it enrolled 68 patients, mean age 73, monitored by 31 physicians. The first phase was an 18-month period in which SMG's baseline experience was documented. The second phase was an 18-month period in which enrolled patients received frequent telephone check-ins with an experienced nurse, who then initiated alerts to physicians when certain complaints or measurements indicated early signs of deterioration. The calculated savings after fees ($700 per patient per year) was approximately $480,000 due to prevented hospitalizations. Unfortunately, because of the financial structure of the hospital risk pools, the savings did not translate into additional income for SMG. Although the program saved almost half a million dollars, other costs pushed expenses over the global budget.

SMG physicians resisted the program because it incurred new costs in lean times. They resented outside commercial "skimmers," third-party intrusion into the doctor–patient relationship, and the implication that existing care was deficient. Physician acceptance was facilitated by the experimental study design, existence of credible previous studies showing improved outcomes in CHF with DM programs, and the time LifeMasters staff spent in visits and presentations. "Physician involvement from the outset was a critical component of the success, and response to physician criticisms greatly strengthened the program," Welly says. However, criticism from some physicians continued regarding cost ("Give me the money instead"), and "false alerts" that increased patient contacts and staff overhead, resulting in reluctance to refer newly identified patients and cynicism regarding SMG's administrative efforts in the quality improvement arena. Welly noted, "Physicians have a hard time understanding the global aspects of these systems. If they get no check, they become angry and consider the system a failure."

Welly joined SMG as the study period was ending. It was his first exposure to a commercial DM program and he was impressed with the results. There was, however, a serious structural flaw—lack of financial rewards at the level of the physicians' offices. The physicians were required to look at the alerts that came in from LifeMasters nurses, and respond to them, with no reimbursement for their time. He recognizes the resources LifeMasters brought that SMG lacked—the experienced personnel and the physical space in this rural area and the information systems. Nonetheless, he doesn't believe SMG would enter into the same partnership now; LifeMasters would have to take financial risk and financially reward the physicians for their cooperation.

Osteoporosis

With the support of a pharmaceutical grant and the technical assistance of a member rheumatologist, SMG developed a program to rationalize osteoporosis screening. SMG mailed osteoporosis patient education materials to all female enrollees above a certain age. Physicians were required to fill out a questionnaire to establish patient risk in order to refer a patient for a bone density study. The patient score on the questionnaire determined which, if any, study would be performed. The cost was $70,000; women at risk received appropriate osteoporosis screening, and inappropriate studies were reduced.

Diabetes

The current age-standardized prevalence of diabetes in the United States is 8 percent, a rising prevalence associated with increases in obesity and sedentary lifestyle. Diabetes is the leading cause of new cases of blindness in adults 20 to 74 years old. Approximately 500,000 hospitalizations per year list diabetes as the primary diagnosis. Cardiovascular disease, kidney failure, amputations, and ketoacidosis are complications that frequently require hospitalization. In 1997, more than 33,000 new cases of end-stage renal disease were attributed to diabetes. Long-term complications of diabetes can be prevented through glucose, lipid, and blood pressure regulation, and early detection and treatment of eye, foot, and kidney abnormalities. Improved patient education and self-management, and the provision of adequate and timely screening services and medical care, can prevent complications.

Last month SMG launched a patient education promotion project supported by a grant from Aventis, a producer of insulin. Using claims data, physician offices were prompted to refer their diabetic patients to the diabetes education program at Sisters Hospital. With grant funds, SMG financially rewarded cooperating physicians and their staffs.

Welly is on the steering committee of the California Cooperative Healthcare Reporting Initiative's (CCHRI) Diabetes Continuous Quality Improvement Project, a statewide collaborative to improve diabetes management. CCHRI is a program of the Pacific Business Group on Health, a large purchaser that negotiates rates with 12 HMOs for 21 companies. The mission of CCHRI is to measure performance and cooperate in quality improvement programs at the level of the physician group. SMG will be one of five medical groups participating in a pilot data-sharing project seeking to improve electronic data exchange between health plans and provider groups to routinely track services to diabetic patients.

CCHRI has developed basic guidelines for diabetes care (Table III.2), endorsed by all the major health plans. Welly's efforts to have the guidelines incorporated into practice are primarily a "consciousness elevation" approach, with frequent communications on the subject. He believes that close to 50 percent of SMG's diabetic patients receive care that fulfills most of the guidelines.

An endocrinologist and internist from Coast Medical Associates worked with SMG's intranet provider, Axolotl, to develop a computer-based

---

TABLE III.2
Components of Diabetes Disease Management

Periodic Physical and Emotional Assessment

- Blood pressure and weight each visit, adjust medications to control blood pressure
- Foot exam—visual exam every visit, pulses and neurological exam annually
- Dilated eye exam annually by ophthalmologist
- Depression screen annually—treat with counseling, medication, and/or referral
- Dental exam twice annually

Self-Management Training

- Assess patient knowledge of diabetes, medications, self-monitoring, and complications
- Home blood-sugar testing by patient, clinician reviews results
- Counsel on weight loss and nutrition, assess progress toward goals, and identify problem areas
- Smoking cessation—screen, advise, and assist
- Physical activity—assess and prescribe activity based on patient's needs/ condition

Laboratory Exams

- Hemoglobin A1C (marker for diabetic control) quarterly if not meeting goals, 1 to 2 times per year if stable, treat with diet and medication.
- Microalbuminuria (marker for early kidney disease) annually
- Blood lipids—treat aggressively with diet and medication; measure quarterly if not meeting goals, annually if stable

decision support diabetes program that would have provided clinical reminders in patient charts. However, because Axolotl is restructuring to focus on Web-based upgrades, the SMG program has been delayed. The Web-based program is expected to be expensive.

SMG collects data on the monitoring of diabetes patients, both to comply with the Healthcare Effectiveness Data and Information Set and for its own quality management. SMG has provided written feedback reports to physicians regarding their performance in diabetes care, but this is difficult using claims data only.

SMG Support for Disease Management (DM)

Welly's involvement with DM is still a fairly lonely crusade. "The physicians don't know what is going on in the larger field." Welly believes it is politically impossible to take money out of patient care revenue to invest in a DM program, whatever the return on investment or guaranteed savings. SMG currently shares financial risk for hospitalizations with HMOs. A budget is negotiated with each HMO based on historical utilization rates and blended with regional utilization rates. The difference in hospital costs above or below budget is evenly divided between SMG and the HMO.

HMOs are insisting medical groups implement disease management. HMOs have an "extremely condescending attitude to physician groups because it takes physicians so long to get anything done," Welly says, so HMOs contract with commercial vendors or have their own DM divisions. Some DM companies are willing to share financial risk with health plans.

Commercial Diabetes DM Programs

McKesson CareEnhance, Pfizer Health Solutions InformaCare, Merck & Co., Inc., Health Management Services, American Healthways, Health Management Corporation Healthy Returns, Cor Solutions, and Matria are a few diabetes DM vendors. The programs are variations on a basic design of population assessment and data analysis, predictive modeling to stratify patients into high and low risk, targeted interventions, physician communications, and tracking utilization data.

Diabetes Healthways uses an engagement model, aggressively contacting patients. The company projects a $1.5 million annual diabetes care savings for an average 100,000-member commercial HMO. A retrospective analysis of 7,000 patients in its NetCare program found a $50 per member per month savings in diabetes treatment costs over 12 months and an 18 percent drop in hospital admissions.

Matria refers to the scientific literature to support claims of clinical effectiveness and economic benefit. The Diabetes Control and Complications Trial concluded that intensive management focused on reducing hemoglobin A1C levels in patients with type 1 diabetes prevented or delayed the onset of complications and significantly reduced the impact of these complications. The United Kingdom Prospective Diabetes Study reached similar conclusions for patients with type 2 diabetes. "A 1997 study concluded that reducing hemoglobin A1C from 9 percent to 7 percent reduced average diabetes-related medical costs by $1,200 per patient," Welly says. However, this study by Gilmer did not compare pre- and post-DM program medical costs; it was a retrospective analysis that found charges for medical care from 1993 to 1995 were closely related to patients' hemoglobin A1C levels in 1992.

As Welly reflected on his recommendation to the board, he wondered whether it was his role to get physician buy-in on DM programs, or whether he should limit his efforts to what was necessary for compliance with HMO contracts. He wanted to be realistic about how much he could expect to accomplish given the low level of integration of the independent physician offices. He wasn't sure whether a DM program would increase SMG revenue, savings, or costs. How would SMG pay for the increased coordination and intensity of services to patients with chronic illness? Welly had been successful with small pharmaceutical grants and hoped to realize larger grants, knowing the large resources of pharmaceutical companies and the incentive they have to fund programs that would increase the sales of their products. He didn't think this presented a conflict of interest, or an ethical dilemma, but wasn't sure he should push for a DM program not knowing with certainty that the funding would be available.

Case Questions

1. Would a diabetes DM program increase SMG revenue, savings, or costs?
2. What is it about the organizational structure and culture of an IPA that facilitates or blocks quality improvement?
3. Should Welly recommend to the SMG board of directors that it contract for a diabetes DM program? Should he recommend that the organization develop its own, with or without a partner?
    • If yes, how could Dr. Welly increase support from SMG physicians and management for DM programs?
    • If no, what should Dr. Welly recommend to the board to improve SMG's diabetes management?
4. Is the diabetes DM program a strategic decision?

Case I
Selling an Evidence-Based Design for Waterford Hospital

Nathan Burt and Ann Scheck McAlearney

Campeon Health is a Midwestern healthcare system composed of five hospitals, ten affiliated hospitals, and an extensive ambulatory care network. Given favorable demographics and a strong bottom line, Campeon Health has recently decided to construct a new hospital in Waterford, a suburb of the larger Grouse Creek metropolitan area. In all, Grouse Creek currently contains three major hospital systems and a children's hospital, but despite steady population growth, new hospitals have been scarce. The Campeon Health facility would be the region's first newly constructed hospital in over 22 years.

The Waterford suburb was considered an ideal site for the new hospital due to the wealth of the surrounding area and the growing population. In fact, Waterford boasted the highest number of children per household for the Grouse Creek metropolitan area. Contributing to the location decision was the fact that Campeon Health currently drew few patients from the Waterford area to its other hospitals due to the presence of closer competitor hospitals. Campeon's projections suggested that Waterford Hospital could draw 70 percent of its patients from among those presently receiving service outside the Campeon Health system. In addition, Campeon predicted that the new hospital would be received favorably by local physicians, including those practicing at other Campeon Health facilities. Planned to be a 90-bed community hospital, Waterford could serve as a feeder hospital for the system's large flagship hospital, Lakeside Hospital, while accommodating the preferences of physicians interested in expanding their practices to include the Waterford community.

The Charge

Prior to breaking ground for the new facility, Katherine Humphries, RN, had been appointed president of Waterford Hospital. Humphries had worked as CEO of another Campeon Health hospital for three years, and had established a strong reputation as a transformational leader. She has been charged by the board of Campeon Health and the Campeon Health CEO to lead the initiative to design, construct, staff, and operate the new community hospital in Waterford. At the present time, the Waterford Hospital site is nothing more than a field, located across the street from an existing Campeon Health ambulatory care center.

Humphries has been given relatively free rein to design the hospital. Humphries's years of experience as a registered nurse and as an operations leader have given her valuable insights into the delivery of care and ways that it can be improved. She is aware that elements of evidence-based design have been shown to improve care quality for patients and workplace climate for caregivers, and she is eager to consider this approach.

Evidence-Based Design

Evidence-based design is being used increasingly by hospitals that are trying to improve staff morale, patients' experiences, and the outcomes of care provided. Evidence-based healthcare designs are specifically used to create environments that are therapeutic, supportive of family involvement, efficient for staff performance, and restorative for workers under stress. Ultimately, evidence-based healthcare designs should result in demonstrated improvements in the organization's clinical outcomes, economic performance, productivity, customer satisfaction, and cultural measures. However, this healthcare design approach is a relatively new concept. The pool of available research and information will rarely fit a hospital's situation precisely, thus requiring critical consideration of specific design modifications and project goals.

In healthcare, the application of evidence-based design is particularly appropriate. Physicians are accustomed to practicing, at least in part, using evidence-based clinical guidelines and measures, thus the notion of applying evidence to facility design may be well received. Further, design principles focusing on the physical characteristics of facilities design that may reduce patient stress and contribute to the healing process appeal to patients and families who are likely familiar with the stressful and often frightening experiences that are common to hospital stays. Hospitals themselves have been shown to benefit economically from reduced costs and increased organizational effectiveness when applying the principles of evidence-based design (Saba and Hamilton 2006).

Evidence-based design principles include many elements of building design, several of which have been demonstrated to be effective. In particular, exposure to sunlight, access to nature through direct access or views, acuity-adaptable rooms, and decentralized nurses' stations are design elements that hold promise. For instance, studies have shown that climate and exposure to sunlight can influence the length of a patient's stay. One research group randomly assigned bipolar patients to sunny rooms and others to rooms with less exposure to sunlight. The patients who were exposed to greater amounts of sunlight had a mean length of stay 3.67 days shorter than the control group. Similarly, patients recovering from abdominal surgery had shorter hospital stays if they had a bedside window view of nature rather than windows that looked out onto a brick wall (Ulrich et al. 2004).

Another promising feature of evidence-based design is the potential for well-designed rooms and buildings to improve clinical outcomes. In fact, the list of examples such as lower rates of acquired infections, fewer medication errors, fewer patient falls, and reduced patient stress are growing (Ulrich et al. 2004). Something as simple as placing an alcohol hand rub dispenser at the patient's bedside can yield significant improvements in practitioners' hand-washing practices, thereby reducing contact infection rates. Evidence-based design can also help to reduce medication errors by focusing on care delivery elements such as lighting, environmental distractions, and workflow interruptions that may increase medication administration errors. Patient falls can also be reduced when patient rooms are well-designed, and good building design can reduce noise levels, thereby reducing stress levels for patients and their caregivers (Ulrich et al. 2004).

Acuity-Adaptable Rooms

A key component of evidence-based design in hospitals is the acuity-adaptable room. While the more common universal patient room has gained popularity because of its potential to accommodate clinical needs and new technologies as future care delivery innovations are introduced, such patient rooms are still used in the traditional clinical manner, necessitating patient transfers between rooms, units, and floors when patient acuity changes. In contrast, the acuity-adaptable room is designed to accommodate a wide range of patient acuity levels, thus reducing the need to transfer patients and change the care delivery workflow (Brown and Gallant 2006).

Acuity-adaptable rooms are private rooms that are composed of a patient area, a staff area, and a family area. Evidence-based design principles are applied to the layout of acuity-adaptable rooms, thus maximizing the likelihood of care improvements to be gained from these principles. For example, a private room is quieter than a shared room, thereby potentially reducing patient and caregiver stress. Space dedicated to a family area permits social contact with family and friends to further improve the healing process (Brown and Gallant 2006). Bathrooms are situated on a headwall with rails leading to them, potentially reducing the likelihood of patient falls. In addition, the accommodation of family and friends within patient rooms on a 24-hour basis reduces the possibility of patients falling, and can also reduce patient stress.

An acuity-adaptable room design helps solve some of the problems with bottlenecks in patient flow that occur daily in most hospitals. These bottlenecks can have several negative consequences, including diversions to other hospitals or warehousing patients in hallways without adequate monitoring and nursing care. Within traditional hospitals, patient flow revolves around nursing units, which are generally organized by diagnosis type. Diagnosis type is, in turn, influenced by three factors: (1) the headwall capability to accommodate lines and gases; (2) the clinical skills of the nurse to treat different levels of acuity; and (3) the historically variable reimbursement from the Centers for Medicare & Medicaid Services (Hendrich et al. 2004). This mix of considerations about diagnosis type and nursing unit results in assignment of patients to units based on the unit's capacity to accept patients with a particular diagnosis and level of acuity. As a result, this traditional nursing unit–centric model contributes to situations where a bed may be available, but it is not the "right" bed for that particular patient. This then causes a patient flow bottleneck. Further, because many patients experience variable levels of acuity during a hospital stay, the nursing unit–centric model may also result in patients being transferred three to six times during the course of their stays (Hendrich et al. 2004). The additional coordination required by multiple transfers then increases the complexity of patient flow within the hospital and further contributes to bottlenecks. Also, as explained by Brown and Gallant (2006), "the transfer process is not a clinically benign process and has been shown to cause physiologic and psychologic distress that could lead to negative clinical outcomes." By targeting areas such as bed placement, communication, and housecleaning efficiency, slight improvements can be made within the current model of care, but a different model must be adopted to permit large gains in quality and efficiency (Hendrich et al. 2004).

A Growing Evidence Base

Improvements in clinical and patient satisfaction outcomes associated with the introduction of acuity-adaptable rooms were starting to be documented. In particular, Humphries was intrigued by two examples reported in the recent research literature where adoption of acuity-adaptable rooms had been linked to positive outcomes. These examples are described in Sidebar III.1.

Decentralized Nurse Stations

Another opportunity that has emerged out of the principles of evidence-based design is to develop decentralized nurse stations. In practice, the layout of hospitals has not changed much in decades, despite the fact that the jobs of nurses, physicians, and other caregivers have changed significantly. According to one recent study, nurses spend approximately 30 percent of their time

SIDEBAR III.1
Examples of Acuity-Adaptable Models in U.S. Hospitals

An Acuity-Adaptable Comprehensive Critical Coronary Care Floor at Clarian Health

Clarian Health, based in Indianapolis, Indiana, switched from a traditional model of care to an acuity-adaptable model in coronary care by building an acuity-adaptable comprehensive critical coronary care (CCCC) floor. The acuity-adaptable CCCC is capable of performing all necessary care in one room, from admission to discharge (Brown and Gallant 2006). Using a pre-post design to evaluate the success of this model, Clarian recorded two years of baseline data and then compared clinical outcomes after CCCC adoption with these baseline data.

During the baseline period, the two units that were to become the CCCC had an average of 200 intra-unit transfers per month. The time spent coordinating transfers, processing paperwork, and transporting the patient were all considered to be non–value added activities that would be better spent in direct patient care. In addition, these 200 handoffs per month elevated the risk of medical errors associated with handoffs.

After moving to an acuity-adaptable model of care, intra-unit transfers were cut by 90 percent (Hendrich et al. 2004). Also noteworthy, medication errors were cut by 70 percent, likely due at least partially to the reduction in patient handoffs and transfers. Finally, patient falls decreased to a national benchmark level, and patient satisfaction increased overall (Hendrich et al. 2004).

An Acuity-Adaptable Model Implemented at Celebration Health

Celebration Health, based in Orlando, Florida, implemented an acuity-adaptable model within its new facility and saw marked improvements in clinical outcomes. In particular, patients' lengths of stay for most diagnosis-related groups (DRGs) declined significantly after introduction of the acuity-adaptable model. Comparing data with another state, Celebration Health reported that the average length of stay for five specific DRGs in its system was 5.4 days, compared to 9.5 days reported in the state of California. Thirty percent of Celebration Health patients with those five DRGs were discharged within four days. These length-of-stay improvements occurred with simultaneous reductions in nursing hours per patient day (Gallant and Lanning 2001).

walking around the hospital, and less than 60 percent of their time on actual patient care (Ulrich et al. 2004).

A typical nursing unit has a central nurse station with the rooms laid out in a double corridor rectangular pattern around the nurse station. This nurse station typically houses a unit clerk, provides an area for nurses to do their chart work, and accommodates the medical records of the unit's patients. A change in the layout of a floor can increase the amount of time nurses are able to be involved in direct patient care by reducing requirements for walking around. In fact, nurses working in a radial unit walk much less than nurses working in a rectangular unit (Ulrich et al. 2004). Nurses on a floor with decentralized nurse stations walk even less than those nurses working in a radial unit, as long as supplies are decentralized as well. This decentralized nurse station model thus presents many opportunities to improve the quality and efficiency of care provided, by reducing the amount of wasted time nurses spend walking around and freeing nursing time to provide direct patient care.

Implementation Challenges

Evidence-based design options such as acuity-adaptable rooms and decentralized nurse stations have tremendous potential to improve the quality of patient care, but there are also substantial challenges associated with implementation. In particular, staffing using an acuity-adaptable model of care can be difficult. Nurses tend to practice within a specialty because they enjoy the specialty. For instance, a critical care nurse is typically very good at handling urgent situations, but often lacks the skills required to manage large numbers of patients, including providing required patient education and communicating with families. Similarly, telemetry nurses are often skilled at managing large numbers of patients, providing patient education, and dealing with patients' families, but they may lack the skills necessary to handle high-acuity patients (Brown and Gallant 2006). Critical care nurses staffed to work in an acuity-adaptable environment with decentralized nurse stations may feel uncomfortable if they do not have another critical care nurse within sight in the event that an emergency arises, or if they want to consult with another comparably trained nurse about a complex patient.

The Role of Technology

Technology can help overcome some of the challenges surrounding implementation of evidence-based design options such as acuity-adaptable rooms and decentralized nurse stations. For instance, in order for a decentralized nurse station to be successful, it must be completely independent of the central nurse station. All required supplies and technology, including computer access, must be available at the decentralized nurse station. Wireless communications, automated patient call and alarms, medication administration, and even linens must be available at the nurse station (Brown and Gallant 2006). Technology solutions can help to support these requirements, but their use has not yet been widespread.

In practice, a robust computerized physician order entry (CPOE) system can help to overcome some of the challenges presented by decentralized nurse stations. A CPOE system that is linked to all areas of the hospital can house test results and facilitate physicians' ordering of required tests and studies while also helping nurses to manage their patients effectively. While a unit clerk in a centralized nurse unit coordinates tests and studies with other departments, a CPOE system eliminates the need for this unit clerk on the nursing floor, thus reducing some of the barriers associated with adopting a decentralized nurse station model.

Technology can also help to improve communications in a decentralized nurse unit model. When patients have high acuity levels, communication between and among nurses may be problematic if nurse stations are decentralized within the hospital. However, technology can help caregivers communicate quickly and thoroughly with each other, even in a decentralized environment. For instance, new technologies such as smart beds, smart pumps, and specific clinical alarms can be adopted to improve patient monitoring and facilitate patient-related communications within this decentralized nurse unit model.

Financial Implications

Construction costs per square foot for an evidence-based design building are not much higher than for a traditional building, but increased costs should be considered. First, overall construction costs would be higher due to the modifications in architectural designs necessary to introduce sunlight within 95 percent of the building, and due to the larger square footage required for acuity-adaptable rooms compared to traditional room sizes. From a design standpoint, introducing sunlight could be tricky for internal spaces. One solution is to build gardens within the core spaces of a building. While such gardens tend to be expensive, they do offer very visible areas for community support, and are often selected due to their ability to contribute to the healing environment. With respect to room size, acuity-adaptable rooms must be able to accommodate a large range of equipment and have space for family members. As a result, acuity-adaptable rooms may be 30 to 50 percent larger than traditional single-occupancy rooms.

From an operating standpoint, any differences in operating costs associated with an acuity-adaptable model of care are still unclear. While the skill sets required for nurses on acuity-adaptable units may be higher, it is possible that higher staff costs may be associated with shorter lengths of stay linked to improved patient well-being. It is also possible that a higher level of management may be required to oversee complicated staffing needs associated with an acuity-adaptable model of care, but this may be offset by less demand for management given a higher level of skill among staff. In contrast to outstanding questions about changes in human resources costs, it is clear that an evidence-based design can reduce costs associated with utilities, since the availability of sunlight throughout the building will reduce electricity costs. Similarly, maintenance and supplies costs are typically reduced due to standardization of equipment and supplies throughout the hospital.

Capitalizing on the Opportunity

Humphries is convinced that an evidence-based design model will be appropriate for the design of Waterford Hospital. Working with the hospital architect and contractor, Humphries has been able to outline an evidence-based design for Waterford Hospital that includes components such as acuity-adaptable patient rooms, decentralized nurse units, and liberal use of windows and open spaces to provide patients and their families with access to nature. The latest version of the architectural drawings features all private rooms for patients, with each room including a family area designed to contain a couch/bed, a refrigerator, and a separate television for the families. In addition, gardens are planned for both inside and outside the hospital, with easy access points for patients, family, and hospital staff. Staff and families will also have access to respite areas, which are spaces individuals can go to relieve stress and deal with difficult situations and decisions. Finally, all patient areas, and 95 percent of other hospital space, are designed to have access to direct or indirect sunlight.

Overall, Humphries is pleased with the preliminary plans for Waterford Hospital, but she knows she has a long way to go to convince hospital staff and physicians accustomed to working in traditional hospital environments that the evidence-based design model is sound and desirable. In fact, moving forward with an evidence-based design is risky if she does not get key stakeholders on board. She knows her next step is to build support for the application of an evidence-based design for Waterford Hospital, but she doesn't have much time.

Case Questions

1. Who are the key stakeholders who must support Humphries's vision for an evidence-based hospital design? How would you obtain their support?
2. What reactions might you predict from physicians regarding the use of evidence-based design at Waterford Hospital? How about from members of the Waterford community? The Grouse Creek community? Other local hospitals and health systems?
3. What challenges do you think Humphries and the leadership team at Waterford Hospital will face as they try to implement an acuity-adaptable model of care?

References

Brown, K. K., and D. Gallant. 2006. "Impacting Patient Outcomes Through Design: Acuity Adaptable Care/Universal Room Design." *Critical Care Nursing Quarterly* 29 (4): 326–41.

Gallant, D., and K. Lanning. 2001. "Streamlining Patient Care Processes Through Flexible Room and Equipment Design." *Critical Care Nursing Quarterly* 24 (3): 59–76.

Hendrich, A. L., J. Fay, and A. K. Sorrells. 2004. "Effects of Acuity-Adaptable Rooms on Flow of Patients and Delivery of Care." *American Journal of Critical Care.* 13 (1): 35–45.

Saba, J., and K. Hamilton. 2006. "The Bottom Line on Evidence-Based Design." Presentation at American College of Healthcare Executives Congress, Chicago. [Accessed online on 4/14/09: http://www.healtharchitects.org/uploaded /ACHE_Presentation_Part_2_Evidence_Based_Design.pdf].

Ulrich, R., X. Quan, C. Zimring, A. Joseph, and R. Choudhary. 2004. Unpublished paper presented at the American Institute of Architects, Academy of Architecture for Health, virtual seminar on healing environments.

Short Case 12
A Proposal for the Restructuring of Wise Medical Center

Anthony R. Kovner

This proposal is written by Sam Spellman, chief operating officer of Wise Medical Center.

Wise Medical Center (WMC), a 700-bed urban hospital, faces the enormous challenge of delivering healthcare in an external environment full of chaos and change. Will the existing organizational structure provide enough agility, adaptability, and swiftness to maintain or surpass its current position in the marketplace (financially sound, clinically respected, etc.)?

I would argue that one response is to redesign our hospital into a manageable number of smaller, more autonomous business entities. WMC would be divided into at least the following businesses, all linked to the whole through a set of accountabilities and organizational structure and support. The businesses would be:

- The Surgical Hospital
- The Private Attending Medical Hospital
- The General Medical Hospital
- The Maternal and Child Health Hospital
- Ambulatory Care
- Psychiatric and Substance Abuse
- Rehabilitation
- Clinical Support (radiology, lab, etc.)
- Corporate Services—with potentially several subcompanies (to include food services, housekeeping, security, training, human resources, information systems, etc.)

Each of the major entities would be led by a chief operating officer or jointly led by a high-level administrative leader and a physician. These leaders would be charged with the integrity, bottom-line performance, quality assurance, development, and implementation of a set of strategic and long-range objectives, and each would be accountable to the central management of WMC.

Sam Spellman convened a meeting of top managers to discuss his proposal for restructuring WMC. Highlights from their discussion follow:

Tony Rivers (vice president of finance): Don't we have enough on our minds without drastically reorganizing patient care services?

Paul Bones (chief of medicine): How are we going to factor in our teaching and research objectives and strategies?

Pam Ewing (VP of nursing): Where does the nursing service figure in all this restructuring? You're going to put the doctors in charge of the nurses, and I'm not sure that doctors ought to be telling nurses what to do or how we can best work together.

Tom Starks (VP of human resources): How are you going to bring the unions into this kind of restructuring?

Lew Oakley (director of planning): Sam, are you suggesting that we could start contracting out a service like our planning department? Wouldn't this create a lot of uncertainty among my staff, who are doing the best possible job that they know how to do?

Carl Smith (CEO): What worries me about your proposal is (1) We're under tremendous pressure to do other things such as raise capital for a new inpatient facility and cut costs to respond to payers. (2) Who else at WMC wants to push for this proposal? (3) Do you medical chiefs really have the skills and experience to run these mini-hospitals?

Case Questions:

1. What evidence is needed to answer Carl Smith's questions?
2. How can the key obstacles to restructuring be overcome?
3. What would you advise Sam Spellman to do? Why? How?

Short Case 13
A Hospitalist Program for Plateau University Hospital

Jeff Weiss

Plateau University Hospital is a large academic medical center in a major urban area. In order to survive in a competitive and economically challenging geographic market, Plateau built upon a strategy of inpatient volume growth. Each time the volume grew, it increased capacity through savings in reduced length of stay (LOS). This allowed the hospital to meet ambitious budgetary goals and realize the desired growth and profit targets.

To accomplish this, Plateau has made some dramatic strides in efficiency over the past five years. However, executives feel that much of the low-hanging fruit has been picked and further progress and additional opportunities for LOS reduction will require greater creativity. When looking at further opportunities to reduce LOS while maintaining their mission to deliver high-quality patient care, Plateau leadership is exploring the idea of building upon their small hospitalist group. Currently, there is a four-person hospitalist group, which manages the inpatients of a small proportion of the hospital-owned office group practices. These hospitalists have a reduced LOS compared to other doctors and are perceived to deliver high-quality and accessible care. Is there more opportunity here?

Plateau leadership has begun to read about the growth in hospitalist programs across the country and has heard about their potential to improve efficiency and quality of inpatient care. On the other hand, they also have heard that these programs have potential problems with hiring and retention as many doctors see them as temporary "burnout jobs" for recent graduates. The current crop of four doctors seems to fit this profile. The four hospitalists have been working a lot of weekends and morale is low. While they are running their own program, they reportedly have insufficient support or leadership.

To take on the challenge of building the hospitalist group, the hospital hires an energetic but inexperienced physician leader. Dr. Angel Young is ambitious, and he realizes he got the job largely because others may not have wanted the position. However, he sees this as a real turnaround opportunity. After the first few meetings with the hospitalist group, Young realizes he has an uphill battle. In spite of the negatives associated with their current situation, the four hospitalists are still resistant to change and appear resistant to Young's new authority.

Young immerses himself in the job and tries to experience the hospitalist role as the four practitioners do. He is a hands-on leader who studied the workflow and processes in which his group operated. He also networks with leaders at other hospitals and joins national hospitalist groups to develop a better understanding of the landscape for this growing specialty. He knows that in order to be successful, he needs support both from hospital administration above and from the four hospitalists below. After a few months, he is able to list the challenges and opportunities associated with building a successful hospitalist program:

Challenges

- Low morale—"ignored," "overworked," "underpaid"
- Difficult personalities—"us versus the world" culture
- Resistance to change
- Revolving door of leaders—"why trust this one?"
- Reputation as "burnout job"
- Lack of administrative structure—no organized schedule, no moonlighting (coverage) pool for nights and weekends
- Loosely supervised and inefficient—no real boss, few metrics, little accountability
- Rapid growth—no strategic plan to recruit and retain hospitalist providers

Opportunities

- Harness institutional need for hospitalist services
- Provide attention to hospitalists/gain trust
- Job redesign—make it sustainable with possibility for upward mobility
- Create room for career development—add academic opportunities, research support
- Create administrative structure—take out of hands of frontline physicians
- Process improvement—remove irritants in the system
- Create proper incentives—bonus plan with quality and efficiency measures
- Utilize information technology capabilities—improve workflow and provide data to drive productivity
- Expansion—infuse new people and attitudes

With support from Plateau administration, Young begins to tackle these challenges and initiate the change campaign. However, Young does not move too quickly and impulsively with respect to change. He knows he needs a few "short-term wins" to begin the cultural change process and build support from both the group and his bosses. Developing a fair bonus plan with proper incentives is an effective early step that garners significant support. In addition, monthly hospitalist lectures are added to the hospital's lecture schedule. This conveys a concern for career development and provides a venue for education and team building among the hospitalists.

Equally important among Young's early steps is quickly building a moonlighting pool. This effort wrestles away a large chip of informal power that the hospitalists previously wielded. Through a new call system and some strategic process improvements, the hospitalists are also able to be more efficient and productive. The number of admissions per FTE increases and the LOS for the hospitalists' patients improves. These positive results attract additional support from hospital administration to help energize the initial push and withstand any resistance around the change efforts.

While the first six months are rough and not without tension and resistance, the initiative seems headed in the right direction. Young works with his hospitalist group to ensure that they maintain their initial momentum by communicating about goals and accomplishments, encouraging teamwork, and creating a strategic vision for the hospitalist service at Plateau University Hospital.

Case Questions

1. What are the challenges a new leader faces when trying to implement change?

2. How can Dr. Young best approach this difficult group of doctors?
3. What are the key elements in building a successful hospitalist program, and how can Plateau build a sustainable model that will be attractive enough to recruit and retain physicians?
4. What kinds of data and metrics might a hospitalist leader need to run his group and track progress and success?
5. What is senior leadership looking for from Dr. Young and his group, and how can they best deliver on these expectations in order to ensure ongoing support and resources for their program?

Short Case 14
Integrating Rehabilitation Services into the Visiting Nurse Service of America

Jacob Victory

Over the last century, the Visiting Nurse Service of America (VNSA) has grown into a national home care entity. Serving 750,000 patients in 15 states annually and employing 25,000 nurses, therapists, social workers, and home health aides, VNSA earns a 5 percent profit margin on a $3 billion revenue base and has a conservative management team that monitors business and care quality targets. These divisions primarily serve the frail elderly, with thriving programs that focus on the homebound long-term care population, targeting the vulnerable Medicaid and dually eligible populations. Growing at an 8 percent rate, VNSA is proud of its current market prominence and of its origins as a nursing-based home care organization.

Indeed, nurses are considered each patient's primary case coordinator, and from the CEO down to the nursing team leaders, nurses dominate the organization's culture and all levels of its decision-making processes, business strategy, resource allocation, and marketing. In fact, all but the Rehabilitation Services division has a nurse at its head.

Rehabilitation Services

VNSA's Rehabilitation Services (Rehab) is the black sheep of the organization. It employs 3,500 physical, occupational, and speech therapists and serves about 65 percent of VNSA's patients. Rehab is considered a pseudo-program, as it was carved out of the larger, skilled nursing–focused agency.

The program reports to the vice president of operations, a clinician who is in charge of a dozen nursing-dominated programs. Yet, it is an ancillary service that is not on the senior staff's immediate radar. In fact, the program is noticed only occasionally, particularly if a therapist is late in serving a "VIP" patient or if there is a perceived "rehab emergency" with an orthopedic patient.

VNSA patients who need rehabilitation services are primarily referred to Rehab by intake nurses and nurse care coordinators. And while the organization has developed nursing teams, led by a nurse manager and clinical support staff, therapists are not integrated into these teams. Although therapists are informally invited to the team meetings, the meeting agendas are strictly nursing-focused, and rehab-specific issues are never addressed. Moreover, Rehab has a thin management staff. Each rehab manager supervises up to 50 therapists (each with a caseload of up to 20 patients), while each nursing manager supervises no more than 10 nurses. In the marketing realm, VNSA's advertisements all focus on nurses providing care, even in scenarios where a rehabilitation need is clearly depicted. This is, after all, a visiting *nurse* organization.

Jeanine Bastian, the new rehabilitation administrator, notices these issues immediately. With over 25 years of experience in running hospital, nursing home, and now home-based rehab programs, Jeanine has a doctorate in occupational therapy and is a fun-loving but no-nonsense leader. She received the mandate to grow Rehab and to bring the program "to the next level" to ensure innovation and market dominance of home-based rehabilitation services. VNSA's president accepts Jeanine's plan to bring in new management talent and a calculated effort is planned to change the culture and mind-set of the Rehab division, particularly since the program has been plagued by poor management over the past decade.

Over the next year, two directors of finance and operations are hired, and a new clinical director who is responsible for quality improvement and staff training and education. New business, financial, quality, and workforce-related metrics are developed and monitored monthly. The clinical staff is reorganized into cohesive teams, and education and retraining sessions are designed to teach clinical best practices. Scorecards are developed to monitor outcomes and service utilization. An informal Rehab-specific profit and loss statement is monitored quarterly to trend revenues and expenses.

The analysis reveals that the program has annual revenues of over $450 million and a net profit margin of 20 percent (the next most profitable program within VNSA has a margin of 4 percent). The finance and operations directors hold the Rehab managers of each state accountable for meeting targets and ensuring growth. Accountability is the new catch-phrase, and 50 percent of Rehab's management team resigns within seven months, complaining about how often "Big Brother" is watching. More seasoned Rehab managers are immediately hired, instilling new management vigor. Though the program has been historically under-noticed, one powerful nurse executive wryly notes in a meeting, "Rehab is sure making some noise these days."

Undeniably, the noise is quite loud. The program enjoys a 22 percent growth in admissions. Bastiane persuades prominent orthopedic surgeons to refer their patients to VNSA, something the business development staff could not do. Better results than the current year are projected, and the program is highly rated with respect to employee satisfaction. There is even talk of marketing a distinct "VNSA Rehabilitation Medicine" program.

Yet, the "noise" is accompanied by what Bastiane calls "success woes," which, ironically, stem from the notable growth. The program is not getting the financial and human resources needed to sustain its growth rate.

First, while it brought in a $90 million profit for the organization, Rehabilitation has no voice in how this profit is allocated. This money is put in an agency-wide pool and used to subsidize the deficit-ridden programs and to fund investments in technology and new clinical programs.

Second, each therapist dictates where and when he or she will serve patients; any change in the service area that the therapists believed they "own" is met with raised eyebrows, veiled threats to leave the agency, and adamant resistance. Now, however, the productivity and service utilization of each therapist is the focus of a major quality improvement initiative, and each therapist is monitored to ensure that targeted weekly visit quotas are met (in order to meet demand). This additional focus has the frontline staff nervous and cautious.

Third, there are not enough management and supervisory staff to monitor the clinicians. The added stress of assigning cases, monitoring utilization, reorganizing into teams, and focusing on quality of care and outcomes wears down an already thinly spread management staff.

Finally, executive administration requests that in addition to growth, the program develop "rehabilitation packages" to sell to managed care companies, orthopedic hospitals, and specific targeted populations such as wealthy, private-paying clientele. Without additional investment in management talent and tools to monitor growth and quality, and given the historically nurse-friendly environment at VNSA, Bastiane and her team have more than a few balls to juggle.

Bastiane chews on her pencil as she leans back in her chair. Her office is quiet—her thoughts are not.

Case Questions

1. How was Rehabilitation Services viewed before Bastiane was named administrator? How is this different from how it was viewed a year after her appointment?
2. What are Bastiane's three key management challenges that she must tackle first?
3. How would you advise Bastiane to better integrate Rehabilitation Services within VNSA?
4. How should Bastiane sell the case to obtain more financial and human resources?
5. How can she influence changing the current "nursing culture" to be more a "clinical culture"?

Short Case 15
Matrix or Mess?

Ann Scheck McAlearney

Carol is very excited about her newest job change. After serving as a quality improvement (QI) manager for the past two years, she will finally be able to put her expertise in both nursing and informatics to use by taking on a new role as a clinical informaticist for the hospital. While it seemed she had been in school forever, her experience as a nurse combined with her undergraduate degree in informatics and plenty of on-the-job training in quality improvement has given her a broad perspective about how information technology could be usefully implemented to improve the quality of care provided at Valley Community Hospital.

This new job, though, while seemingly a great fit on paper, also makes Carol a bit nervous. In her prior role in QI she had reported to a single director. Her new position gave her a second boss, the director of information systems (IS) for the hospital. In a so-called matrix design, Carol reports to both directors, and is responsible for satisfying them both.

In fact, the IS department as a whole is a matrixed department within the hospital. This organizational design for IS had been introduced because of the combination of functional and project responsibilities involved in each IS initiative. The functional areas of the department, such as budgeting, hiring, and training, are consistent, regardless of project. However, IS project responsibilities vary based on the nature of the project and the other hospital

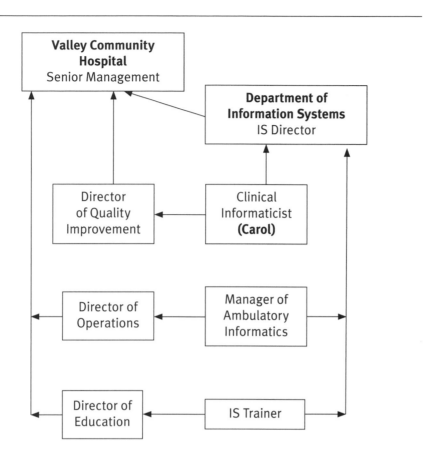

FIGURE III.6
The
Information
Systems
Department's
Matrix Design

department(s) involved. For instance, a project to install a new drug delivery system for the hospital would have particular project-related needs associated with working with the department of pharmacy, as well as IS department needs related to staffing, accounting, and so forth. As a result, each IS manager always reports to two directors, the IS director and another hospital director, based on the clinical or other operational departments served. One prominent example Carol was aware of was that the manager of ambulatory informatics reported to both the director of IS and the director of operations for the hospital. Even the IS trainers have two bosses, as they report to the IS director and the director of education for the hospital. Figure III.6 shows examples of these reporting relationships, as well as where Carol's new role fits.

To Carol, this matrix arrangement for IS and QI seems to make sense given the shared goals and objectives of clinical informatics and QI within the hospital. Yet she suspects issues could arise. Carol wants to make sure she is clear about each of her boss's expectations of her and her new role, but she isn't sure how to make this transition from her original single boss to a dual reporting relationship.

Case Questions

1. What issues will Carol likely face in reporting to two bosses?
2. Does the matrix organizational design make sense for this hospital's IS department, or would another design be more appropriate? What would you propose?
3. What strategies can Carol use to perform well in her new role without feeling pulled in two directions?

IV

PROFESSIONAL INTEGRATION

In the United States, the physician is
not so much part of the hospital as the
hospital is part (and only one part) of the
physician's practice.
—*Eliot Freidson*

Among the factors that have been associated
with good nursing performance are: flattening
of organizational structures; increased
professional status for staff nurses associated
with shared governance and increased autonomy
over practice and the practice environment; and
effective communication between nurses,
physicians and administrators.
—*Jack Needleman, Ellen Kurtzman, and Kenneth Kizer*

COMMENTARY

The integration of clinician and organizational goals is one of the key challenges facing managers in healthcare organizations today. The issues have become more complex as a larger number of physicians work for hospitals (e.g., hospitalists) and nurses aggressively pursue their goals, including more independence. The overriding goal that integrates each group's aim is improved patient service. For this to be a sufficient motivator, healthcare organizations must be held accountable for patient outcomes and service, with consequences (such as top managers losing their jobs) if standards are not met. These issues affect various types of organizations—hospitals, nursing homes, group practices, visiting nurse organizations, and health maintenance organizations—in different ways.

The issue can be framed in more standard labor relations terms, where managers negotiate contracts with unions or professional organizations representing workers. Hundreds of thousands of health workers are unionized, though relatively few physicians and nurses. There are over 200 different healthcare occupations, including many highly trained professionals other than physicians and nurses, such as optometrists, dentists, podiatrists, pharmacists, and physical therapists. For reasons of space, we shall concentrate here on relations between hospitals and physicians and nurses.

Hospitals and Physicians and Nurses

A study of the key drivers of physician loyalty concluded that clinical quality, efficiency, and convenient access were at the center of the physician agenda, with most hospitals not meeting physician standards as to operational efficiency and staff competency (Healthcare Advisory Board 1999). A more recent study found that fixing physician–hospital relationships is difficult, for several reasons: (1) financial incentives reward poor performance; (2) improvement efforts must confront decades of culture and tradition; and (3) there are never enough resources. The authors conclude that what physicians are concerned about are the core clinical services the hospital provides them and their patients (VHA Research Series 2004).

Lake (2007) posits eight domains of the nursing practice environment that combine factors related to job satisfaction and professional practice. These include autonomy; a philosophy of clinical care emphasizing quality; status of nursing, including empowered nursing leaders and organizational participation by nurses; recognition of and advancement based on nurse preparation and expertise; professional development; and supportive or collaborative relationships with managers, physicians, and peers (Lake 2007).

Some divergence among hospital and physician and nurse (and between physician and nurse) objectives is normal, and often helpful to hospital goals. Physicians and nurses are concerned with the best possible care for their patients. Managers are concerned with the best possible care for all patients and potential patients. A lack of divergence here may indicate a lack of sufficient manager, physician, or nurse response on behalf of their respective constituencies. If the divergence is too great, the result may be suboptimization, as physician and nurse objectives are achieved at the expense of hospital objectives or vice versa. But who will pay for achievement of all these goals? The managers say there isn't enough money to meet all the objectives of physicians and nurses. The physicians and nurses are often not persuaded by managers that there isn't enough money, particularly given the high salary many top hospital managers collect.

Physicians and nurses can expect from hospitals the following: a reasonable income and lifestyle, professional recognition, and participation in decision making (Griffith and White 2002). Of course, all workers want these kinds of working conditions; many of us cannot achieve them. What is a reasonable income anyway, relative to whose income? Some physicians and nurses can never get sufficient professional recognition. Some physicians and nurses do not want to participate in hospital decision making; others want to participate too much, given their limited skills and experience and given certain conflicts of interest. Bottom line, an important part of the manager's job is managing the expectations of physicians and nurses so that they will get a clearer, more realistic view of these issues. The goal is for all parties to see and hopefully move toward more of a win-win situation, although not at the expense of patients or of the tax- and premium-paying public.

Marketplace Considerations

These days, larger organizations are capturing more and more market share, in the hospital business, the group practice business, the nursing home business, the visiting nurse service business, and the health maintenance organization or insurance business. The size of firms selling to healthcare organizations is increasing. These firms include pharmaceutical and medical supply manufacturers, information hardware and software firms, outsourcing firms—such as dietary, laundry, emergency services, pharmacy, and physical therapy—and management consultants. Professional organizations representing physicians and nurses and other professionals do not seem to have similarly expanded their market share over the last ten years.

Larger organizations justify their increasing market share based on their capability to deliver superior outcomes in quality of care, cost of care, or access to care. Government and insurance companies have begun to reward provider organizations based on performance. Evidence is required to justify these claims. But certainly healthcare organizations are more likely to continue to grow and prosper when they do a better job in recruiting and retaining doctors and nurses, presumably because they have systems and supporting services and governance that result in higher quality patient care and better service to patients.

References

Griffith, J. R., and K. R. White. 2002. *The Well-Managed Healthcare Organization*, 5th edition. Chicago: Health Administration Press.

Healthcare Advisory Board. 1999. *The Physician Perspective: Key Drivers of Physician Loyalty.* Washington DC: Healthcare Advisory Board.

Lake, E. T. 2007. "The Nursing Practice Environment: Measurement and Evidence." *Medical Care Research and Review* 64 (2): 104S–22S.

VHA Research Series. 2004. *Physician Hospital Relationships: Forging the New Covenant.* Irving, TX: VHA.

THE READINGS

Cohn, Friedman, and Allyn posit that the silo mentality of leaving patient care to the doctors (and nurses) and finance and operations to the managers is doomed to fail in a fast-changing environment. They encourage managers to focus on improving clinical outcomes and allowing doctors (and nurses) to participate in resource allocation to achieve organizational goals. They suggest that patients and families should be at the center of everyone's concerns, which would make cultural change possible.

Griffith and White suggest that improved performance following the above approach will be increasingly recognized by customers, courts, and accrediting and payment agencies as the standard for all hospitals (and healthcare organizations) to achieve. Easy to say, difficult to achieve. The challenge for managers is how much to risk being out in front, making necessary changes that do not have a positive return on investment within one year (and which may not really work as planned in your institution at this particular time with these particular stakeholders). If enough managers do not step up, necessary change will not take place. And when revolutions occur, much that is good may be lost in the turmoil that follows.

The Tectonic Plates Are Shifting: Cultural Change vs. Mural Dyslexia

Kenneth Cohn, Leonard H. Friedman, and Thomas R. Allyn
From *Frontiers of Health Services Management* 24 (1), Fall 2007

Summary

In response to a rapidly changing healthcare marketplace, a variety of new business models have arisen, including new specialties (hospitalists), selective care (concierge medicine), and joint ventures (ambulatory surgical centers, specialty hospitals), some with hospitals and others with independent vendors. Since both hospitals and physicians are feeling the squeeze of rising expenses, burdensome regulations, heightened consumer expectations, and stagnant or decreasing reimbursement, the response to global economic competition and the need to improve clinical and financial outcomes can bring physicians and hospitals together rather than drive them further apart.

In response to perceived threats, physicians and hospital executives can engage in defensive reasoning that may feel protective but can also lead to mural dyslexia, the inability or unwillingness to see the handwriting on the wall. The strategies of positive deviance (finding solutions that already exist in the community rather than importing best practices), appreciative inquiry (building on success rather than relying solely on root-cause analyses of problems), and structured dialogue (allowing practicing physicians to articulate clinical priorities rather than assuming they lack the maturity and will to come to consensus) are field-tested approaches that allow hospital leaders to engage practicing physicians and that can help both parties work more interdependently to improve patient care in a dynamically changing environment. Physician-hospital collaboration based on transparency, active listening, and prompt implementation can offer sustainable competitive advantage to those willing to embark on a lifetime learning journey.

> "If you don't like change, you're going to like irrelevance a whole lot less"
> —Erik Shinseki, Retired U.S. Army Chief of Staff

When leaders fail to appreciate what is happening in their environment, their misperception can originate from fatigue, information overload, conflicting priorities, unwillingness to listen, preexisting mental models, subconscious biases, and unclear communication (Cohn and Barker 2006). A significant barrier to environmental awareness comes from defensive reasoning: when confronted with a potential threat or embarrassment, people protect themselves by blaming others (Argyris 1994).

A consequence of defensive reasoning is mural dyslexia, the unwillingness or inability to read the handwriting on the wall (Zinkham 1999). Because the healthcare landscape is rapidly changing, healthcare leaders must be able to differentiate significant signals of environmental change from background noise. The tectonic plates on which healthcare delivery currently rests (both the business and mental models) are in motion, and the rumbling is increasing. An unwillingness or inability to see what is going on can have serious consequences for healthcare leaders, their organizations, and most importantly, their patients and communities (Cohn 2005, 39–45).

Healthcare leaders need to discern the handwriting on the wall relating to the economic implications of the evolving relationship between hospitals and physicians and to embrace cultural change as an opportunity rather than a threat. This article will help leaders apply different frameworks, even though increasing influence and sense of control by admitting uncertainty and welcoming new insights and collaborators may seem counterintuitive.

In the article, we briefly analyze forces promoting this rift from a historical perspective and then discuss retail, wholesale, and collaborative strategies to offer a perspective that can reduce defensive reasoning and mural dyslexia. With each collaborative strategy, a brief case presentation shows how theory can play out in the real world.

Enabling Forces

In the 1990s, as payers moved financial decision making from physicians to third-party intermediaries, control shifted from providers to payers. Today physicians and hospitals compete with one another for patients and their associated reimbursement and collaborate on joint projects, resulting in a number of new alliances.

Some of the enabling forces that have exacerbated rifts between physicians and hospital leaders include:

- Global economic pressure for heightened operational efficiency. Forced to compete in a global market in industries where the wage and benefit structure is much lower than in the United States, U.S. firms are driven by the rising cost of healthcare to relocate their production capacity overseas (Friedman 2005). Hospital executives, who change jobs every three to five years, may see the effects of globalization in a variety of settings, but physicians, who tend to remain localized, attribute economic deterioration to local incompetence (Cohn and Peetz 2003).
- Outpatient migration. The shift of care from inpatient to outpatient settings is one of the most dramatic ways that healthcare has changed over the last two decades. This shift results from a number of factors, including cost pressures, changes in Medicare reimbursement, consumerism, minimally invasive procedures, and improved drugs and home monitoring devices (Galloro 2001). Because patients are rarely admitted to the hospital the day before elective procedures, process inefficiency becomes more readily apparent and less easy to correct in time to avoid disrupting physicians', patients', and families' schedules. In many states, especially those in which new construction does not require a certificate of need, physicians have invested in and developed focused factories (Herzlinger 1999). These specialty hospitals and ambulatory surgery centers improve physicians' ability to see and treat patients and increase revenue at a time when reimbursement has been stagnant and office expenses have been increasing. However, these facilities have siphoned off low-cost patients from hospitals, leaving hospitals with inpatients with multiple medical comorbidities requiring higher staffing ratios and additional resources.

Such specialty centers also draw valued operating room staff from the hospital, as these providers are eager to be freed of the burden of night and weekend call (Cohn, Gill, and Schwartz 2005).

- Changing sociology. An effect of the outpatient migration process is that fewer physicians spend time in the hospital, which can undermine the sense of community that once existed with physicians as well as administrators. With the use of hospitalists, key internists and family practitioners no longer come to the hospital and, in many communities, have resigned their hospital privileges. Without proactive programs to involve community physicians, those physicians' feelings of ownership and responsibility for community hospitals will diminish (Cohn, Litten, and Allyn 2006). This situation may intensify as the concept of hospitalists extends to trauma surgery, orthopedics, obstetrics, and neurology (Health Leaders 2007a).

- Regulation and the burden of undercompensated care. Many of the complex and conflicting healthcare regulations make hospitals enforcers, essentially pitting hospital leaders against physicians. For example, although the Emergency Management Treatment and Labor Act (EMTALA) was revised in 2003, it still puts hospitals in the middle between federal law and physicians who are pushing back against the burdens of providing emergency care (Griffen 2007). The rising burden of unreimbursed care has led physicians to push for pay-for-call stipends, which limits the ability of hospitals to fund replacement of aging equipment and facilities (Griffen 2007). Uncompensated care is never free (Weissman 2005).

- The expanding oversight of the federal government. Medicare, for example, which initially increased physicians' incomes when first established, has decreased reimbursement and added complexity that requires specialized assistance to avoid criminal penalties (Cohn and Peetz 2003). Complex regulations and their attendant bureaucracy increase physicians' feelings of being over-monitored and underpaid and limit their willingness to collaborate with hospital leaders, even though hospital executives are not responsible for the regulations.

- Evolving work models. As imaging has become digital and transmission of large quantities of data has become more rapid, analysis has become globalized, for example, the night-time reading of imaging studies. Cardiologists, vascular surgeons, and radiologists compete for minimally invasive vascular procedures; radiologists' reliance on physician and hospital patient referrals make them vulnerable to disruptive innovation (Christensen et al. 2006). As radiologists attempt to negotiate exclusive agreements for vascular procedures, maintain high wages and long vacations, and have the hospital pay for night coverage, one can expect radiologists' relations to the hospital and to other physicians to come under pressure.

New Business Models

Clearly, complexity has increased for physicians and job satisfaction has decreased because of increased workload, decreased reimbursement, and feelings of powerlessness and disenfranchisement. The physician's role as captain of the team has diminished. Furthermore, physicians feel that administrators trained in bottom-line management have treated their services as undifferentiated commodities and have trampled a sacred trust among physicians, patients, and families (Zuger 2004). In a survey of 1,205 physicians (Steiger 2006), the top causes for low physician morale were declining reimbursement, loss of autonomy, red tape, patient overload, and loss of respect perceived as devaluation of physician services and time. Nearly 60 percent considered leaving the practice of medicine because of discouragement with practice environment, and nearly 70 percent know at least one person who has stopped practicing as a result of low morale. The consequences of low morale were: fatigue (77 percent), burnout (66 percent), marital discord (32 percent), depression (32 percent), and suicidal ideation (4 percent).

Thorough training in technique and judgment has not prepared most physicians to deal with the challenges of working in rapidly changing institutions, building consensus, and resolving conflict (Cohn and Peetz 2003). The word "administration" serves as a lightning rod for their multi-factorial discontent and leads some to work outside hospital boundaries to gain control of schedules, personnel, and operations affecting their time.

As no taxonomy neatly fits the rapidly changing healthcare setting, we offer the following caveats to the discussion that follows:

- We have focused on new business models rather than new physician roles because some business models like retail mall clinics do not use physicians but may affect the income of primary care physicians, either positively by allowing them to spend more time with patients and bill for more complex evaluation and management, or negatively by taking away lucrative sources of income, like school physical examinations.
- We have arbitrarily divided new business models into wholesale and retail strategies, admitting that the two categories may overlap.

Wholesale Strategies

As healthcare professionals feel the squeeze of rising expenses amid stagnant reimbursement, one strategy that physicians have used is to invest in ventures that will allow them to bill for the technical as well as the professional component of services delivered. Such "wholesale strategies" take the form of ambulatory surgical centers, outpatient imaging centers, and specialty hospitals. Not-for-profit hospitals can be at a disadvantage compared to outside vendors because of the complex regulations governing charities and the laws governing financial interactions between physicians and hospitals, such as the Stark Laws, which prohibit enrichment from self-referral in designated health services, and anti-kickback laws, which generally prohibit rewards for referrals. Where feasible, we recommend a proactive strategy, based on dialogue, collaborative conflict to attack problems rather than people, and containment, that is, agreeing to table the issue for later discussion rather than allowing a stressful situation to lead to blaming (Cohn 2005, 17–23). The rationale for this unconventional approach is outlined in the section titled "The Dance of the Blind Reflex."

Retail Strategies

Business models that entrepreneurs have chosen in response to new trends include the following categories; each category includes a brief assessment of its impact on hospitals and physician-hospital relations (admittedly, the effects may vary according to the response of individual people, organizations, and local and state regulatory agencies).

Concierge Medicine

Concierge medicine is based on annual membership fees that allow primary care physicians (PCPs) the opportunity to reduce their number of patients, dependence on insurance, and economic uncertainty. Although concierge medicine can decrease the number of PCPs available to care for unassigned patients after they leave the hospital setting, concierge physicians visit the hospital to care for their inpatients and thus can remain an active part of the hospital community.

Hospitalists

Hospitalists are physicians who specialize in caring for inpatients, and they thus free PCPs to focus on their office patients. The number of hospitalists is expected to grow to 20,000 by 2010 (Williams 2004). The freeing of PCPs puts pressure on the hospital to link to its base of PCPs by using hospitalists as ambassadors and by offering continuing education programs, Internet-based conferencing, and even financial collaboration projects such as medical office building and equipment leasing coinvestment projects (Cohn, Litten, and Allyn 2006).

This is an incredibly important development. How the hospital relates to community physicians who no longer come to the hospital is crucial to capturing and retaining market share. Poor hospitalist-PCP communication, particularly at the time of discharge, leads to suboptimal clinical outcomes and undermines PCP–hospital relations (Kripalani et al. 2007).

Retail Mall Clinics

At storefront clinics, patients can shop while waiting for nurse practitioners who can perform basic services, such as administering vaccinations or diagnosing sore throats, bladder infections, and earaches (Christensen et al. 2006). The level of competition remains dynamic, with PCPs potentially caught in the middle between territorial specialists and clinics that offer convenience and quick turnaround times. It may be too early to predict the effect on physician–hospital relations; however, storefront clinics offer an opportunity to decrease emergency room congestion and thus allow ERs to provide better service to patients truly in need of emergency care. The question remains as to where patients will go for care beyond the scope of the clinic—hospitals and physicians need to develop strategic, proactive alliances with the owners and healthcare providers of these services. Alternatively, hospital leaders can develop community-based resources, such as their own mall clinics, to take the pressure off their ER facilities.

Telephone Medicine

Companies such as TelaDoc offer 24/7 telephone access to family practitioners, on-call specialists, and emergency physicians. TelaDoc also maintains a patient's medical record electronically (Health Leaders 2007b). These services offer new employment models for physicians who want or need to work in predictable shifts, for example, in order to care for young children. As with the mall clinics, hospitals would be well served to partner with rather than compete with these providers to increase patients' likelihood of seeking out a particular physician or hospital for subsequent care.

Health Tourism

Health tourism is another developing retail strategy. As an example, prices in India average 10 to 33 percent of surgical fees in the United States, and approximately 200,000 foreigners traveled to India for care in 2005 (Mannan 2006). This figure is expected to grow 15 percent per year. Any loss of income can be expected to strain relations further between physicians and hospital leaders, as each group points fingers at the other without understanding the context.

The Dance of the Blind Reflex

Both physicians and non-physician healthcare leaders focus on the part of the system that is directly in front of them; the other parts rest outside their consciousnesses (Cohn, Gill, and Schwartz 2005). Members of a section or a department have limited or no knowledge about what is going on in the rest of the system or non-system of fragmented care. Therefore, these participants do not see the enabling role they play in the conditions that they deplore. This inability to see the whole system results in what Oshry (1996) refers to as the "dance of blind reflex," which is made up of five interlocking parts:

1. People at the top of the organization feel *burdened* by unmanageable complexity.
2. Those at the bottom of the organization feel *oppressed* by insensitive higher-ups.
3. People in the middle feel *torn* and become weak, confused, and fractionated.
4. Physicians, patients, and families feel *righteously done-to* by an unresponsive non-system of fragmented care, which irritates hospital leaders who feel that their efforts are underappreciated.
5. Nobody sees his or her part in creating and sustaining any of the above conditions.

In this dance, blame is freely shared. To call a halt to the dance of blind reflex, we must first work to see the systems that we occupy. Not only do we have systems (i.e., a collection of component parts acting interdependently [Cohn 2005, 30–38]), but the systems also have us.

Making Sense of Systems

Our ability to see and make sense of systems encounters three obstacles—"how to," "want to," and "able to" (Friedman, King, and Bella 2007). All three of these obstacles are connected through "defensive reasoning" (Argyris 1994), which kicks in when we perceive others attempting to blame us or when we sense that we are part of the problem. We revert to defensive reasoning when we feel embarrassed, threatened, incompetent, or under scrutiny. We then seek to shift the blame elsewhere and hide that we are defending ourselves (Friedman, King, and Bella 2007). The field-tested frameworks described below offer an alternative to the status quo that improves the practice environment and decreases physician-hospital tensions.

Alternatives to the Systems that Have Us

The remainder of this article explores the use of frameworks and associated case presentations to work smarter rather than harder, act more interdependently than independently, and create an environment that supports learning and improving clinical outcomes rather than assessing blame. Engaging practicing physicians is key to the economic performance of hospital leaders and their organizations (Cohn 2005, 17–23).

Dealing with Physician-Hospital Competition

To work with the systems that have us, break the dance of the blind reflex, and reduce defensive reasoning, we recommend a proactive strategy, based on dialogue, mutual respect, and collaborative conflict to attack problems rather than people (Sidebar IV.1). For example, if the goal of physician-hospital financial collaboration is to create something of value that benefits patients, physicians, and the hospital, collaboration requires win-win agreements that enlarge the economic pie rather than divide decreasing shares. Both parties gain if physicians act as owners rather than clients, increasing admissions and revenue and pointing out ways to improve processes and outcomes. A spectrum of collaboration opportunities, from service contracts to medical office building/real estate to joint ventures is possible for parties (Cohn 2005, 12–16) if they:

- share information widely to build transparency and trust,
- work proactively to develop a shared vision of care that will benefit physicians, patients, and the hospital, and
- rapidly identify and remove system roadblocks to effective and efficient care, which is key to retaining physician loyalty

Positive Deviance

One way to overcome system roadblocks involves using positive deviance (PD), a bottom-up approach to organizational change based on the premise that solutions to problems already exist within the community. It encompasses intentional behaviors that depart from the norms of a group *in honorable ways* (Weber 2005a). PD seeks to identify and optimize *existing* resources and solutions rather than obtain external resources to meet those needs. Keys to the PD method include (Weber 2005a):

- self-identification as a community by members of the community; that is, people see themselves as working toward the same goal;
- mutual designation of a problem by community members, rather than identification through a top-down approach;
- inclusion of community members on the leading edge who have managed to surmount a problem;
- an analysis of meritorious behaviors that enable outliers (positive deviants) to achieve success; and
- the introduction and adoption of meritorious behaviors elsewhere in the organization.

SIDEBAR IV.1
Field-Tested Strategies for Dealing with
Physician-Hospital Competition

- Appeal to physician champions to discuss with colleagues the advantages of reinvesting profits within the community rather than lose them to out-of-town investors.
- Build on known hospital strengths, such as familiarity and comfort to patients; experience with regulatory agencies; access to capital and land; participation advantages in purchase of expensive, rapidly obsolescing high-tech equipment; and market power to obtain bundled reimbursement from payers for cutting-edge services.
- Come to know the most valuable physicians proactively by visiting them at least quarterly and learning what hospital executives can do to add value, especially regarding improving processes.
- Use collaborative conflict to attack problems rather than one another; avoid hot-button words, such as "you," "always," "never," "but," "why," "just," "cost," and "I disagree."
- Engage in active listening by giving the other party full attention, being aware of the importance of body language and tone of voice, suspending judgment, and empathizing to understand the other person's point of view.
- Practice a five-step approach during difficult negotiations (Ury 1991):
  1. Go to the balcony, where you can escape mentally to clarify thoughts about both parties' interests and reflect on the next steps.
  2. Step aside—emotional jujitsu—to enable you to listen, acknowledge, defuse anger, and find areas of agreement on which to build.
  3. Reframe, letting the problem be the teacher to foster a team-based approach, with phrases such as, "What would you recommend to help *us* solve this problem?"
  4. Build bridges, which allows both sides to save face and satisfy mutual interests.
  5. Make it difficult to say no, which helps to decrease the risk of failure and reassures both parties that the goal is mutual satisfaction rather than unilateral victory.
- When negotiations break down, agree to meet again in several weeks rather than blame the other side for failure.

Note: Adapted from Cohn 2005, 17–23.

The following case study shows how a community hospital applied the principles of PD to improve communication and collaboration (Weber 2005b).

Case Study:
Wrestling with Readmissions

Waterbury Hospital Health Center is a 234-bed Connecticut community teaching hospital that invited Jerry Sternin, the founder of the positive deviance approach, to speak at grand rounds in autumn of 2004. As the staff discussed the application of PD to healthcare settings, they identified communication as their most pervasive challenge. Dr. Anthony Cusano and nurse Bonnie Sturtevant designed a telephone survey to learn whether recently discharged patients were following their prescribed regimens successfully.

To their surprise, 80 percent of patients were taking their medications incorrectly. For example, one patient, told to take a pill every other day, took it only Tuesday and Thursday, incorrectly assuming that weekends did not count. Another patient, sent home with a variety of new prescriptions, did not take a necessary medication he already had at home because he did not receive a new prescription for it. Additional patients did not fill a prescription because of expense, but did not inform their physicians and thus never learned of more affordable alternatives.

The investigators analyzed the 20 percent who exhibited no medication errors and learned that patients who were taking their medications correctly received an educational call from a nurse shortly after discharge. Nurses who were making the phone calls found the results so startling and the corrective process so satisfying that they told colleagues, who volunteered to make phone calls to recently discharged patients. Within a few months, they had reached over 150 patients and had expanded the calling process to include new interns and residents (Weber 2005b).

Case Analysis

Prior to the intervention, Waterbury Hospital readmitted two patients per month on average for failure to adhere to post-discharge medication plans (Weber 2005b). Dr. Cusano noted,

> The patients getting the calls love to know that someone cares about them, and it
> makes the staff feel good about what they are doing. We realized that people who

were getting the calls were close to 100 percent on doing the right things. It turns out that the phone call itself is the solution. So we had to find a way of getting it done for everyone: If everyone on staff makes one phone call a month, we can contact every discharged patient. If communication is the issue, positive deviance showed us that it is also the answer.

The power of PD lies in its bottom-up process. Frontline care providers rather than the CEO determine where to direct their efforts. They invest effort in figuring out which approaches will yield the best results. Sternin felt that organizational resistance to identifying and following other institutions' best practices was similar to transplant rejection in that it stimulated more conflict than collaboration (Pascale and Sternin 2005). What healthcare professionals discover for themselves, they own (Weber 2005b).

This case study and analysis were also discussed in Cohn, K. 2006. *Collaborate for Success! Breakthrough Strategies for Engaging Physicians, Nurses, and Hospital Executives.* Chicago: Health Administration Press, 117–19.

* * * * * *

Appreciative Inquiry

Appreciative inquiry (AI) is a technique that focuses on building on success (Ludema et al. 2003). It is based on the premises that people respond favorably to positive reinforcement and that sharing stories of past successes generates more energy and less defensiveness than analyzing problems and attributing blame. We encourage hospital executives to apply AI especially when root-cause analysis becomes mired in defensive reasoning. Healthcare leaders can incorporate AI into their daily practice in the following ways (Studer 2003):

- making rounds and giving positive reinforcement to physicians, nurses, and allied healthcare professionals when patients express satisfaction or delight;
- asking people, "What is going well for you?" rather than making problems the focus of rounds;
- during evaluations, asking, "Would you like to write a note to anyone who was particularly helpful to you?" and having notecards and envelopes in the room.

The following case study demonstrates the relevance of AI in a healthcare setting.

Case Study:
Physicians and Hospital Leaders Build on Successful Crisis Management

While the CEO was out of town, contamination of a Northeastern community teaching hospital's water supply was discovered. Routine testing showed small quantities of a microorganism capable of causing systemic illness in immunocompromised patients arising from an old shower head. Rapid repeat testing confirmed that the contamination was not a result of laboratory artifact and raised the question that the hospital water supply might be contaminated. Physicians and management representing infectious diseases, oncology, pediatrics, and the offices of the vice president of medical affairs, patient care services, operations, and public relations cleared their schedules and formed a command post from which to receive and communicate information rapidly and often. They shut off the existing water supply and made arrangements for emergent resupply of fresh water while they researched ways to determine the extent of the contamination, remove the source(s), and purify their water delivery system. They calmly briefed the CEO and board of directors and then medical staff, employees, the press, and local community agencies to offer assurance that they had identified a problem and they were in the process of remedying it. In addition, they stepped up monitoring of susceptible patients. Within three days, the team had replaced the old shower heads and purified the water system. No patient morbidity or mortality occurred as a result of the contamination.

In discussion of the situation afterward, some participants felt that the departmental culture created silos that made it difficult to obtain interdepartmental cooperation except in times of crisis; however, all agreed that the shared values, camaraderie, and pride they felt from their rapid and effective handling of a potentially life-threatening contamination episode gave them a sense of accomplishment on which they built during future challenges.

Case Analysis

Physicians and hospital leaders can use AI to overcome defensiveness, turf battles, negativism, change fatigue, and slow response time. Professionals prefer being inspired to being supervised. Generally, it is quicker and easier to build on wins than to try to persuade people to abandon established approaches to perceived problems (Weick 1984). Story-telling, which is an integral part of AI, decreases the inhibiting effects of hierarchy on an organization, uses metaphors to summarize important points and make them vivid, and provides vignettes that are remembered more readily than facts.

This case study was also discussed in K.H. Cohn, M.D. Araujo, and S.L. Gill. 2005. "Appreciative Inquiry." In *Better Communication for Better Care: Mastering Physician-Administrator Collaboration*, by Cohn, K., 25–27. Chicago, Health Administration Press. Used with permission.

★ ★ ★ ★ ★ ★

Structured Dialogue

Structured dialogue is a process that helps a group of practicing physicians articulate their collective, patient-centered self-interest and feel a sense of shared ownership in improving physician-hospital relations. For example, structured dialogue can help physicians improve physician-physician communication, understand more fully the complexity of hospital operations, and articulate clinical priorities for their communities and their practices (Cohn, Gill, and Schwartz 2005).

Unlike hospital-centric change efforts, the structured dialogue process is led by a medical advisory panel (MAP) of high-performing, well-respected clinicians who review and recommend clinical priorities based on presentations by the major clinical sections and departments. Contrary to the apprehensions of some hospital executives, the recommendations generally include performance improvements and minor expenditures that support these improvements, rather than a list of capital-intensive budget items. In return for giving physicians a say in clinical priority setting, the hospital is able to enlist physicians to attend meetings and outline their priorities. We encourage hospital executives to use this method when they tire of clinicians shooting down hospital executives' suggestions for reform and want to focus the mirror on physicians' efforts to set clinical priorities. Benefits of effective physician-administrator dialogue are illustrated below.

Case Study:
What to Do Next?

George (a pseudonym) was an industrial engineer by training. He used a precise, step-by-step approach that his direct reports mirrored and had always been known as a turnaround CEO who came in, stopped the bleeding, and left the hospital in much better shape within five years.

Eight years after becoming the CEO of a community teaching hospital, however, he felt stuck. He had tried the latest theories, including reengineering and rapid-sequence change processes, without success. Deficits increased, staffing decreased, and morale plummeted. With the encouragement of his marketing senior vice president who had witnessed a successful structured dialogue process at her previous job and the approval of physician leaders, he appointed two clinically talented and highly regarded physicians to be cochairs of a 13-member MAP. The cochairs, not administration, picked the remaining members to represent outstanding medical staff practitioners from other departments.

The charge to the MAP was to engage physicians to analyze and recommend priorities to improve care for the community, physician-physician communication, and physician-administrator collaboration. Over the next six months, they heard recommendations from all major clinical areas to improve care for the community over the next three to five years. The MAP chose a time span of three to five years to stretch participants' imagination and encourage them to think about the future rather than the past. The panel's report listed approximately 100 recommendations from physician presenters that fell within four overarching themes:

1. Improve service to patients and their families.
2. Enhance physician-physician communication.
3. Implement clinical protocols in all major diagnostic-related groups to save money, limit variation, and improve quality and safety.
4. Develop coordinated diagnostic and treatment centers.

Although these recommendations seem conventional to outsiders, the structured dialogue process represented the first time that the hospital administration had obtained a consensus report from its most talented clinicians. Furthermore, each recommendation derived from issues and opportunities raised in clinical section presentations. Previously, hospital leaders received feedback mainly from their "squeaky wheels."

Over the next two years, physicians, nurses, and administrators worked together to implement over 90 percent of the panel's recommendations. The remaining 10 percent were no longer relevant because of rapidly changing marketplace conditions. The structured dialogue process improved patient and employee satisfaction; increased surgical volume, market share, and operating margins; and groomed new medical staff leadership. George is now a sought-after speaker who explains how collaboration with practicing physicians was key to his hospital's turnaround.

Case Analysis

During the structured dialogue process, physicians engage in face-to-face dialogue with one another and hospital leaders and learn to view their individual practices within a larger context, thus abandoning the dance of the blind reflex described earlier (Oshry 1996). A physician wrote:

> Our report represented the first time that the hospital received a consensus report from practicing physicians about what the hospital should do in the future. Before, the process involved squeaky wheels pursuing individual agendas.
>
> We evolved from a self-interested view of what the hospital should do for us as physicians to a more empowered view of how the hospital could employ limited resources to improve care for our community. Through the process of discovery, we began to think and act more as long-term partners and co-owners than short-term customers and renters.

Hospitals of varying size have used the time-tested, structured dialogue process successfully by meeting the following three prerequisites:

1. Physicians and hospital executives must be interested in exploring how they can improve care for their community.
2. Practicing physicians must recognize the benefit of making time to prepare for and attend meetings based on their need to use their time better, increase practice revenues, improve processes of care, and/or leave a lasting legacy, becoming physician champions (Boxes IV.1 and IV.2).
3. Hospital administrators and the board must agree a priori to make every effort to implement the physicians' carefully thought-out recommendations, even if the physicians' suggestions represent a change in the hospital's business model.

BOX IV.1
Description of a Physician Champion

- Creates a safe environment for learning
- Presents and discusses clinical data with practicing physicians
- Increases institutional transparency by sharing information
- Minimizes physician-hospital battles
- Helps to build trust
- Through the process of discovery, acts like an owner
- Leaves a lasting legacy

BOX IV.2
Ways to Cultivate and Nurture Physician Champions

- Make effective communication a high priority, using face-to-face communication to build trust
- Share information for mutual advantage in a customized manner
- Be proactive and get to know the champion in non-crisis settings
- Find common perspectives inside and outside the hospital
- Show that you value the champion's time
- Focus on achieving large goals in small, measurable steps
- Celebrate victories as a team
- Move from disagreement to creative abrasion to become an organization that fosters learning (Cohn et al. 2006)

This case study and analysis was also discussed in Cohn, K. 2006. *Collaborate for Success! Breakthrough Strategies for Engaging Physicians, Nurses, and Hospital Executives.* Chicago: Health Administration Press, 2–9.

* * * * * *

Conclusion and Recommendations

Ironically, the forces that are pushing physicians and hospital executives apart may be what ultimately reunite them (Cohn, Gill, and Schwartz 2005). Both are experiencing rapid change and uncertainty, being squeezed by the disparity between reimbursement and rising expenses, and receiving pressure from a variety of experts to collaborate to improve quality and safety. As Waldman, Hood, and Smith (2006) point out, both groups agree on the "who," since they live in the same communities and share the same patients; they also generally agree on the "why," as they are both attracted to healthcare careers to make a difference in the lives of patients and their families. The "how" is the basis of dynamic interchange between physicians and hospital executives. Despite the shifting tectonic plates, the mission of most doctors and hospitals remains to provide compassionate care for patients.

The silo mentality embodied in "Let the docs deal with patient care and leave finance and operations to the administrators," is destined for failure in a rapidly changing environment. A more suitable approach is embodied in the report by Malcolm and colleagues (2003) on cultural convergence. They wrote that a key reason that New Zealand had improved healthcare outcomes was that integrated district health boards have encouraged managers to shift from a preoccupation with resource management to improving clinical outcomes and allowing physicians to embrace a clear role in stewarding resources to achieve the board's goals. That both groups have minimized the gap between physician and managerial cultures and moved to a more Copernican view that puts patients and families at the center of the universe should give us hope that cultural change is possible, with dividends for physicians, administrators, hospital employees, and especially patients and families.

Sternin wrote that it is often easier for people to change their viewpoints by implementing reforms than to change their actions by changing their viewpoints (Dorsey 2000). To that end, we offer ten steps to take now to engage physicians and improve patient care:

1. Encourage practicing physicians to articulate future clinical priorities, as discussed in the structured dialogue section, to increase their sense of shared ownership and improve clinical outcomes.
2. Include doctors who are users of radiology, anesthesiology, pathology, and emergency services when drawing up contract specifications and monitoring performance to improve service; physicians may pay lip service to administrators but listen to other physicians who refer patients to them.
3. Establish a hotline for process improvement issues that is tracked at least monthly in senior management meetings to make sure that the communication loop is closed (Stubblefield 2005).
4. Treat the top 20 percent of physicians as partners, and visit them at least quarterly, regardless of their irascibility (Cohn, Gill, and Schwartz 2005).
5. Ask "go-to" docs, "What can we take off your plate?" at least semiannually to monitor and reduce burnout (Cohn, Panasuk, and Holland 2005).
6. Map out steps of policies and procedures to improve effectiveness and refine handoffs especially when people complain that they need more workers to accomplish tasks. Many times, staff creep is a result of work-arounds created by inefficient processes that can be identified and improved by putting each step on a Post-it note and asking members of a group to remedy the gap between what could and should be happening compared to what is actually occurring.
7. Have the chief information officer and programmers participate in rounds periodically with physicians to see how physicians struggle with information technology and how they could use their time more productively.

8. Develop a hospitalist surgical service to off-load call burdens for physicians and diminish the need to pay stipends to physicians for carrying a beeper.

9. Celebrate and reward all healthcare professionals who exceed their job descriptions to care for patients; if culture trumps strategy, stories of such professionals can become the basis of a positive culture that strives to improve outcomes and service to patients and family (Ludema et al. 2003).

10. Establish a pool with fines for using hot-button words (such as "you," "always," "never," "but,") and killer phrases (such as "Let's appoint a committee to study that some more") and use the money collected to support a worthwhile service or celebration (Cohn 2005, 17–23).

References

Argyris, C. 1994. "Good Communication That Blocks Learning." *Harvard Business Review* 72 (4): 77–85.

Christensen, C. M., H. Baumann, R. Ruggles, and T.M. Sadtler. 2006. "Disruptive Innovation for Social Change." *Harvard Business Review* 84 (12): 94–101.

Cohn, K. H. 2005. *Better Communication for Better Care: Mastering Physician-Administrator Collaboration.* Chicago: Health Administration Press.

Cohn, K. H., T. R. Allyn, R. Rosenfield, and R. Schwartz. 2005. "Overview of Physician Ventures." *American Journal of Surgery* 189 (1): 4–10.

Cohn, K. H., D. B. Panasuk, J. C. Holland. 2005. "Workplace Burnout." In *Better Communication for Better Care: Mastering Physician-Administrator Collaboration* by K. H. Cohn, 56–62. Chicago: Health Administration Press.

Cohn, K. H., S. L. Gill, R. W. Schwartz. 2005. "Gaining Hospital Administrators' Attention: Ways to Improve Physician-Hospital Management Dialogue." *Surgery* 137 (2): 132–40.

Cohn, K. H., and M. E. Peetz. 2003. "Surgeon Frustration: Contemporary Problems, Practical Solutions." *Contemporary Surgery* 59 (2): 76–85.

Cohn, K. H., and J. Barker. 2006. "Improving Communication, Collaboration, and Safety Using Crew Resource Management." In *Collaborate for Success: Breakthrough Strategies for Engaging Physicians, Nurses, and Hospital Executives* by K. H. Cohn, 33–44. Chicago: Health Administration Press.

Cohn, K. H., D. Litten, and T. R. Allyn. 2006. "Maintaining Collaboration Between Hospitalists, the Hospital, and Primary Care Providers." In *Collaborate for Success: Breakthrough Strategies for Engaging Physicians, Nurses, and Hospital Executives* by K.H. Cohn, 21–32. Chicago: Health Administration Press.

Cohn, K. H., T. R. Allyn, and R. Reid. 2006. "The Challenges and Opportunities of Collaborating with Creatively Abrasive Physicians." In *Collaborate for Success: Breakthrough Strategies for Engaging Physicians, Nurses, and Hospital Executives,* by K. H. Cohn, 11–20. Chicago: Health Administration Press.

Dorsey, D. 2000. "Positive Deviant." [Online article; accessed 10/14/05]. http://pf.fastcompany.com/magazine/41/sternin.html.

Friedman, L., J. King, and D. Bella. 2007. "Seeing Systems in Healthcare Organizations." *Physician Executive*, in press.

Friedman, T. 2005. *The World is Flat: A Brief History of the Twenty-First Century.* New York: Farrar, Straus, & Giroux.

Galloro, V. 2001. "Promise and Peril: Cancer Care." *Modern Healthcare* 31 (25): 74–76.

Griffen, F. D. 2007. "A Perfect Storm: ED Crisis and the On-call Surgeon." *Contemporary Surgery* 63 (2): 73–76.

HealthLeaders Leadership Review. 2007a. "Low Comp Creates Challenges for Neurology." *HealthLeaders Media* 8 (2):1–3.

HealthLeaders Physician Compensation Report. 2007b. "Market Strategy: Competition—Just a Phone Call Away." *HealthLeaders Media* 26 (2): 1.

Herzlinger, R. 1999. *Market-Driven Healthcare: Who Wins, Who Loses in the Transformation of America's Largest Service Industry.* New York: Perseus Books.

Kripalani, S., F. LeFevre, C. O. Phillips, M. V. Williams, P. Basaviah, and D. W. Baker. 2007. "Deficits in Communication and Information Transfer Between Hospital-Based and Primary Care Physicians: Implications for Patient Safety and Continuity of Care." *JAMA* 297 (8): 831–41.

Ludema, J. D., D. Whitney, J. Bernard, and J. Thomas. 2003. *The Appreciative Inquiry Summit: A Practitioner's Guide for Leading Large-Group Change.* San Francisco: Berrett-Koehler.

Malcolm, L., L. Wright, P. Barnett, and C. Hendry. 2003. "Building a Successful Partnership Between Management and Clinical Leadership: Experience from New Zealand." *British Medical Journal* 326 (7390): 653–54.

Mannan, M. 2006. "Boom Time as Health Tourism Hits New High." [Online article; cited 9/4/06]. www.thepeninsulaqatar.com/Display_news.asp?section=World_News.

Oshry, B. 1996. *Seeing Systems: Unlocking the Mysteries of Organizational Life.* San Francisco: Berrett-Koehler.

Pascale, R. T., J. Sternin. 2005. "Your Company's Secret Change Agents." *Harvard Business Review* 83 (5): 73–81.

Steiger, B. "Doctors Say Morale is Hurting." *The Physician Executive* 32 (6): 6–15.

Stubblefield, A. 2005. *The Baptist Health Care Journey to Excellence: Creating A Culture That WOWs!.* Hoboken, NJ: John Wiley & Sons, Inc.

Studer, Q. *Hardwiring Excellence.* 2003. Gulf Breeze, FL: Fire Starter Publishing.

Ury, W. L. 1991. *Getting Past No.* New York: Bantam.

Waldman. J. D., J. N. Hood, and H. L. Smith. 2006. "Hospital CEOs and Physicians—Reaching Common Ground." *Journal of Healthcare Management* 51 (3): 171–87.

Weber, D. O. 2005. "Positive Deviance, Part 1." [Online article; retrieved 10/9/05]. *Health and Hospital Networks* www.hhnmag.com.

Weber, D. O. 2005. "Positive Deviance, Part 2." [Online article; retrieved 10/9/05]. *Health and Hospital Networks* www.hhnmag.com.

Weick, K. E. 1984. "Small Wins: Redefining the Scale of Social Problems." *American Psychologist* 39 (1): 40–49.

Weissman, J. S. 2005. "The Trouble with Uncompensated Hospital Care." *New England Journal of Medicine* 352 (12): 1171–73.

Williams, M. V. 2004. "The Future of Hospital Medicine: Evolution or Revolution?" *American Journal of Medicine* 117 (6): 446–50.

Zinkham, R. 1999. "To Be or Not to Be? How Hospitals and Doctors Should Decide Whether to Reinvest in or Divest of their Group Practices. [Online article; retrieved 1/9/07]. http://www.venable.com/publications.cfm

Zuger, A. 2004. "Dissatisfaction with Medical Practice." *New England Journal of Medicine* 350 (1): 69–75.

The Revolution in Hospital Management

John R. Griffith and Kenneth R. White
From *The Journal of Healthcare Management* 50:3, May/June 2005

Executive Summary

Five healthcare systems that have either won the Malcolm Baldrige National Quality Award in Health Care or been documented in extensive case studies share a common model of management: they all emphasize a broadly accepted mission; measured performance; continuous quality improvement; and responsiveness to the needs of patients, physicians, employees, and community stakeholders. This approach produces results that are substantially and uniformly better than average, across a wide variety of acute care settings. As customers, courts, and accrediting and payment agencies recognize this management approach, we argue that it will become the standard for all hospitals to achieve.

This article examines documented cases of excellent hospitals, using the reports of the three winners of the Baldrige National Quality Award in Health Care and published studies of other institutions with exceptional records.

* * * * * *

Excellent organizations demonstrate long-term results that satisfy most or all of their stakeholders. This article examines documented cases of excellent hospitals, using the reports of the three winners of the Malcolm Baldrige National Quality Award in Health Care and published studies of other institutions with exceptional records (see Table IV.1). These reports show that the organizations share many management practices.

TABLE IV.1 Characteristics of Systems and Hospitals Studied	Hospital or Healthcare System	Documentation	Size	Scope of Service	Locations
	Baptist Hospital, Inc.	Baldrige National Quality Award Application, 2003	$158 million revenue; 492-bed urban hospital	Tertiary and referral care	Pensacola, Florida
	Catholic Health Initiative	Case study; *Thinking Forward* book	$6 billion revenue; 47 "market-based organizations" of one or more hospitals	Ranges from "critical access" hospitals to tertiary centers; includes long-term and palliative care	64 communities in 19 states
	Intermountain Health Care	IHC annual reports; Harvard Business School Case 9-603-066	$3 billion revenue; 20 hospitals and clinic facilities	Ranges from rural clinics to Intermountain Medical Center, a tertiary medical teaching center	27 communities in Utah and Idaho
	SSM Health Care	Baldrige National Quality Award Application, 2002	$2 billion revenue; 21 general and specialty hospitals with clinic facilities	Acute, long-term, rehabilitative, and palliative care	7 markets in Missouri, Illinois, Wisconsin, and Oklahoma
	St. Luke's Hospital	Baldrige National Quality Award Application, 2003	$308 million revenue; 482-bed suburban hospital	Tertiary and referral care	Kansas City, Missouri

While these are certainly not the only excellent institutions, their achievements have been successfully applied in a wide variety of settings, generating results that are substantially superior to those of typical hospitals. Their approach has now been tested in over 100 diverse American communities, suggesting that it is an appropriate model for most U.S. hospitals and healthcare systems.

The Malcolm Baldrige Health Care Criteria for Performance Excellence (2004) provide a template that shows how this management approach has been built into day-to-day actions that produce excellence in quality, cost, financial stability, and physician and worker satisfaction. The Baldrige criteria in general are deliberately designed to cover a broad range of businesses and strategies and organized in seven sections that emphasize leadership, strategy, patient relations, worker relations, information management, operations, and results.

Leadership

Leadership is "how senior leaders address values, directions, and performance expectations, . . . focus on patients and other customers and stakeholders, empowerment, innovation, and learning. . . . also . . . governance and . . . public and community responsibilities" (Malcolm Baldrige Healthcare Criteria 2004).

The Baldrige expects leaders to establish universal two-way communication practices and to use them to deploy organizational values and performance expectations. Leading hospitals now do the following:

1. Use mission, vision, and values statements as central referents to describe the organization to its publics, attract compassionate workers, focus ongoing dialog, and test propositions for change. SSM Health Care (SSMHC 2002) has a "Passport" for every employee that states its mission, vision, and values. St. Luke's Hospital's (SLH 2003) "Very Important Principles" card lists its strategic goals. Catholic Health Initiatives (CHI) keeps its values—"Reverence, Integrity, Compassion, and Excellence"—constantly in the mind of its associates by including them on badges, posters, and other printed media (Griffith and White 2003).
2. Use several hundred measures and benchmarks to provide each responsibility center with multidimensional measures of performance (Griffith and White 2002; Simmons 2000). Baptist Hospital, Inc. (BHI 2003) aggregates more than 75 measures to 14 for governance reporting. SLH (2003) aggregates 86 broadly used measures to a color-coded scorecard of 27 for senior leadership.
3. Report promptly and often publicly. Important performance measures are reported daily, biweekly, and monthly so that all managers and most employees know exactly where they stand. Both BHI (2003) and SLH (2003) stress 90-day action plans. BHI claims, "The agility inherent in 90-day review . . . gives BHI an advantage in its highly competitive environment." SSMHC (2002) reports 49 measures monthly and 14 more quarterly. At SSMHC " . . . specific goals and objectives . . . are posted in [each] department. Posters provide a visual line of sight connection from SSMHC's mission to department goals."
4. Use the measurement system to shape two-way communication. Performance improvement teams (PITs) identify, test, and implement process changes that drive next year's goals. A hospital may have a dozen or more teams redesigning processes. PITs are facilitated and supervised

by a senior management group (BHI 2003; SLH 2003; SSMHC 2002; Griffith and White 2003). SLH (2003) claims its performance management process "produces a set of specific, measurable behaviors that exemplify the core values for each and every SLH employee." The values, the scorecard, and continuous quality improvement (CQI) converge to empower workers and lower-level managers. A culture is created that requires senior management to listen to and respond to frontline concerns (BHI 2003; SLH 2003; SSMHC 2002; Griffith and White 2003).

5. Attract and retain effective team members. Leading organizations monitor satisfaction, turnover, and safety routinely for physicians and employees. All have formal and informal listening activities such as forums and walking rounds. SLH has an "administrator on call" 24 hours a day/7 days a week and an "open door policy." The "service value chain" concept—satisfied workers produce satisfied customers and improved overall performance—has been widely accepted (Heskett, Sasser, and Schlesinger 1997). BHI pioneered the service value application to hospitals, and along with SSMHC have won national awards for employment practices. CHI is implementing the concept at several sites, pursuing a "Spirit" model that focuses employee education on a new topic each month (Griffith and White 2003). SSMHC (2002) is implementing an accountability-based professional practice model "to give nurses and other employees greater decision-making authority." As of 2004, all hospitals have implemented the model in nursing, and many have implemented it in all clinical services (Friedman 2004).

6. Use financial incentives to reward goal achievement, supplementing the recognition and celebration included in CQI and the service value chain. BHI and SLH use a merit increase program with individual objectives and a detailed review. CHI offers substantial cash incentives for managers. At least one CHI site provides performance-based awards for all workers. Intermountain Health Care (IHC) allows its managers to earn bonuses that meet national pay standards (Griffith and White 2003).

The Baldrige asks how senior leaders create "an environment . . . that fosters legal and ethical behavior" (Malcolm Baldrige Healthcare Criteria 2004). BHI (2003) leaders are required to attest that they "have no knowledge of violations of Baptist's high standards." CHI and SSMHC use an audit system that makes the internal auditor accountable to an outside agency. CHI supplements the audit with quarterly certification of reports by its local CEOs and CFOs. It has a similarly sophisticated compliance process, designed as much to create effective relationships as to prevent violations of the law (Griffith and White 2003). SSMHC uses the model compliance plan proposed by the Office of Inspector General as a foundation but "goes beyond compliance . . . to ensure that SSMHC values are reflected in all work processes. . . .

KPMG has identified SSMHC's corporate review process as a best practice nationwide" (SSMHC 2002).

The Baldrige application asks how the organization "addresses its responsibilities to the public [and] practices good citizenship." Leading hospitals and systems have identified and measured their community contribution (Catholic Health Association 2001) and made their information public (see each organization's web sites). SLH has established a joint venture in cancer care with its largest competitor, HCA. In Portland, Oregon, four healthcare organizations have linked with state and county health departments to establish a collaborative network (Griffith 1998). BHI (2003) collaborates with a competitor to run clinics.

The Baldrige is also concerned about how the hospital "contributes to the health of its community." The best hospitals have established effective processes for contributing to promote healthy behavior and to prevent illness. They have promoted alternatives to acute care, such as chronic disease management and palliative care (Griffith and White 2003). The American Hospital Association's "Healthy Communities" movement has taken hold as a priority in winning hospitals. SSMHC (2002) launched a systemwide "Healthy Communities" initiative in 1995, and it also has a committee to foster environmental awareness at each local site. In Kearney, Nebraska, CHI established an award-winning collaboration with local industry, government, and religious organizations. The model has increased in popularity and gained commitment while sharing the cost of the program with other organizations (Griffith and White 2003). BHI (2003) sponsors a Partnership for Healthy Communities and "Get Healthy Pensacola" program. . . . [E]nrollees can earn prizes or discounts arranged with local businesses. . . . "

Strategic Planning

According to the 2004 Malcolm Baldrige Health Care Criteria, strategic planning is "how your organization develops strategic objectives and action plans. . . . how your chosen strategic objectives and action plans are deployed and how progress is measured."

The Baldrige application expects the components of continuous improvement—goals, empowerment, analysis, and revision—to be imbedded in the culture. Change is the rule. The strategic process is about how alternatives are selected and implemented through a plan with explicit goals and timetables.

Leading institutions do the following:

1. Begin an annual cycle with a review of mission, vision, and values, both to keep these current and to reinforce them as core criteria to guide their strategy.

2. Undertake a rigorous, multifaceted environment review of threats or opportunities presented by the market, technology, critical caregivers, competitors, and regulation. They explicitly integrate financial needs and resources. Support from system corporate offices has helped many hospitals.

3. Use retreats to build consensus around the implications of the facts and the appropriate strategic responses.

4. Set goals based on systematic analysis of benchmark and market data as well as local history.

5. Use task forces or PITs to change performance. PITs have broad participation, clear charges and deadlines. The plans they develop have explicit timetables and performance expectations.

6. Empower member units by delegating authority.

7. Build plan achievement targets into managers' goals and incentives.

SLH has evolved a particularly comprehensive strategic process. As shown in Figure IV.1, it is based on three dimensions of "roll out" (SLH 2003):

• From strategic (level 1) concerns through several levels of accountability (levels II through IV)
• From long-term to short-term (90 day) action plans.

FIGURE IV.1

SLH Leadership for Performance Excellence Model

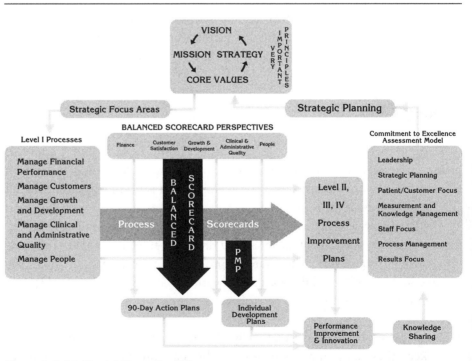

Source: St. Luke's Hospital, Kansas City, MO.

- From strategic goals to process improvement to individual development plans.

Measures, goals, and process improvement plans are articulated at each step of each dimension. The strategy roll out itself is improved by feedback from each of the three dimensions.

Figure IV.2 shows the 90-day tracking mechanism at the senior management level. At SLH, it is in color: blue, green, yellow, and red for four

FIGURE IV.2

SLH Hospital Scorecard Sample Template

Category	Key Measure	Qtr Year	Target 10	Stretch 9	8	Goal 7	6	Moderate 5	4	Risk 3	2	1	Raw Score
FINANCIAL	Total Margin												6
	Operating Margin												4
	Operating Cash Flow												5
	Days Cash on Hand												7
	Cost per CMI Adjusted Discharge												6
CUSTOMER SATISFACTION	Would Recommend (IP;OP;ED)												7
	Overall Satisfaction (IP;OP;ED)												8
	Longer Than Expected Wait Time (IP;OP;ED)												7
	Responsiveness to Complaints												4
	Outcome of Care												9
	IP Active Admitting Physician Ratio												9
	OP Admitting Physician Counts												5
GROWTH & DEVELOPMENT	**Community IP Market Share												6
	Eligible IP Market Share - Draw Zips												5
	Eligible IP Profitable Market Share - Draw Zips												3
	IP PCP Referral - Ratio - Draw Zips												6
	OP Referral Counts Draw Zips												10
CLINICAL & ADMINISTRATIVE QUALITY	***IP Clinical Care Index												8
	***OP Clinical Care Index												7
	***Patient Safety Index												6
	***Operational Index												7
	***Maryland Quality Indicator Index												8
	***Infection Control Index												5
	***Medical Staff Clinical Indicator Index												8
	Net Days in Accounts Receivable (IP/OP)												6
PEOPLE	Human Capital Value Added												4
	Retention												10
	Diversity												7
	Job Coverage Ratio												8
	**Competency												10
	**Employee Satisfaction												7

** Indicates annual measure.   ***Detail in Appendix B

						Overall Score	7
Exceeding Goal		1 Qtr	2 Qtr	3 Qtr	4 Qtr	Goal	7
Goal	Overall Score	7	7			Stretch	10
Moderate							
Risk							

For performance to be scored greater than Level 1, the performance value must meet or exceed the scoring criteria within a Level.

Source: St. Luke's Hospital, Kansas City, MO.

levels of goal achievement. Managers can "drill down" for run charts, goals, and benchmarks. Similar reports go to the "level" managers of Figure IV.1.

The processes for strategy are not substantially different from those used at IHC and Henry Ford Health System a decade ago (Griffith, Sahney, and Mohr 1995). The difference, as IHC executives noted at the time, is implementation. Focused on the results, leaders implement the process with both vigilance and rigor. Vigilance allows them to spot opportunities and threats faster. A network of informed and committed agents uncovers new ideas. A rich background to evaluate them develops quickly. Rigor protects them from the usual causes of bureaucratic delay. Denial, special interests, and paralysis by analysis simply are not acceptable in leading institutions. The loop is closed by the short-term plans.

Focus on Patients, Other Customers, and Markets

This criterion is about "how your organization determines requirements, expectations, and preferences of patients . . . and markets. . . . builds relationships . . . and determines the key factors that lead to . . . satisfaction, loyalty, . . . retention, and . . . service expansion" (Malcolm Baldrige Health Care Criteria 2004).

The Baldrige application expects solid and expanding relationships with patients, families, physicians, other healthcare providers, students, insurers, employers, patient advocacy groups, the community, and government agencies. The leaders systematically do the following:

1. Refine a comprehensive system of "listening and learning tools" using focus groups, community need surveys, patient and other customer satisfaction surveys, reports from PITs, meetings with physicians, and industry market research. BHI is "obsessed" with patient care and customer satisfaction, surveying every inpatient and one of eight outpatients. Scores are near the 99th percentile in the nationwide data (BHI 2003).

    SLH creates a "patient path," a patient-friendly format of the care plan that explains timing and purpose. All employees are empowered and expected to resolve complaints. Each patient is assigned to a patient advocate (PA) who visits patients on their first, fifth, and tenth day, and more frequently if needed. Many of the PAs are bilingual and serve as translators (SLH 2003).

2. Assess opportunities for improving service and clinical quality. Through environmental scanning, one of SMHC hospitals discovered an opportunity to satisfy an increased demand for heart services as a result

of the dissolution of a physician group. The hospital then opened the first heart hospital in its community, for which the hospital received an "Innovator of the Year" Award (SSMHC 2002).

3. Analyze performance to identify what contributes to patient loyalty. The SSMHC planning staff provides monthly reports to each entity that identify trends and opportunities in patient loyalty. For example, classes about particular diseases or conditions, support groups, and e-health information empower patients to proactively manage their disease/condition and therefore build loyalty (SSMHC 2002).

4. Meet requirements of physician partners and build physician loyalty. SSMHC (2002) hospitals have physician liaisons and other staff members who focus on physician relations, recruitment, and retention. BHI and SLH (2003) survey physicians annually and hold periodic interviews and focus groups. BHI (2003) implemented a "Physician Action Line," which allows members of the medical staff to give BHI leaders feedback. When BHI leaders found out that a common physician irritant was not being able to locate nurses quickly, they issued wireless phones to nurses. BHI also trains physician office staffs and assists with office patient satisfaction surveys.

5. Treat employers as important customers. BHI surveys community employer groups to assess satisfaction, attitude, and needs. In focus groups with employers, BHI (2003) discovered a desire to encourage healthy lifestyle and responded with an incentive-based healthy lifestyle program for workers.

6. React immediately to customer complaints with a standardized process of response, tracking, follow-up resolution, and pattern analysis. BHI (2003) maintains a customer loyalty team that focuses on making things right when responding to complaints. Complaints are addressed within 24 hours at SLH (2003), and SSMHC (2002) uses a software management program for tracking complaints developed by one of its hospitals.

7. Celebrate extra effort for the customer, and "recover" from service errors. All of the Baldrige winners describe service recovery processes that focus on listening to the customer and recommending problem solutions. Employees at BHI (2003) are empowered with spending guidelines for resolution of problems that involve lost items, delays, or complaints concerning physicians. Extra effort by employees is explicitly rewarded with written acknowledgment, celebration, and gifts. CHI's "Complaints as a Gift" program emphasizes that complaints are an opportunity to make things better (Griffith and White 2003). Dominican Hospital (DH 2003) tracks compliments for communication to employees, physicians, and key stakeholders and celebrates results with individual employees.

8. Search outside the healthcare industry to learn about maintaining customer loyalty and building customer relationships. BHI's (2003) Standards Team, a subcommittee of the Culture Team, actively pursues best practices in leading nonhealthcare organizations.

Measurement, Analysis, and Knowledge Management

This criterion is defined as "how your organization selects, gathers, analyzes, manages, and improves its data, information, and knowledge assets" (Malcolm Baldrige Health Care Criteria 2004).

The Baldrige scores knowledge as a resource that is slightly more important than the human resource. The points are equally divided between "measurement and analysis of organizational performance" and "information and knowledge management."

"Measurement and analysis" require definitions, input, verification, standardization, archiving, and analysis of large volumes of data from multiple sources. The management challenge is to develop, maintain, and use these data to improve performance. The leading institutions follow these steps:

1. Build medical-records coding and data, billing, materials management, cost accounting, satisfaction surveys, and human resources data so effectively and reliably that they are taken as a given. CHI and SSMHC use their internal audit function to ensure the accuracy of critical nonfinancial measures (Griffith and White 2003; SSMHC 2002).
2. Benchmark and compare to best practice. No goal is set without benchmarking. SLH (2003), for example, uses six outside commercial sources for comparisons, including survey companies, financial analysts, and market analysts plus VHA, Maryland Quality Indicators, and the Missouri PRO. SLH and BHI are signed up for the Centers for Medicaid and Medicare Services' "7th Scope of Work" initiative that goes beyond the Joint Commission's "Key Measures" (SLH 2003; BHI 2003). SSMHC (2002), which believes "external visits are key to the benchmarking process," has a guide book on its intranet that describes sources and uses of benchmarks.
3. Provide internal consultants to help PITs analyze the relationships between measures, identify trends, and prepare forecasts. Improvement proposals are expected to provide quantitative forecasts of all relevant measures, and accepted proposals are expected to achieve the forecasts. IHC's Institute for Healthcare Delivery Research has been central to several significant process changes (Bohmer, Edmondson, and Feldman 2003).
4. Use a formal structure to improve the data processing resource and the selection and definition of measures. SSMHC (2002) and BHI

(2003) use an information council, including senior management and representation from users and information specialists. Ad hoc information management teams develop and evaluate specific measurement and knowledge programs. They bring in technical expertise, listen for implementation issues, and create specific short-term and long-term plans. SSMHC (2002) and CHI (Griffith and White 2003) use a farm system—required, standard, and nonstandard—that allows individual units to experiment with new measures.

5. Involve line management in knowledge management. The leaders have invested heavily in managerial effort, worker training, and data warehouses over a period of years. They believe these investments have paid off, and they plan to continue a high level of investment.

The 2004 Baldrige Health Care Criteria state, "Information and knowledge management . . . examines how your organization ensures the availability of high quality, timely data . . . for all your key users." The criteria address needs, not methods. They do not demand an electronic medical record or even computerized patient order entry. The leaders do the following:

1. Build the process management and general business capability ahead of their clinical information systems. They have emphasized using standard commercial software and the information it produces rather than developing modifications.
2. Use web technology to put management information at the caregivers' and the managers' fingertips. BHI (2003) claims that it "provides a 'no secrets' environment with organizationally educated, knowledgeable employees." All employees and physicians are encouraged to access the BHI intranet for information.
3. Expand electronic medical record capability. Access to clinical information is now a high priority. IHC has the most comprehensive electronic medical record, which was developed over several years (Griffith and White 2003). BHI's information system covers order entry and some results reporting. SLH has only recently moved to an electronic order entry, results, and communication system.
4. Emphasize reporting to physicians. SLH has built a system to supply discharge summaries, key findings, EKG results, and cardiac imaging to referring physicians. It is also developing an electronic intensive care unit monitoring and reporting system, allowing intensivists in the flagship hospital to care for patients in smaller institutions. SLH and CHI are working actively on telecommunications with rural hospitals and patients (SLH 2003; Griffith and White 2003).
5. Keep data secure and confidential to meet HIPAA (Health Insurance Portability and Accountability Act) requirements. Permanent committees

supervise confidentiality policies and access. SLH has an extensive firewall system, hourly tape backups of critical data, and a disaster recovery process.

This strategy emphasizes measures and users, as opposed to hardware and technical capability. The leaders show that when the strategy is pursued for a few years, it results in a situation where people "understand where the numbers are coming from and move on to improving . . . operations" (Griffith and White 2003). From that emerges a culture that is evidence based, quantitative, and committed to continuous improvement. CHI has shown substantial results in only three years, with a modest investment in hardware (Griffith and White 2003). IHC's managers believe its cost accounting system and deliberate collaboration with physicians are as important to success as its medical record technology (Bohmer, Edmondson, and Feldman 2003).

Focus on Staff

This focus is defined as "how your organization's work systems and staff learning and motivation enable all staff to develop and utilize their full potential. . . . and maintain a work environment . . . conducive to performance excellence and to personal and organizational growth" (Malcolm Baldrige Health Care Criteria 2004).

The Baldrige expects human resource practices that attract and retain competent and satisfied employees and that continuously improve their skills. The work environment must develop staff, volunteers, students, and independent practitioners by aligning their expertise and efforts with the organization's overall strategy. The leading institutions do the following:

1. Strive to identify and keep good employees as the core of the human resources strategy. BHI's (2003) employee turnover rate has declined from 31 percent in 1997 to 13.9 percent in 2003. The percent of staff reporting positive morale has risen from 47 percent in 1996 to 84 percent in 2001. In 2002 and 2003, BHI was ranked in the top 15 in *Fortune*'s 100 Best Companies to Work For in America. SSMHC's (2002) all-employee turnover rate fell from 21 percent in 1999 to 15 percent in 2002. SLH's (2003) employee retention approaches 90 percent. All three exceed the Saratoga Institute's median, which is about 70 percent in 2002.
2. Create human resources systems that foster high performance. Job descriptions, career progression, motivation, communication, recognition, and compensation are well-designed, integrated processes. Selection, training, and on-the-job reinforcement of knowledge and skills are tied to individual and organizational objectives and action

plans. Explicit policies provide ways to recognize employees, physicians, and volunteers. An executive career development program identifies and develops future leaders (SSMHC 2002). SLH (2003) uses matrix accountability to manage work and jobs, emphasizing multidisciplinary teams and committees to enhance a patient-focused delivery model.

3. Emphasize organizational learning and adaptation to change. These organizations provide more than 40 hours training to each employee per year, with managers receiving almost twice as much as hourly workers. SLH (2003) appointed a chief learning officer in 2003 to identify learning needs for all staff, volunteers, and physicians. BHI's (2003) commitment to tracking the learning investment in business results led to its recognition as a "Top 50" learning organization by *Training* magazine in 2003.

4. Continually improve staff well-being, motivation, benefits, and workplace safety. To attract and retain the women who comprise 82 percent of its workforce, SSMHC (2002) offers flexible work hours, work-at-home options, long-term care insurance, insurance coverage for legally domiciled adults, retreats and wellness programs. Its workers regard its tuition assistance and student loan repayment programs as differentiating SSMHC from its competitors. At SLH (2003), factors that determine employee well-being, satisfaction, and motivation are uncovered through formal surveys, open forums with senior leaders, targeted focus groups, senior leader "walk rounds," "stay" and "exit" interviews, and a peer-review grievance process.

5. Promote a diverse workforce. SLH (2003) has focused intensely on ensuring that its workforce reflects the diversity of the community, including diversity training for all employees and "lunch and learn" sessions about diversity-related topics. Minority managers and professional staff have increased from 3 percent in 1998 to almost 10 percent in 2002. SSMHC (2002) has used a diversity mentoring program to increase minorities in professional and managerial positions from below 8 percent in 1997 to 9.2 percent in 2001, part of a larger diversity program that was recognized as a national best practice in 2002 by the AHA. Both SLH and SSMHC substantially surpass the healthcare industry average of 2 percent.

Process Management

Process management deals with "your organization's process management, including key health care, business, and other support processes for creating value" (Griffith and White 2003).

The Baldrige approaches organizations as a large set of work processes. Each process is described and monitored by performance measures that usually cover availability, cost, quality, customer satisfaction, and worker satisfaction. The benchmarks, goals, and stakeholder opinions from the strategic planning criterion are used to identify opportunities for improvement. A performance improvement council commissions PITs to pursue the most promising opportunities. Table IV.2 shows the scope of process improvements among Baldrige winners. Because of page limitations of this journal, the processes listed are the applicants' best examples. They include both outpatient and inpatient activities, although they focus on the expensive episodes. Prevention and chronic disease care remain frontiers, but many activities that generate general waste and quality problems are addressed.

The leaders' process management programs do the following:

1. Change the culture of their organizations from professional judgment to measured performance. Nursing, medicine, human resources, and accounting are not evaluated on the opinion of their professional leaders; rather, they are evaluated by performance measures.

2. Support a service line structure that organizes accountability around groups of patients with similar needs, rather than the traditional functional silos. The service lines integrate inpatient and outpatient activity.

3. Pursue all important opportunities. The leaders have the capability to support many teams simultaneously. They have no sacred cows, where history or authority protects a process from review.

4. Decision of whether performance is "good" or "not good enough" is based on comparison to goal. Any measure, from the post infarction mortality rate to days of accounts receivable, is "good" if it achieves a previously negotiated goal. The goal is often moved forward each year, based on benchmark or, in some cases such as incorrect surgical sites or medication errors, on zero defects.

5. Listen extensively to supplement the measures. Qualitative information from customers, workers, and other stakeholders is broadly sought and sensitively analyzed.

6. Revise processes based on careful analysis of qualitative and quantitative information, "outside the box" search for alternatives, and study of the work of others. Like the measures, the processes are compared to similar situations elsewhere. Learning from others is a way to speed improvement and reduce its risks. SSMHC (2002) has "collaboratives," and CHI has "affinity groups" of managers that perform similar jobs across their systems (Griffith and White 2003). SSMHC, CHI, and IHC participate in Institute for Healthcare Improvement programs to share best practices (IHC 2004).

Direct Care Processes	Site	Results
Implementation of hospitalists	BHI	Substantial reduction in length of stay, and 34 percent decrease in cost of inpatient care
Clinical pathways	SLH	~60 percent of patients assigned treatment protocols
Medication errors and patient falls	All	Decreased substantially
Heart-risk screenings	BHI	More than doubled in three years
Patient and Customer Focus		
Patient satisfaction	BHI	Increased to, at, or near the 99th percentile (inpatients, outpatients, LifeFlight)
Referrals from primary care physicians	SLH	Improved by one-third
Admitting-physician satisfaction	SLH	Improved by one-quarter
Patient volumes	BHI	Six-year growth in admissions, out-patient, emergency department use
Cardiology and orthopedic market shares	BHI	Increased by one-third
Clinical Support Processes		
Precision of blood chemistry results	SLH	"outperforms national stretch targets"
Electronic diagnostic reporting to attending physicians	SSMHC	Increased fivefold
Mammogram turnaround	SSMHC	Four days to one day
Lab tests/adjusted discharge	SLH	"among the lowest in the nation"
Other Support Processes		
Financial		
Bond rating	SSMHC	Rating achieved by only 1 percent of U.S. hospitals
Current ratio	BHI	Steady increase, exceeds Moody's median
Days in accounts receivable	SLH	Reduced by more than half, now below COTH top quartile
	BHI	Reduced by two-thirds and dropped below Moody's median
	SSMHC	Increasing
Operating margin	SLH	Increasing trend, exceeds COTH top quartile
	SSMHC	Increasing trend, matched top quartile of Catholic systems

TABLE IV.2

Examples of Successful Process Improvement from Baldrige Winners

(*continued*)

TABLE IV.2
(*continued*)

Other Support Processes	Site	Results
Return on assets, equity	SLH	Increasing trend, exceeds COTH top quartile
Cash collections	SLH	Increased by one-third (SSMHC and BHI reported similar progress)
Days cash	SLH	Imporved by one-half
	SSMHC	Improved to exceed top quartile of Catholic systems
Net income per FTE (adjusted)	SLH	Improved by half, exceeds consultant's benchmark

Productivity

Operating expense per adjusted patient day	SSMHC	Declined from 1999 through 2002
FTEs per adjusted discharge	BHI	Substantial reduction
	SSMHC	Reduced, below Catholic systems top quartile
Supply cost per discharge	SLH	Moved below COTH benchmark
Costs per hire	SLH	Reduced by two-thirds, below consultant's benchmark

Human Resources

Employees trained on compliance and ethics	SLH	100 percent
OSHA incidents	SSMHC	Reduced by 40 percent
Employee satisfaction	BHI	"Best in class" in 1999, improved subsequently
	SLH	Steady improvement
	SSMHC	Approached consultant's "best in class"
Employee turnover/retention	BHI	Improved to "best in class"
	SLH	Improving, exceeds national benchmark
	SSMHC	Improving, top quartile of consultant's data
Employees terminating because of dissatisfaction	SLH	Declining
RN vacancy rate	BHI	Reduced to one-fifth of regional average
Special-effort recognition	BHI	Increased by one-third
Workers' compensation rating	BHI	Improved to "best in class"
Lost-time injuries and claims	SSMHC	Declining, well below OSHA averages

(*continued*)

Other Support Processes	Site	Results
Needle sticks	BHI	Reduced by one-third, less-than-half national average
	SLH	Exceeds national benchmark
Back incidents	SSMHC	Declining
Training hours per employee	SSMHC	Increasing by two and one half times the reported industry average
Advanced CQI training	SSMHC	Increasing
Training effectiveness—demonstrated skill	SSMHC	Improving
Return on training investment	BHI	Exceeds national "Top 100"
Employees' performance on personal improvement goals	SLH	Steadily increasing
Employee health survey results	SLH	High-risk employees improved
Diversity in managerial/professional positions	SLH	Improving, exceeds local population and national average
	SSMHC	Improving, exceeds national average

Service Quality

Patient room work orders—ten-minute response	BHI	"Best in class"
Employee suggestions	BHI	Increased both submitted and implemented
Registration information accuracy	BHI	Decreased errors by one-third
Medical record completions	BHI	Decreased noncompliance by half
DRG coding errors	SLH	Reduced by two-thirds
Baldrige assessment scores	SLH	400 to 600, before winning award
Admission wait time	SLH	Improving
"Single call" elective admission	SLH	Tenfold growth
Information system availability	SLH	99.9 percent (SSMHC reported 99.5 percent; BHI reported "best in class")
Information system customer satisfaction	SSMHC	Improving
Supply-order accuracy	SLH	Over 99 percent
Charity care provided	SSMHC	Increasing

TABLE IV.2
(*continued*)

7. Train improvement team leaders. Team leaders get "meeting in a box" tools, analytic skills, money to travel to comparison sites, and funds for experimentation.

8. Monitor improvement teams closely. Timetables and interim goals are set. Rigorous analysis is expected. Constructive advice on complex situations and conflict resolution assistance is available from senior management.

Organizational Performance Results

According to the 2004 Health Care Criteria, this criterion refers to "performance and improvement . . . relative to those of competitors and other organizations providing similar health care services."

The measurement focus of leading hospitals allows them to document their achievements, which, in turn, has led to a number of awards. The Baldrige winners exceed national medians in more than 75 percent of their reported measures.

Discussion and Conclusion

These institutions' achievements set a new standard for performance accountability and excellence that we believe is a revolution in hospital management. Simply put, they have shown how to run healthcare organizations substantially better than is typical. Similarly, they have documented the processes that produce excellence. The new norm will not be overlooked in boardrooms, reimbursement negotiations, bond rating agencies, accrediting reviews, and courts. Just as medicine now follows guidelines for care, successful managers will use evidence and carefully developed processes to guide their decision making. Healthcare systems and hospitals that copy these processes can expect to do well. Their stakeholders—patients, trustees, physicians, nurses, payers—will be pleased. As word spreads, other stakeholders will demand no less.

Professional excellence for hospital management will become the ability to use these processes and match or exceed these numbers. Hospital managers, across the nation and at all levels, face a substantial challenge.

The evidence suggests that the challenge can be met in only a few years. Although IHC and SSMHC began their quality journeys before 1990, BHI began intensive employee training in 1997 and CHI achieved success in just three years. As Sister Mary Jean Ryan (2004), president and CEO of SSMHC, says, "the Baldrige criteria also establish a path to meet that challenge." The first four leadership steps—mission, measures, prompt reporting, and two-way communication—are the right beginning.

Revolutionary change includes profound shifts in organizational culture. Governance becomes proactive rather than reactive. It turns to ongoing cooperation instead of negotiated settlements. The concepts of professional domains—the board's, the physicians', the nurses'—gives way to dialog about the cost and quality per case; it is a fundamental shift in perspective from inputs to outputs, from tradition to results, from static to dynamic. Management is now dually accountable—upwards for results, downwards for supporting and training associates and teams. The approach is firmly grounded in learning and rewards; it is not punitive or coercive. Collaboration has become the key word at all levels. Teams collaborate to improve care, support units collaborate to meet caregiver needs, and the organization as a whole collaborates with stakeholders to further mutual aims.

References

Baptist Hospital, Inc. (BHI). 2003. Baldrige Award application. Pensacola, FL: BHI.

Bohmer, R., A. C. Edmondson, and L. R. Feldman. 2003. "Intermountain Health Care." HBS Case9-603-066. Cambridge, MA: Harvard Business School Publishing.

Catholic Health Association 2001. *Community Benefit Program*, St. Louis MO: CHA. Also see http://www.chausa.org/RESOURCE/COMMBENEFIT PROGPROMO.ASP.

Dominican Hospital (DH). 2003. Baldrige Award Application. Santa Cruz, CA: Dominican Hospital.

Friedman, P. 2004. Personal interview, September 3.

Griffith, J. R. 1998. *Designing 21st Century Healthcare*. Chicago: Health Administration Press.

Griffith, J. R., V. K. Sahney, R. A. Mohr. 1995. *Reengineering Healthcare*. Chicago: Health Administration Press.

Griffith, J. R., and K. R. White. 2002. *The Well-Managed Healthcare Organization*, 5th edition. Chicago: Health Administration Press.

———. 2003. *Thinking Forward: Six Strategies for Highly Successful Organizations*. Chicago: Health Administration Press.

Heskett, J., W. E. Sasser, and L. Schlesinger. 1997. *The Service Profit Chain*. New York: The Free Press.

Institute for Healthcare Improvement (IHC). 2004. [Online information; retrieved 6/30/04.] http://www.qualityhealthcare.org/IHI/Topics/Improvement/ ImprovementMethods/Literature/LessonsfromtheBaldrigeWinnersin HealthCare.htm.

Malcolm Baldrige Health Care Criteria for Performance Excellence. 2004. [Online information; retrieved 2/27/04.] http://baldrige.nist.gov/HealthCare_ Criteria.htm.

Ryan, M. J. 2004. "Achieving and Sustaining Quality in Healthcare." *Frontiers of Health Services Management* 20 (3): 3–11.

St. Luke's Hospital (SLH). 2003. Baldrige Award application. Kansas City, MO: SLH.

Simmons, R. 2000. *Performance Measurement and Control Systems for Implementing Strategy*. Upper Saddle River, NJ: Prentice Hall.

SSM Health Care 2002. Baldrige Award application. St. Louis, MO: SSMHC.

Discussion Questions on Required Reading

1. At the organizational level, what can top management do and how can they work to bring about the revolutionary change urged by Griffith and White?
2. How will professional domains—the board's, the physicians', the nurses'—give way to dialogue about the cost and quality per case?
3. Describe current policy as to how healthcare organizations act to recruit and retain doctors and nurses who work in the organization. Suggest changes to current behavior to improve recruitment and retention results.
4. What are some of the opportunities available to managers to better integrate the goals of physicians and nurses with those of the organization?

Required Supplementary Readings

Blumenthal, D. 2002. "Doctors in a Wired World: Can Professionalism Survive Connectivity?" *The Milbank Quarterly* 80 (3): 525–46.

Griffith, J., and K. White. 2007a. "Nursing Organization." In *The Well-Managed Healthcare Organization,* 6th edition, 253–92. Chicago: Health Administration Press.

———. 2007b. "The Physician Organization." In *The Well-Managed Healthcare Organization,* 6th edition, 203–52. Chicago: Health Administration Press.

Lake, E. T. 2007. "The Nursing Practice Environment: Measurement and Evidence." *Medical Care Research and Review* 64 (2, Suppl.): 104S–22S.

Discussion Questions for Required Supplementary Readings

1. How does organizational structure influence physician and nurse integration with healthcare organizational goals?
2. What are the causes of physician and nurse dissatisfaction in hospitals, and what can hospital managers do to improve physician and nurse morale?
3. How do organizational mission and goals influence clinician integration?
4. How does payment of clinicians influence clinician integration with organizational goals?

Recommended Supplementary Readings

Aiken, L. H., S. P. Clarke, D. M. Sloane, J. Sochalski, and J. H. Silber. 2002. "Hospital Nurse Staffing and Patient Mortality, Nurse Burnout, and Job Dissatisfaction." *Journal of the American Medical Association* 288 (16): 1987–93.

Delbecq, A. L., and S. Gill. 1985. "Justice as a Prelude to Teamwork in Medical Centers." *Healthcare Management Review* 10 (1): 45–51.

Freidson, E. 1989. *Medical Work in America*. New Haven, CT: Yale University Press.

Kilo, C. M. 1999. "Improving Care Through Collaboration." *Pediatrics* 103 (1): 384–92.

Lake, T., K. Devers, L. Brewster, and L. Casalino. 2003. "Something Old, Something New: Recent Developments in Hospital-Physician Relationships." *Health Services Research* 38 (1 Part II): 471–88.

Liedtka, J. M., and E. Whitten. 1998. "Enhancing Care Delivery Through Cross-Disciplinary Collaboration: A Case Study." *Journal of Healthcare Management* 43 (2): 185–203.

Maister, D. H. 1993. *Managing the Professional Service Firm*. New York: Free Press.

Needleman, J., E. T. Kurzman, and K. W. Kizer. 2007. "Performance Measurement of Nursing Care: State of the Science and the Current Consensus." *Medical Care Research and Review* 64 (2, Suppl.): 10S–43S.

Numerov, R., M. N. Abrams, and G. S. Shank. 2002. "Retention of Highly Productive Personnel Now at Crisis Proportions." *Healthcare Strategic Management* 20 (3): 10.

Tucker, A. L., and A. C. Edmondson. 2003. "Why Hospitals Don't Learn From Failures: Organizational and Psychological Dynamics that Inhibit System Change." *California Management Review* 45 (2): 55–72.

VHA Research Series. 2004. *Physician Hospital Relationships: Forging the New Covenant*. Irving, TX: VHA Inc.

Wynia, M. K., S. Latham, A. Kao, J. W. Berg, and L. Emanuel. 1999. "Medical Professionalism in Society." *New England Journal of Medicine* 341 (21): 1613–16.

Young, G. J., M. P. Charns, J. Daley, M. G. Forbes, W. Henderson, and S. F. Khuri. 1997. "Best Practices for Managing Surgical Services: The Role of Coordination." *Healthcare Management Review* 22 (4): 72–81.

THE CASES

The case studies in this section emphasize the many aspects of professional integration that healthcare managers are challenged to consider. First, the "Physician Leadership: MetroHealth System of Cleveland" case describes the overhaul in management/medical staff relations brought about by new leadership. Of note is this leadership's successful effort to compete in the Cleveland market as a public hospital. The "Managing Relationships: Taking Care of Your Nurses" case shows the importance of integration with other clinical professionals, particularly nurses, to both patient care delivery and organizational performance.

Today, while the medical profession still retains most of the basic and legally enforced monopoly over the key functions of healthcare as primary authority in diagnosing and treating health problems, many things are changing. The basis of their decision making has been experience and clinical judgment. Increasingly, this informal unchallengeable mode of decision making is being replaced, however, under physician supervision, by "evidence-based" medicine, and even "evidence-based management." This includes data gathering that is based on population-based reasoning, clinical decision analysis, cost-effectiveness analysis, clinical paths, guidelines or algorithms, process improvement thinking, outcomes analysis, statistical process control, quality-of-life measurements, and comparative cost analysis.

Physicians can rely on numerous sources of power in dealing with managers, including the protection afforded them by organizations or through negotiated contracts. Physicians may use the authority based on their knowledge to demand resources from managers such as additional staff, space, and equipment. Physicians are often respected by the public, certainly more than healthcare managers. They may have access to board members and community leaders who are their patients. Their power may stem from the ability to unite and to withdraw their services from organizations whose behavior is unacceptable to them.

Physicians expect recognition, acceptance, and trust from managers, and they expect that their livelihood will not be threatened by managerial initiatives. Physicians are concerned about their status and power compared to other occupational groups, to other physicians within an organization, and to physicians working at competing institutions. They want to determine their own working conditions and to be provided with support services adequate to house, feed, and care for their patients. Physicians do not like to waste time in endless or frequent meetings, and they expect to be consulted if organizational policy changes will affect them.

Many of these seem to be reasonable expectations. Why, then, do physicians feel that expectations are not met by the organization and its managers? Other physicians may be competing for limited resources of funds, space, and staff; demand may change for one specialty compared to others. The manager may have a different concept of time waste. To the physician, completing records represents time unreimbursed or ambulatory care not delivered. To the hospital, it is required for necessary cash flow. Sometimes events move too quickly to permit adequate consultation, or there is a lack of communication among physicians and lay managers.

For example, a manager may ask the chief of staff, a department head, or the medical board for approval of implementation of a risk management program, provision of financial guarantees to recruit family practitioners, or appointment of a new chief of emergency medicine. Medical officials may give informal approval and get back to physicians in each department for further discussion and recommendations for action. In the interim, however, time, money, and skilled personnel may no longer be available. Even after policies are agreed upon, the manager may find that medical leadership has misinterpreted what was agreed to at joint meetings. Following implementation of new policies, physicians may personally object, and subsequently provide care of poor quality. Yet they may fail to understand why managers do not honor what seem to them to be legitimate requests. Further, as physicians are independent contractors, they may have goal conflicts with organizations within which they practice.

Similarly, the manager expects recognition, acceptance, and trust from the physician. Managers expect physicians to be concerned about organizational goals such as cost containment and quality improvement. Managers expect physicians to fulfill specific organizational commitments agreed to in advance, such as punctual attendance at hospital meetings. The manager does not expect to be attacked personally when she and a physician disagree. She expects respect for her organizational role and responsibility for internal coordination of activities and adaptation of the organization to external pressures. The manager expects physicians not to waste the manager's time but instead, for example, to try to solve a problem first with the involved department head whose lack of timely response to the physician's request may, after all, be reasonable. The manager expects to be consulted if an action by a physician will affect the organization's goal attainment or system maintenance.

Many of these expectations seem reasonable. Why then don't physicians meet them? Physicians may not view the manager as she views herself. Physicians may view the manager as a supporter of their medical work rather than as an organizational coordinator or integrator. They may see the manager as working *for* physicians rather than *with* them to attain organizational goals. Many physicians may fear the manager because of increasing dependence on the organization for their livelihood. Managers, because of their influence on budget allocation and their control of information, may affect the physician's access to scarce resources.

If physicians can discredit the manager, the manager will have less power over them. Physicians are accustomed to giving orders, not to taking them. If the manager is actively attempting to increase revenues and decrease expenses, physicians can surely find fault. (The manager did not consult sufficiently with them, she did not consult sufficiently in advance, or she has favored certain other departments with respect to allocation of budget and staff.) Further, physicians may object to the manager's tone, style, travel schedule, number of assistants, size of office, or amount of salary.

Physicians will often disagree with the manager over policy. For example, physicians at Alpha Hospital may decide that expensive equipment will help in their daily practice, and note that surgeons at neighboring Beta Hospital are getting more sophisticated equipment. Alpha Hospital's policy of providing services to the chronically ill will therefore not help surgeons stay competitive or increase their incomes. Or physicians may have a conflict of interest with the hospital; extra nursing staff will reduce the operations surplus or lead to operations deficits.

There is often no effective organizational responsibility system for most physician behavior. Physicians can take "cheap shots" at the manager if they are not effectively accountable to anyone in the organizational structure for incurring costs or ensuring quality and access. Non-paid physician department chiefs and committee chairs are usually more interested in maintaining their physician networks of patient referrals than in achieving organizational goals. Physicians work long hours and they consider the competing and conflicting clinical and professional demands on their time more important than certain organizational obligations, even those to which they have agreed in advance.

Finally, physicians may distrust the manager, find the manager incompetent, or dislike the manager personally. This may be because of the manager's actions or inaction, ranging from failing to gain board approval for a CT scanner to responding inappropriately to low nursing morale. Increasingly physicians are being hired as managers by healthcare organizations, in part because they are more likely to be obeyed than non-physician managers. Many physician managers quickly learn, however, that, to the extent they are paid by the organization and no longer practice medicine, they are increasingly viewed by many physicians as one of "them," rather than as one of "us."

Given the inherent difficulties, what opportunities do managers have to perform effectively and yet maintain decent working relationships with physicians? Is this even possible? Managers can exchange scarce resources of money, staff, and space with physicians in return for assistance in goal attainment. Managers can order physicians to implement decisions, calculating that physicians lack the power to resist effectively. Managers can persuade physicians to act in the long-term interest of the organization, the patient, and the consumer. The manager has a limited amount of political "chips" to spend, just as she has a limited amount of organizational funds available. The manager can invest in political power by building good informal relationships with key physicians, or she can spend power in making decisions opposed by key physicians or groups. Timing, tone, body language, and judgment are all important for the manager whose tenure may well vary conversely with activism.

The manager has resources available that the physician lacks. She may have influence with the governing board regarding long-range planning decisions, influence on appointment of physicians to paid and unpaid positions or access to grants and gifts, and influence on rates of physician remuneration. The manager may have special knowledge useful in advising physicians on business and personal problems and in doing personal favors for them. The manager has information concerning results of implementing proposed strategic initiatives at other healthcare organizations.

Even as physicians have authority for patient care decisions, the manager has authority for support decisions, based on expertise in, for example, marketing and compliance with government regulation. Often competitive and regulatory requirements can be interpreted by managers to rationalize decisions that will benefit patients and consumers at the expense or inconvenience of physicians. The manager may also accrue a certain authority because of long tenure in a position, having gained the trust of physicians with similar tenure. When a manager has gained such trust, others will back critical decisions or disagree in private or in advance, without personal attacks.

The manager can persuade physicians of the justice or advantage of policy or administrative decisions. Of course, some physicians will not wish to be persuaded. It is not difficult to wake up someone who is sleeping, but it is hard to awaken someone who is pretending to be asleep.

The manager can help physicians obtain the resources they need, which may be in the organization's interest as well. The manager may delay implementation of what physicians oppose until a more favorable future time. Above all, the manager must know what she is doing, be sure of her facts, and be conservative in her forecasts. As in other fields, nothing succeeds like success or fails like failure, and often the failing manager will not be given a second chance.

Both the long and short cases in this section present various issues that might confront a manager working with physicians and other clinical professionals in a healthcare organization. All the cases generally focus on clinical leadership and the need to bring along the clinicians sooner rather than later.

Case J
Physician Leadership:
MetroHealth System of Cleveland

Anthony R. Kovner

As of fall 1998, key changes shaping the Cleveland health system included the following: increasing concentration in the hospital market, expansion of high-end medical services, health plans facing stiff price competition and internal administrative difficulties, and employers not pursuing aggressive purchasing strategies (Center for Studying Health System Change 1998). Three local institutions—the Cleveland Clinic, University Hospitals Health System (UH), and the former Blues plan, Medical Mutual of Ohio—retain dominance in the market.

Market Description

The Cleveland Clinic owns 40 percent of the hospital beds in Cuyahoga County, Ohio (population 2.2 million) and 30 percent in the broader six-county primary metropolitan statistical area (see Figure IV.3), compared with UH's 11 percent. While the two local not-for-profit hospital systems have grown, the two for-profit systems have lost market share over the last two years. MetroHealth, the county's public hospital, continues to be the leading provider of charity care and Medicaid services (see Figure IV.4). Metro retains a close relationship with the Cleveland Clinic, participating as a lead member of the Cleveland Health Network (CHN).

Cleveland has been viewed as a specialty-oriented healthcare market with considerable excess hospital capacity. The expiration of Ohio's certificate-of-need law has resulted in new construction and technology investments by hospitals. Clear competition also exists among health plans. Premium levels have been flat or have declined during the past year. Most plans share the same broad provider networks. Purchasers (employers) have not increased their demands for highly managed care insurance products nor turned to direct contracting to get more control over costs and quality.

Medicaid plans are having financial difficulties. The state's payment rates have declined and competition among the plans has increased. The number of Medicaid plans is expected to decline further as the state implements enrollment floors in each county, under which only plans that enroll 10 percent or more of the eligible population will be allowed to contract with Medicaid. MetroHealth is Ohio's largest provider of Medicaid services.

FIGURE IV.3
Cuyahoga County Hospitals

BF   UHHS Bedford
CC   Cleveland Clinic
DC   PHS Deaconess
EU   Euclid
FV   Fairview
HC   Hillcrest
HR   Huron
JW   St. John W. Shore
LU   Lutheran
LW   Lakewood
MM   Marymount
MH   MetroHealth
MS   PHS Mt. Sinai
PM   Parma
ME   PHS Mt. Sinai East
SM   St. Michael
SL   St. Luke's
SV   St. Vincent Charity
SP   South Pointe
SW   Southwest
UH   University

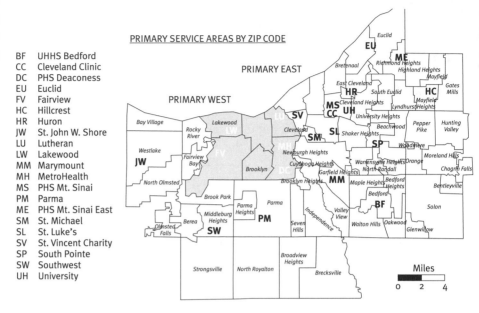

Reprinted with permission of MetroHealth.

FIGURE IV.4
Map of MetroHealth Facilities

Ⓗ   Acute Care & Rehab
★   Skilled Nursing Facilities
●   Community Health Centers
◆   Satellites

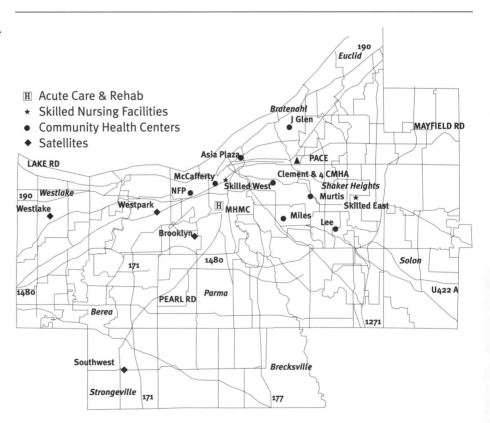

Reprinted with permission of MetroHealth.

Overview of the MetroHealth System

The mission statement of the MetroHealth System is as follows:

> The MetroHealth System commits to leadership in providing healthcare services that continually improve the health of the people in our community. We offer an integrated program of services provided through a system that encompasses a partnership between management and physicians and reflects excellence in patient care supported by superior education and research programs. We are committed to responding to community needs, improving the health status of our region, and controlling healthcare costs.

Metro is licensed to operate 680 beds, of which 524 are staffed and in use. Metro also operates two skilled nursing centers with an additional 490+ beds, a network of 16 ambulatory care centers offering primary care services in various locations, and three substance abuse treatment centers. The medical center's 41-acre campus is located on the near west side of the city of Cleveland, approximately two miles from downtown. All facilities are fully accredited.

Since 1914, Metro has been a major teaching affiliate of Case Western Reserve University and provides 40 to 50 percent of all clinical hours for university medical students. Grant funding for Metro's Center for Research and Education from the National Institutes of Health was more than $10.8 million in 1997, up from $3.8 million in 1992.

Cuyahoga County provides financial support for Metro through annual appropriations from a portion of the proceeds of two voted property tax levies for health and human services and, from time to time, its general fund. Metro trustees are appointed jointly by the Board of County Commissioners and the senior judges of the probate and common pleas courts. They serve without compensation for six-year overlapping terms and may be reappointed upon the expiration of their terms. By law, the composition of the trustees must be bipartisan with equal representation from the two major political parties.

Metro houses a Level I (highest level of complexity) trauma center, serving as the regional burn center for northeast Ohio and northwest Pennsylvania. The neonatal intensive care unit is one of three Level III (highest level of complexity) nurseries in Cleveland. The Center for Rehabilitation is a distinct 143-bed acute rehabilitation center, one of the largest in the country. Metro operates Metro Life Flight, the nation's second busiest aeromedical transport service, with four owned helicopters.

Two-thirds of Metro's 21,536 discharged patients (excluding normal newborns) live in its primary service area, whose population is approximately 500,000. In 1996, Metro accounted for 9.18 percent of the 193,802 county patients (excluding normal newborns) discharged from Ohio hospitals. In

TABLE IV.3

Indicator	1995	1996	1997
Staffed Beds	532	532	524
Occupancy Rate*	65.5	58.6	56.9
Occupancy Rate**	64.8	58.4	57.2
Licensed Beds	728	728	728
Occupancy Rate	47.9	42.9	41.0
Discharges	21,603	19,913	18,036
Patient Days	127,180	113,868	108,863
ALOS (no newborns)	5.9	5.7	6.0
Newborn Bassinets	48	48	48
Number of Births	3,823	3,910	3,719
Newborn Days	10,010	9,755	10,531
ALOS (including newborns)	5.4	5.2	5.5

MetroHealth Medical Center Utilization Statistics, 1995–1997

*Excludes newborns
** Includes newborns
NOTES: Effective May 13, 1996, 29 rehabilitation beds were changed to skilled nursing beds.
1. Staffed beds, 1995–1997 all exclude nursery bassinets. However, 1996 and 1997 include 29 subacute beds.
2. Licensed beds include 48 nursery bassinets and the 29 subacute beds. (In 1995 the 29 beds were rehabilitation.)
3. The discharges and patient days for 1996 and 1997 exclude both newborn and subacute activities.

the primary service area, which alone accounted for 46.4 percent of all discharges in the county, Metro captured the largest share of the market at 16.7 percent. Metro was a market leader in burns (70.7 percent), rehabilitation (58.3 percent), neonatology (19.2 percent), and obstetrics (18.5 percent). Metro provided more than 500,000 outpatient visits in 1997 (see Table IV.3 for Metro utilization statistics).

Metro's medical staff is organized into 16 major departments, each with a full-time chair. There are more than 350 employed physicians in each of these departments, as shown in Table IV.4, and more than 300 residents. Total medical staff includes 238 associate staff, 193 adjunct or affiliate staff, plus 71 bioscientific, emeritus, or honorary staff members. Metro employs 5,562 full- and part-time employees, including the active medical staff. Approximately 2,000 of these employees are union members.

Relationship Between Management and the Medical Staff

Metro's CEO, Terry White, has previous leadership experience at Lutheran Hospital, University Hospital of Cleveland, and University Hospital of Cincinnati. He has been the MetroHealth CEO for five years. According to Mr. White, organizations are made up of people, structure, and process. In 1994,

Department	Active Staff
Anesthesiology	18
Dentistry	7
Dermatology	4
Emergency Medicine	19
Family Practice	27
Medicine	95
Neurology	2
Ob-Gyn	21
Orthopedics	14
Otolaryngology	2
Pathology	9
Pediatrics	52
P M & R	18
Psychiatry	21
Radiology	24
Surgery	31
Total	364

TABLE IV.4
Number of Physicians by Major Medical Departments (as of July 22, 1998)

the hospital lacked such proper structure and process. Since then, Mr. White has been developing a grand alliance with the medical staff to have one rather than two management groups. He has tried, in his direction of the institution, to create a culture incorporating physician leaders. Going beyond the tokenism of board representation or the installation of a medical director, he has tried to build a physician-driven organization, with medical leadership and accountability.

When Mr. White started at Metro, a high-quality medical staff was in place, functioning under an employment model. This model had 17 different medical departments, with separate practice plans, and no oversight and accountability. Chairs were responsible for more than $100 million of budget, half of which came from practice revenue and half from hospital subsidy. The senior medical officer position was short-tenured and the occupants were neither respected nor empowered. The credentials of chief medical officers were mediocre in research and in business. No one wanted a really strong person to occupy this post. Under the previous CEO, the chairs had direct access to the CEO for most key management decisions.

In 1995, the interim chief of staff retired, and Mr. White hired a national search firm to recruit a successor. The search committee, led by a physician who was not a department chair, was composed of "physicians of the future," rather than being chair-dominated. Dr. Melinda Estes, who was finally selected as chief of staff, had unassailable credentials (including an MBA), a great number of publications, impeccable training as a neuropathologist, and her own research lab; in addition, she was the first woman on the board of governors at the Cleveland Clinic, where she was also associate chief of staff. Dr. Estes was articulate, with good interpersonal skills.

Mr. White wants Metro to be a physician-led organization; therefore, he sees his job as empowering the chief of staff to do this. She is in charge of the medical staff, and the department chairs—who are not allowed to make end runs to the CEO—report to her. In addition, the MetroHealth Management Council (MMC) was created. Before any major recommendation goes to the governing board, it must be agreed to and processed by the MMC. (See Appendix IV.1 for the MMC management protocol.)

What Mr. White has asked of physicians in return is accountability—that they support the institutional mission and be accountable for it. For the first time, the budget for 1999 integrated medical and hospital revenues by service. Results for physicians are measured in terms of productivity rather than revenues—otherwise, practice plans could be successful but slip into providing a lower standard of care for non-paying patients.

Mr. White sees his main CEO functions as helping develop Metro's vision and strategy, managing the board relationship, supporting the organization and fundraising, and building a structure to accomplish the Metro mission. He carries out his duties as CEO through a goals-and-objectives process.

Participation in Managed Care

Metro has approximately 35,000 covered lives in managed care, approximately two-thirds of whom are women and children covered by Ohio's mandatory Medicaid program. More than 12,000 covered managed care lives are not on Medicaid. Metro employees have a fee-for-service insurance program and managed care contracts with all the major insurance companies. Metro is part of the CHN network for managed care contracts, which was set up with the Cleveland Clinic. Being part of a network has also enabled economies in purchasing, as Metro is able to access Premier, a multi-hospital organization that negotiates national contracts with suppliers for a broad range of products. Collaboration with other providers has also involved clinical services. For example, Metro was losing $1.7 million annually on renal inpatient services until it formed a joint venture with another provider of renal services. The partnership has resulted in a $400,000 annual surplus, which enables Metro to capitalize satellite centers, which results in more people served in a more cost-effective way. By gaining control of these costs, Metro's 1998 costs were below those in 1994.

Metro is the largest Medicaid provider in Ohio, both in terms of fee-for-service and managed care. Managed care revenue makes up less than 20 percent of total Metro revenue. (Metro still has a large fee-for-service

Medicaid business because of turnover of beneficiaries who lose eligibility in the Medicaid program and because the disabled are not yet included in the mandatory program.) A number of competitors in this market have either pulled out or gone bankrupt, and only four HMOs in Cuyahoga County cover Medicaid managed care beneficiaries.

Metro receives full-risk capitation under its Medicaid HMO contracts. HMOs administer payment for services rendered by other providers to Metro Health Services members. Metro receives the net premium less HMO management fees, which average 15 percent of the premium. The state and county have retained vendors to manage enrollment. Metro is losing money on Medicaid managed care because of a variety of factors, including utilization, inadequate premiums, and high HMO administrative costs. Metro is losing 10 to 15 percent on every contract, but providing services to these beneficiaries is part of Metro's public mission; therefore, it must continue these contracts.

Metro's managed care panel includes 107 primary care practitioners and 366 specialists. Before contracts are negotiated they are reviewed by the MMC. Metro issues quarterly statements and reports on inpatient utilization, showing where they are losing money. Metro views the Medicaid managed care capitation rate set by the state as too low. In addition, the utilization targets that form the actuarial premises for these premiums are not realistic, given the population served. Metro's Utilization Committee now has data on a per-doctor level, which may, in the future, be related to physician compensation.

Development of Ambulatory Care Networks

Eight of Metro's satellites are in the city and four are in the suburbs, in addition to ambulatory care provided at the main hospital site. These satellites were developed to expand access and support managed care penetration for all payers. Set up to work like private practice models, the suburban satellites grew 20 percent in 1998. Patients are attracted to their own physicians, who are employed by Metro, and who often have roots in the community. The suburban satellites break even and the urban centers lose money.

Physicians under managed care are under pressure to be more productive. Base salary is now structured so that part is variable based on relative value units delivered. The physician leadership in ambulatory care is integrated within the system leadership structure, sits on all committees, and is involved in future planning. The medical operations unit provides support to the physician leadership in ambulatory satellites. Ambulatory care is a competitive market, with other hospital systems locating new sites to funnel off paying business from the Metro satellites.

Regarding ambulatory care strategy, Dr. Harry Walker, the medical director for the Center for Community Health, put it this way: "It's hard to be successful if you lock yourself into being only a public hospital. We can't lose the mission, but economic realities have to be co-equal. We must be efficient even where we are losing money, so as to use precious resources to the best advantage." Dr. Walker finds physicians more committed now to the defined strategic goals of the organization. "There is a challenge in staying alive in a competitive market, facing up to reality, but physician leaders have been brought in who want the system to work. There is a higher trust level now, more of a shared responsibility; before, there were two separate decision-making groups—medical and administrative."

Keeping Financially Healthy

Metro financials are healthy (see Table IV.5 for 1995–1997 comparative data) and have improved since 1995. Comparing 1997 to 1995, occupancy is down 13 percent (to 57 percent), discharges are down 16.5 percent, and inpatient days are down 14.4 percent. However, total outpatient visits are up 12 percent, and gross revenues are up 1.7 percent. This total includes a 21 percent increase in commercial insurance revenues. Net revenues are down 0.25 percent. Total gross revenues were $341 million and charity and bad debt costs were almost $44 million, a 13.6 percent decrease from 1995. Metro received a $17.8 million governmental subsidy in 1997. This subsidy will be $24 million for 1999.

Healthcare is a large part of the Cleveland economy. According to surveys, Metro has a positive image with the public, and residency programs have a good image with those seeking residencies, as reflected in the match results. Although many people in the greater Cleveland area may not know that Metro is a public hospital, MetroHealth lags in awareness by the public and favorableness relative to its primary competitors. The system approach with satellites has improved its image. Metro's primary care community is mainly the working poor, rather than the unemployed. And it is not located in an area with many competing hospitals of comparable clinical stature and capability.

Several of the current top Metro managers came from the Cleveland Clinic. Physicians working at Metro are proud of their mission and excited by taking cases that others don't want. But Metro cannot just rely on government status and subsidies, and physicians understand this—1999 was the first year in which medical and administrative budgets were integrated. Department chiefs became accountable, fiscally, for their whole product line.

One result of the integration was to change physicians' schedules to enhance productivity. For example, in surgery, schedules were changed from whatever surgeons wanted to what maximizes revenue utilization and level

TABLE IV.5
MetroHealth
Medical Center
Comparative
Data,
1995–1997

	1995	1997	% Change
Number of Staffed Beds	532	524	−1.50%
Number of Births	3,823	3,595	−5.96%
Occupancy Rate	65.50%	56.92%	−13.10%

Discharges*	1995	1995 %	1997	1997 %	% Change
Medicare	5,372	24.87%	4,330	24.01%	−19.40%
Medicaid	8,753	40.52%	7,177	39.79%	−18.01%
Commercial Insurance	4,672	21.63%	4,560	25.28%	−2.40%
Self-Pay	2,806	12.99%	1,969	10.92%	−29.83%
Other					
Total Discharges	21,603	100.00%	18,036	100.00%	−16.51%

Inpatient Days	1995	1995 %	1997	1997 %	% Change
Medicare	41,175	32.38%	31,758	29.17%	−22.87%
Medicaid	46,611	36.65%	38,392	35.27%	−17.63%
Commercial Insurance	29.699	23.35%	30,556	28.07%	2.89%
Self-Pay	9,695	7.62%	8,157	7.49%	−15.86%
Other					
Total Inpatient Days	127,180	100.00%	108,863	100.00%	−14.40%

	1995	1997	% Change
Total Emergency Department Visits	58,176	51,445	−11.57%
Total Outpatient Department Visits	560,670	628,328	12.07%

Total Outpatient Visits	1995	1995 %	1997	1997 %	% Change
Medicare	79,110	14.11%	96,386	15.34%	21.84%
Medicaid	196,235	35.00%	223,371	35.55%	13.83%
Commercial Insurance	141,233	25.19%	177,691	28.28%	25.81%
Self-Pay	144,092	25.70%	130,880	20.83%	−9.17%
Other					
Total Outpatient Visits	560,670	100.00%	628,328	100.00%	12.07%

Gross Revenues (in thousands)	1995	1995 %	1997	1997 %	% Change
Medicare	$82,651	24.64%	$79,707	23.35%	−3.56%
Medicaid	$118,588	35.35%	$109,519	32.09%	−7.65%
Commercial Insurance	$85,499	25.48%	$103,550	30.34%	21.11%
Self-Pay	$48,750	14.53%	$48,527	14.22%	−0.46%
Other					
Total Gross Revenues	$335,488	100.00%	$341,303	100.00%	1.73%

Net Revenues (in thousands)	1995	1995 %	1997	1997 %	% Change
Medicare	$74,421	28.07%	$71,786	27.14%	−3.54%
Medicaid	$85,163	32.12%	$72,967	27.59%	−14.32%
Commercial Insurance	$61,504	23.20%	$67,495	25.52%	9.74%
Self-Pay	$2,115	0.80%	$2,570	0.97%	21.51%
Medicaid DSH	$30,905	11.66%	$31,852	12.04%	3.06%
Local Gov. Appropriation	$11,012	4.15%	$17,800	6.73%	61.64%
Total Net Revenues	$265,120	100.00%	$264,470	100.00%	−0.25%

Uncompensated Care Costs (in thousands)	1995	1995 % of Costs	1997	1997 % of Costs	% Change
Charity Care and Bad Debt Costs	$50,846	16.33%	$43,918	14.68%	−13.63%

*These data do not include subacute discharges or newborn days and discharges.
SOURCE: NAPH Survey for both years. Only reflects the Medical Center activities.

scheduling. Prior to the schedule changes, a surgeon had a daily clinic schedule, which was never filled, and all the patients were directed to show at 1:00 p.m. Now the surgeon is scheduled for one or two afternoons and the schedule is full.

For medical operations support, departments are organized into a small number of clusters. One such cluster is surgery; ENT; orthopaedics; anesthesia; cardiology; and pulmonary. The operations manager is taking scheduling away from medical secretaries into a central scheduling system. Waiting lists are being reduced. Because of better scheduling, for example, the wait for eye exams has been reduced to three to four weeks from six to eight. Physicians stay later, allowing for three additional appointments per physician each afternoon. Metro collects only 30 percent of billings from the surgical cluster patients, and the new operations manager is working on improving pricing and coding with the help of a consultant.

Developing Information Systems

Metro is making a big transition to more modern systems. Previously, individual departments had their own information systems. They are now installing an integrated system (except for inpatient care) that will cost $20 million over the next three years. The Information Systems Committee started out searching for a purely clinical system and instead replaced a number of systems, looking for one vendor to replace the paper records. They chose Epic Systems as the new vendor because its system included scheduling for physicians and ancillaries, professional billing, managed care referrals and authorizations, and an electronic medical record.

The new system was justified on financial terms to the Metro board based on labor savings. But the new system will also be more accurate, produce information in a timelier way, help Metro satisfy external data requirements, and provide clinical decision support. An intensive training program will have to be conducted for physicians, who have recently been surveyed. According to Dr. Estes, most physicians have some experience with information systems and are not opposed to implementing the new system.

Measuring Quality, Improving Outcomes, and Increasing Patient Satisfaction

Metro is part of the Cleveland Health Quality Choice outcomes measurement program, in which hospitals play a more active role in managing length of stay. As a result of government mandate, attending physicians must be personally involved in care, so Metro has transitioned from a resident-based to an attending-driven model.

Metro has a quality department and a case management department that do concurrent quality and financial reviews of patient stay. Quality and utilization committees collect these data and share them with the relevant department. If multiple departments are involved, the physician in charge of quality improvement addresses the issue. For example, one such issue was communication of abnormal findings in x-ray. Radiologists didn't call the requesting doctor in all cases. The quality department did a root case analysis of the problems. Now physician-to-physician verbal communication is required to close a radiology file. Metro has an open communication system regarding errors, and the Quality Improvement Committee looks at how to improve the processes. For example, patients receiving anti-coagulation medicine were being dosed too heavily and the process was not being monitored carefully enough. An interdisciplinary initiative was launched and three to four protocols were reduced to two with a single pharmacy-based mixture instead of one mixed by a nurse according to physician order.

The director of the quality department spends 10 percent of his time on this function, and there are 12 FTEs in the quality department. Case management has 35 to 40 FTEs. Each year the Quality Improvement Steering Committee reviews the prior year's accomplishments and has a prioritization session for the next year (see Appendix IV.2 for Quality Improvement Steering Committee minutes, 1998 Performance Improvement Selection grid, Performance Improvement Initiatives 1998 and 1999, and Quality Improvement Report Schedule). The top quality improvement priority last year was customer service, specifically, and developing an organizational culture to support customer service. Next year the committee is planning to focus on improving emergency department throughput.

The quality department reviews medical records to meet managed care requirements and reviews ambulatory care charts quarterly. An ombudsman directs complaints to supervisory staff for response. The most frequent complaint was rudeness by employees, which led to the customer service program.

Physician leadership is directly involved in improving patient satisfaction. For example, the new chief of pediatrics found long waits and dissatisfaction in the clinics, with idle time in the morning and overcrowding in the afternoons. Residents were canceling sessions to take elective courses. Now after residents schedule sessions, they can be canceled only 45 days in advance. The number of schedulers was increased and they were moved to the patient care area. A nurse advice line was installed, which improved service to patients regarding prescription refills. As a result of improved scheduling, more pediatric services are provided by appointment rather than as walk-ins.

The chief is now working on extending hours of operation in the evenings and on Saturdays. He says, "I've had administrative support. I have faculty support to do what is good for the patient. We are not compromising education. I lead by example, doing clinics myself, and once a month being on inpatient service. So I know what the problems are."

The Role of Medical Leadership

In addition to being chief of staff, Dr. Melinda Estes is the senior vice president for medical affairs. Dr. Estes has worked in the Cleveland market for 15 years, and has been at Metro for two. (See Figure IV.5 for an organizational chart of the department of medical affairs.) She is supported by four associate chiefs of staff in the following areas: inpatient services, ambulatory care, managed care and utilization, and professional staff affairs. Only four of the chairs who were there when she was hired remain two years later.

In 1997, Dr. Estes found that the quality of physicians was excellent but many had a "victim mentality." Data for effective management was lacking. "We didn't know who we were admitting, how long they were staying, who was taking care of them, and how well we were billing. We had the information somewhere, but not in usable form." Multiple decision-making groups were meeting in parallel fashion, including the multispecialty group practice, the faculty business office, and the physician-hospital organization. The physicians were not taking responsibility for making decisions.

Department chairs, always key leaders at Metro, are now leaders of the institution as well. The new philosophy is (1) departmental business is everyone's business; (2) the office of medical affairs is looking at what departments are doing; (3) the leadership is to deliver bad news without blaming scapegoats; (4) department chairs understand and craft the institutional vision, and must buy into and sell that vision; and (5) department chairs must understand their business—operationally, fiscally, and strategically. Dr. Estes has begun to set clear expectations.

For example, when she came, "no one would send anyone they knew" to the department of dentistry. The area was physically dirty, faculty providers rarely, if ever, provided care, the support personnel were rude and unhelpful, little attention was paid to billing, revenue collections were low, it was a 9 a.m. to 3 p.m. operation, and their phone abandonment rate (callers hanging up when no one answered) was 70 percent. Dr. Estes reviewed performance with the chair and set expectations using Medical Group Management Association standards for benchmarking, as adapted by standards at the dental school. She set modest expectations, moving from three to five patients per dentist during a four-hour shift. There was no progress over six weeks. She

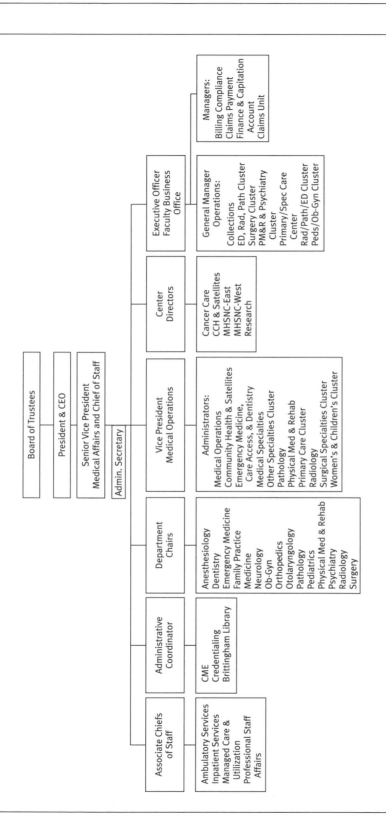

FIGURE IV.5
The MetroHealth System Organization Chart (Medical Affairs)

was visited by two young faculty dentists who said they could "clean matters up." She shared their recommendations with the chair, who replied that the department was functioning optimally and that Dr. Estes didn't understand dentistry. She asked him to step down as the chair. An interim chair was appointed and dentistry is now one of Metro's most productive, respected, and profitable departments. Metro employees now use it. This was accomplished over 12 to 14 months, with a unionized workforce.

The medical operations group provides support to the departmental chairs. Between 75 and 80 people work in this group, which serves as the administrative side for the medical groups. Previously these staff had worked in the individual departments. The group has seven cluster departments for administrative purposes, each headed by an administrator. These staff changes were made in a budget-neutral manner.

Dr. Estes chairs the MetroHealth Management Council (MMC). This group makes policy, develops strategy, and has fiscal responsibility. The MMC has seven physicians and three hospital managers (the CEO, the chief financial officer, and the chief nursing officer). The vice president for medical operations provides administrative support and is a non-voting member. The president of the medical staff is ex officio. (They have never had to take a vote.) Dr. Estes selected a balance of primary care and specialty care physicians to serve on this committee, all acknowledged leaders who think institutionally. The chiefs of surgery and medicine are on the MMC, as are the chief of radiology, the chair of pediatrics, the chair of ob-gyn, the director of community health, and the director of ambulatory care. There are two women.

Since August 1997, the MMC has had three all-day retreats, the last one addressing educational affiliations: what to get from them, and how to renegotiate affiliation contracts. The CMO sets the agenda for MMC meetings. After each meeting, executive summaries are sent to the department chairs. These summaries are discussed at monthly medical staff meetings and by the medical executive committee. Dr. Estes attends departmental meetings, as invited, at least once a year. She holds quarterly lunches with 12 different physicians whom she usually doesn't otherwise see, and walks around and tours departments by design. She writes 15 to 20 personal notes a week to physicians recognizing service or effort and communicates with physicians by e-mail and by appointment. Dr. Estes believes that to be effective, the physician leader must communicate, communicate, communicate; be a problem solver; and be proactive in leading change.

Reference

Center for Studying Health System Change. 1998. *Community Report Cleveland, Ohio*. Washington, DC: Center for Studying Health System Change.

Vision

The MetroHealth Management Council (MMC) will play a key leadership role in establishing and maintaining the MetroHealth System (MHS) as a highly competitive, cost-effective and compassionate provider of improved healthcare to the Cuyahoga County and northern Ohio community. This will be accomplished in a setting that continues to support health education and research.

Mission

The MMC will define and oversee the implementation and evaluation of MHS healthcare initiatives including strategic, financial, and operational practices. It will also develop and maintain an effective partnership between healthcare provider and hospital economies.

Objectives

Activities of the MMC will be consistent with the established vision and mission and will focus on:

1. Definition of strategic business opportunities, ventures, and partnerships.
2. Identification and prioritization of opportunities that will lead to cost and operational improvements.
   - Set priorities for the allocation of resources.
   - Review and approve budgets.
3. Initiation and oversight of ad hoc committees established to analyze operational change, develop market opportunities, and prepare business plans for recommendation to the MMC.
   - The MMC will define the initial mission, objective, and charge for ad hoc committees. This may be subsequently refined by the ad hoc committees and approved by the Management Council.

Committee Composition

The MMC will be chaired by the senior vice president and chief of staff and will be composed of seven physician staff, the president of the medical staff, and three hospital representatives.

As of July 24, 1997, members of the MMC are:

Melinda Estes, MD Chair	Chris McHenry, MD
Errol Bellon, MD	Les Nash, MD
Roxia Boykin, RN	Greg Norris, MD
Pat Catalano, MD	Richard Olds, MD
Ann Harsh	Harry Walker, MD
Mark Malangoni, MD	Terry White

Governance and Process

The chairperson of the MMC is responsible for setting the agenda for each meeting. Other processes will function as detailed below and as graphically illustrated.

A. Member Terms

   a) The senior vice president for medical affairs will chair the MMC.
   b) The chief executive officer, chief financial officer, vice president for patient care services, and the president of the medical staff will be permanent members of the council.
   c) The chairperson annually at the first meeting of the MMC in July will appoint all council members, excluding those indicated in b) above.

(continued)

d) Members are expected to attend all council meetings and the attendance of alternates will not be allowed.

B. Reporting

a) The MMC will report through the CEO to the board of trustees.

C. Communication of MMC Meetings and Activities

An objective of the council is to communicate its activities to all levels of the organization. The council will communicate through a single outgoing communication that will be in the form of an executive summary. Other forums of communication will include:

- MHS Medical Leadership Council
- MEC
- Department meetings
- Town hall meetings
- Management meetings

Minutes will be maintained for the use of the council.

Communication from MHS staff to the MMC should flow through the members of the council with any MHS staff having the opportunity to communicate to the council.

D. Committee Meeting Process

a) An executive session will be used for sensitive issues as determined by the chairperson.
b) Reports of other committees.

Formation and Process for Standing and Ad Hoc Work Groups and Task Forces

The chairperson of the MMC is responsible for establishing standing and ad hoc work groups and task forces, assigning a chairperson for the committee and identifying an initial charge and focus for the work groups or task forces. In the case where a member of an ad hoc work group or task force is not a member of the MMC, the MMC chair will assign a member of the MMC to be the primary interface to the ad hoc work group or task force chair.

Communication through an MMC representative is designed to ensure consistent communication and to facilitate requests for information or other resources that may be required by the work groups or task forces. The MMC will set standard of performance for the work groups or task forces and will monitor and adjust implementation strategies as necessary.

A. Responsibilities of Ad Hoc Work Group and Task Force Chairs

a) Communicate and refine the work groups' or task forces' mission and charge with members.
b) Ensure that a meeting schedule is established and meetings are held.
c) Ensure that minutes are recorded.
d) Work with group to establish list of deliverables and time frames.
e) Apprise the MMC of critical issues and report to Management Council as requested by the Management Council.

B. Evaluation of Work Group and Task Force Rcommendations:

The MMC will evaluate all work group and task force recommendations. Once these recommendations and plans are accepted by the MMC, the designated representative will be assigned for oversight of implementation.

APPENDIX IV.1b
Graphical
Representation
of MMC
Decision
Process

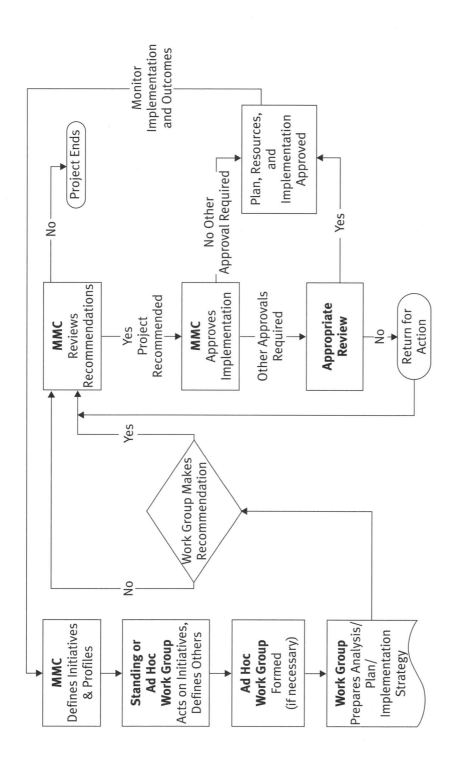

APPENDIX IV.2a

MetroHealth
System Quality
Improvement
Steering
Committee
Minutes

MetroHealth System Quality Improvement Steering Committee	1/21/99 1:00 PM–2:30 PM K-101 ← NOTE: Change in Location for 1999 Meetings

Meeting Called by: Brendan Patterson, MD

Attendees:	S. Amin	M. Legerski	J. Schlesinger
	B. Averbook, MD	T. Lukens, MD	D. Smith, MD
	R. Blinkhorn, MD	M. Malangoni, MD	J. Tomashefski, MD
	R. Boykin	R. Olds, MD	W. West
	B. Brouhard, MD	A. Petrulis, MD	T. R. White

Please Bring: *Minutes, Agenda, Attachments*

AGENDA

	TOPIC	PRESENTER	TIME
1.	Approval of minutes—November 19, 1998		2
2.	Tentative Report Schedule—1999 (Attachment A)	B. Patterson, MD	5
3.	Brainstorming & Multi-voting - PI Priorities for 1999 (See 1998 Priorities—Attachment B)	Group	30
4.	Evaluation of Program—1998 (Attachment C)	S. Amin	5
5.	ORYX • Indicator Selection • Data 3rd Q 1998 (Attachment D)	R. Boykin S. Amin	5
6.	P & T Report	B. Averbook, MD	5
7.	Ethics Report	D. Smith, MD	5

Reports/ Discussion Topics	Frequency per Year	1/21/99	3/25/99	5/27/99	7/22/99	9/23/99	11/18/99
Benchmark Data							
• Cleveland Health Quality Choice Reports	x2			X			X
• ORYX Data	x2	X			X		
• Anthem Report Card	x1				X		
Accreditation Committee	PRN						
Customer Service Performance Improvement Team	x2			X			X
Ethics Reports	x2	X			X		
External Request Oversight Activities	PRN						
Infection Control Reports	x2		X			X	
Mortality Summary	x1			X			
P&T Reports	x2	X			X		
Pathology Quality	x2		X			X	
Risk Management Reports	x3		X		X		X
Safety Report	x4		4th	1st		2nd	3rd
Transfusion Review Summary (include as part of Pathology Quality Report in 1999)	x1						
Utilization Management Reports	x2		X			X	
PI Priorities	x1 & PRN	X					
Evaluation of Program	x1	X					
QI Plan Review	x1	X					
Plan for Next Year	x1						X
PI Initiative Updates	PRN						
New Business	PRN						
Total No. Scheduled Reports		6	5	4	5	4	5

APPENDIX IV.2b

MetroHealth System 1999 Quality Improvement Steering Committee Report Schedule*

*If emergency discussion/actions required when regular report is not scheduled, add as an agenda item under new business.

APPENDIX IV.2c

MetroHealth
System 1998
Performance
Improvement
Selection Grid

Selection Criteria (factors considered during brainstorming & multi-voting processes)		
A. Accomplish mission & goals; actualize vision (Strategic Priorities 1–7)		
B. Hospital-wide function not currently being assessed (Strat. Pr. 2,4,7)		
C. Current or previous compliance issue (Strategic Priorities (1,4,7)		
D. UR, RM, QC, Infection Control issue (Strategic Priorities (1–3)		
E. High cost or significant savings potential (Strategic Priorities 3)		
F. Benchmarking information available (Strategic Priorities 4,7)		
G. Evidence of variations in practice (Strategic Priorities 1,4)		
H. External customer expectation/need (Strat. Pr. 1,5)		
I. New process or problem-prone activity (Strat. Pr. 2,4,7)		
J. Strong internal interest (Strategic Priorities 1–7)		
K. High Volume		
L. High risk		
Total Points		

Potential projects identified by MHSQISC members during brainstorming session (February 1998)

Potential Projects	**MULTI-VOTING RESULTS*** (3 points if selected as highest priority 1 point if 3rd highest priority 0 points if not selected as one of the top 3 choices)
Customer Service (Int. & Ext.)	23 points
Error Management/Root Cause	14 points
Specific Disease Management	12 points
Ambulatory Operations	7 points
Presurgical Evaluation	5 points
Abnormal Labs/Communication	3 points
Billing Issues	2 points
Surgical Waiting Area	0 points
Transportation/East Side	0 points
ORYX/SB50/Sentinel Events	
JCAHO	

CONFIDENTIAL/QA PURPOSES   *Based on responses from 11 individuals

APPENDIX IV.2d
MetroHealth
System Quality
Improvement
Steering
Committee
Performance
Improvement
Initiatives,
1998*

Committee Oversight Activities
- Set performance improvement priorities for 1998 (2/98, 4/98)
- Restructured committee membership and reporting relationships (4/98)
- Developed tentative reporting structure for activities in 1999 (11/98)

Customer Service
- Developed an improvement team to address customer service issues (2/98)
- Identified key deliverables (7/98)
- Developed timeline to accomplish identified strategies/tasks (9/98)

Data Review
- Cleveland Health Quality Choice (4/98, 6/98, 11/98)
- Mortality summary data (5/98)
- Transfusion appropriateness data (5/98)
- ORYX indicators (11/98)

Ethics Committee
- Provided several patient care consultations (9/98)
- Participated in ethics-related educational activities (9/98)
- Discussed/made recommendations regarding ethical concerns of "do not resuscitate" policies/procedure, informed consent, advance directives, managed care

Joint Commission
- Notified that the Joint Commission Type I Recommendations were addressed satisfactorily (2/98) & of revised Joint Commission grid score (4/98)
- Had a mock Joint Commission survey by a consulting team (7/98)
- Received results of mock survey & developed action plan (9/98)

Infection Control Committee
- Summarized reorganization activities of employee health program (9/98)
- Reviewed data regarding care of inpatients with pulmonary tuberculosis in 1997 (9/98)

Informed Consent
- Formed a subcommittee to address informed consent issues (5/98)
- Identified methods to document informed consent (7/98)
- Identified educational needs (7/98)
- Classified major vs. minor procedures needing informed consent (11/98)

Managed Care
- Anthem
  - Notified that actions taken in response to 1996 Report Card were accepted (2/98)
  - Collected & submitted required data for 1997 (4/98)
  - Notified of passing 1997 Report Card score (5/98)
  - Collected & submitted required data for 1st half 1998 (11/98)
- Cleveland Health Network
  - Provided results of medical record audits, office site reviews, & long-term care site review (5/98)
  - Explored alternative methodologies for conducting required medical record audits & office site reviews (7/98)

Pathology Quality Committee
- Implemented new reporting structure for related committee activities (Tissue Committee, Transfusion Committee, Point of Care Testing Committee, & Departmental QI Committee) (9/98)

(*continued*)

APPENDIX IV.2d

(*continued*)

- Evaluated the performance of INR testing in a proposed anticoagulation clinic (9/98)
- Implemented efforts to reduce wastage of fresh frozen plasma & platelets (9/98)
- Implemented a new mechanism to improve turnaround time for specific test results in pediatrics (9/98)

Pharmacy & Therapeutics Committee
- Revised restriction policy for pharmaceutical representatives
- Implemented corrective actions relative to administration of heparin (11/98)

Risk Management
- Coordinated activities to:
  - Reduce frequency and severity of patient falls (4/98, 7/98, 11/98)
  - Reduce elopements from the emergency department (4/98)
- Conducted critical incident reviews with corrective actions for:
  - Administration of heparin (4/98, 7/98, 11/98)
  - Antibiotic administration in the operating room (5/98)
  - Administration of conscious sedation (7/98)
- Clarified appropriate use of terms "sentinel events" and "critical incidents" (7/98)
- Shared plans for a "mock trial" educational session in 1/99 (11/98)

Safety
- Reviewed the annual summary of activities for all Environment of Care components (4/98)
- Summarized capital expenditures to remove physical barriers & improve ADA compliance (5/98, 11/98)
- Noted activities aimed at reducing employee injuries (5/98, 7/98, 11/98) & exposure to latex products (7/98)
- Clarified staff roles regarding the use of restraints in conjunction with patient care (5/98)
- Noted reduction in general liability claims due to efforts by Facilities Engineering to correct hazards on grounds & by Logistics Department to train staff in safe/defensive driving (5/98)
  - Training of staff (5/98)
  - Revision of emergency preparedness & disaster planning (7/98, 11/98)
- Shared activities to integrate Life Flight safety into general safety activities (5/98) and results of inspection of the helipad by the Cleveland Fire Department (11/98)
- Summarized activities taken to improve safety within the physical plant (7/98, 11/98)
- Addressed storage practices in the Quad & the basement of Bell Greve buildings (7/98)
- Noted results of inspection by state of Ohio OSHA that was conducted in response to an employee complaint regarding air quality in the Quad (7/98, 11/98)

Utilization Management
- Provided denial data for delegated utilization management plans (11/98)

*As documented in 1999 minutes from MetroHealth System Quality Improvement Steering Committee.

Case Questions

1. What are the most important factors at MetroHealth that affect physician–management relations?

2. What are some of the ways in which integration of physicians relative to the goals of a hospital system can be effectively measured?
3. To what extent does the payment system at MetroHealth influence physician performance?
4. In what ways is Dr. Estes a successful physician leader?
5. To what extent is physician commitment to organizational mission and strategy key to MetroHealth's success in the marketplace?
6. To what extent is physician commitment to organizational mission and strategy key to MetroHealth's relative success in the marketplace?

Case K
Managing Relationships:
Taking Care of Your Nurses

Anthony R. Kovner

Recently, a patient was transferred to the pediatric cardiac intensive care unit (PCICU) at Children's Hospital, a 250-bed hospital across the street from North Division, one of five hospitals in the University Health System. This 12-year-old boy had had a cardiac arrest on the pediatric floor of a community hospital in a neighboring state. An otherwise normal child, Charlie needs a heart transplant, lots of medications, and a battery of tests. In the process, Charlie's family watched and waited in the operating room as a ventricular assist device was placed. Charlie's parents now sit in his room and listen; they overhear everything and want to know, for example, why the monitor beeps or doesn't beep. Children's Hospital does more heart transplants than any other such hospital in the United States, and completed 27 last year.

Betsy Cline, the patient care director of the PCICU, which has 14 beds, has held this post for two years. (See Figure IV.6.) The unit has an $8 million budget. Cline has worked at Children's Hospital for 16 years. She spends 50 percent of her time on patient safety, 25 percent on staffing and recruitment, and 20 percent with nurses in relation to their satisfaction with the work and with families relative to their satisfaction with care. Ten percent of Cline's time is spent on administrative duties. According to Ms. Cline, "What I like is working with exceptional nurses who are very smart and do what it takes with limited resources. However, we don't always feel empowered, despite the existence of shared governance, a structure I help to coordinate."

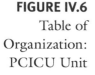

FIGURE IV.6
Table of
Organization:
PCICU Unit

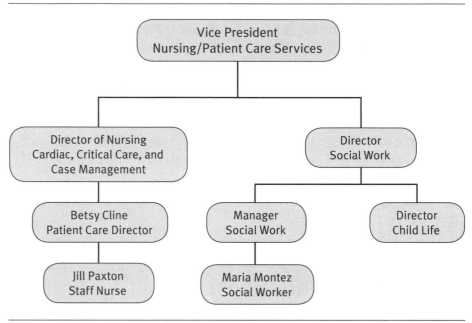

Relationships with Nurses on the Unit

Nurses on the unit work three days a week, 12 hours a shift. Cline says, "we did an employee opinion survey that went to all employees on the unit, 50 people in all, but only 13 responded. Some of them weren't sure who their supervisor was. The employees aren't happy but our patients are happy." She adds that "my name is on the unit, not the medical director's. If anything goes wrong with the unit, they blame it on nursing. Yet I'm brushed off by people whom I have to deal with outside of the unit. For example, we have a problem with machines that analyze blood gases. I spoke with the people there about the technology. This was four weeks ago. It's a patient safety issue. I sent them e-mails. I need the work to get done. The staff don't feel empowered if I'm not empowered. This goes for other departments as well. For example, respiratory therapy starts using a new ventilator without informing us. We have never seen this machine nor have we been in-serviced on it. They don't phone or e-mail. So I make the decision that we're not going to use the machine. With surgeons, when I tell them to wash their hands, they roll their eyes. It takes tremendous energy to deal with this."

"We have too many meetings. Some weeks I spend 70 percent of my time in meetings, from 10 a.m. to 5 p.m. For many meetings, I cut my appearance short or don't go. Evaluations and bonuses are insignificant in influencing my behavior. Last evaluation I had been running two intensive care units with no administrative support and no orientation to my job and they gave me a $4,000 bonus, which was nothing."

Jill Paxton, RN, age 25, is a clinical nurse in the PCICU where she has worked for six months; she has been at the hospital for nine months. Paxton spends 40 percent of her time dealing with patients and families—turning, suctioning, changing dressings; 30 percent talking with physicians—negotiating plans of care and medication plans; 20 percent in medications administration and conversations with the pharmacy; and 10 percent on miscellaneous activities. She has worked on the day shift for only three weeks now but was also on days for three months during orientation. Paxton says she is challenged to get the core services she needs. If she has to give a 2:00 p.m. medication, she would like the medication by 1:00 p.m. but she gets it by 4:00 p.m., even if she calls. She finds it difficult to coordinate services from a child life specialist—a specialist who breaks down medical terminology to children, such as "what's about to happen to you," and who also deals with siblings. Paxton can't find the cardiac transplant consultant when she needs her and doesn't have her pager number. Paxton's main satisfaction comes from educating the people she's working with, repairing children and seeing them go home, and helping the families.

Paxton comments that Cline is "good about getting stuff if you ask her. She deals with a lot. Cline goes around and talks with families, provides continuity, helps out when we're short. Lately she's not been so stressed out and is more accessible. When we were short, Cline and the patient educator admitted patients and helped with codes and patient deaths. Cline gets respect from the nurses, but she doesn't trust us enough. For example, she asks us why we were sick and to bring a doctor's note. Cline is spread thin. There is no assistant director, so the nurse educator helps her. Cline took the job having had no management experience."

Relationships with Families

Cline says, "I'm clear with them in orienting families to the unit, to how we do our job. We treat families with respect. Families watch me, and mentoring of nurses is important."

Paxton agrees that the unit generally does a good job supporting families. She says, "families are kind and happy. There is a problem with turnover of doctors and residents, who aren't here two days in a row. The plan of care can get lost with attendings when they change every week. Families are told of different outcomes and recovery times. Families get stressed out and are often far from home. I listen to them and ask, 'do you have any questions?' 'what do you want to see done?' and 'do you have any questions for the doctors?' I ask them if they want to participate in rounds. Sometimes we just listen. When families can't come in they can call me every two hours as we have an in-house phone that accepts outside calls."

A survey of families in a California hospital about their experiences and their suggestions for improving the quality of end-of-life care found that:

- Parents want to be involved in the decision-making process
- Isolated incidents are extremely painful (e.g., poor communication, feeling dismissed)
- Delivery of difficult news is an issue—families found it important that a familiar person deliver this news (one caregiver in charge)
- A language barrier is an issue—families felt isolated and under-informed
- Bereavement follow-up is helpful and appreciated
- Pain management is an issue—parents describe anguish witnessing a child in pain
- There is a need to support siblings
- Families' interactions with staff are as important as medical aspects of treatment.

Cline and Paxton feel that families are a very important part of what they do, that the unit has special structures and processes to involve families, and that what they are doing is generally working. But they lack concrete ways of measuring unit performance in this regard.

Relationship with Social Work

Cline says, "There is a hospital social worker who deals with heart transplants. This service is fragmented and I have difficulty getting her to come to the unit. I will go to her director or my director if I have to. I understand she has other responsibilities, but she needs to come to rounds, to deal with issues around getting nurses for home care. Of course, social workers can't wave a magic wand."

Maria Montez, the unit social worker, has worked in the PCICU for ten years. She spends 75 percent of her time on the floors with families. She works from 9:30 a.m. to 5:30 p.m. five days a week and there is social work coverage at other hours. The kinds of issues Montez deals with are requests for a visiting nurse; medications and associated education; ordering oxygen; ordering a special intervention team at home if there is a need to assess; and physical, occupational, and speech therapy. If a patient is dying, she discusses with nursing what they can do together when crises come up.

Montez says she has a good relationship with Cline, and that she orients the new nurses to social work. Montez respects the work that nurses do. "We're invited to each others' rounds. The work is so intense, there are so many patients. We've reached a level of understanding; if there's a problem it's not personal, it's what we're all going through. We discuss each of the 37 patients in the three ICUs once a week at an interdisciplinary conference." Montez concludes that "if I could advise the hospital administrator, I would tell him or her to take care of your nurses."

On November 15, 2006, Betsy, Jill, and Maria had lunch in the cafeteria of Children's Hospital. They discussed what "taking care of your nurses" really means from a hospital point of view. A summary of highlights of their discussion follows:

Cline: I don't know. Why should "taking care of nurses" be any different from taking care of any of the clinicians who are working under stress in the hospital? Oh, I'm sure the hospital administrators would say we pay the nurses enough. I think the hospital should do more to reward the patient care directors. None of us got into this business to do management, and they aren't really giving me the tools to do what needs to get done for our patients.

Montez: Staff is doing all we can for the patients and the families, and we're providing good care. I think things are fine as they are if we could be sure that we won't be short staffed, and if other departments would respond better to our requests to help our patients.

Paxton: But Maria, don't you agree that sometimes nurses get stressed out and that this isn't good for those nurses, the other nurses, the patients, the families, or the hospital? How do you determine what's "stressed out"? Well, it automatically flows from the number of patients, the complexity of the treatments, and the numbers of the staff and support staff. Families can tell you when the nurses are no longer providing the services at the level or quality they were providing before.

Cline: I wonder what more I can do as a manager to deal with this problem. I think our regular nursing staff has a pretty good deal here, if you want to work with these patients. And we're provided generally with the support to take good care of these patients and families. Nurses work three days on and four days off. Four days off is a lot of time to recover from stress, I think. Maybe after a number of months working in the unit, our nurses should work with patients who are less acutely ill. But I'm not sure everybody wants to do that.

Case Questions

1. What are the most important things that Betsy Cline can do to "take care of her nurses" who work in the pediatric cardiac intensive care unit?
2. What are the priorities for Jill Paxton?
3. How can nurses in the PCICU judge whether the unit is doing an adequate job supporting families?

4. What would you say are the present strengths and weaknesses of Betsy Cline's performance as a patient care director?
5. What specific advice would you give to the hospital administrator to "take better care of your nurses"?

Short Case 16
Complaining Doctor and Ambulatory Care

Anthony R. Kovner

You are the assistant director for ambulatory services. An attending physician complains, "The clerks are no good in this clinic, and neither is the director of nursing." What do you say to him? Assume that the physician is an important customer.

Later during the week, he is still not satisfied. Now *you* are the problem. What do you do now?

Short Case 17
Doctors and the Capital Budget

Anthony R. Kovner

You are the hospital CEO. Doctors on the capital budget committee can't agree on which equipment to recommend for purchase and for how much. They are way over budget. What do you say to them?

Short Case 18
Doctors and a New Medical Day Care Program for the Terminally Ill

Anthony R. Kovner

You are the hospital CEO. Medical staff is opposed to the hospital's providing needed day care to the terminally ill, which is forecasted to break even financially. They say this is not what the hospital is supposed to do, and that it will actually or potentially compete with their business. What do you say to them?

Short Case 19
Average Length of Stay

Anthony R. Kovner

You are the hospital CEO. Two of the doctors consistently keep too many of their patients in the hospital longer than the average length of stay for several diagnosis-related groups. They say their patients are older and sicker and that they're practicing higher-quality medicine. What do you say to them?

Short Case 20
Building the Office of the Medical Director

Gary Kalkut

New York General Hospital (NYGH) is a large, urban, academic medical center with a 120-year history of serving its community. The majority of its patients are insured by government programs; 20 percent of the population in its service area is uninsured. It has consistently attracted superior faculty drawn by the community-focused mission and the excellence of its academic programs. Despite the adverse payer mix, NYGH has been one of the few health systems in the metropolitan area that has been financially successful. The medical center has invested significantly in information technology for clinical and business systems, added 400,000 square feet of new clinical space including a children's hospital, and refurbished aging infrastructure.

The success of NYGH has been driven by inpatient efficiency and volume. The CEO has said that when he arrived "patients used to stay for the season." Now, case-mix adjusted length of stay is the lowest in the region due to implementation of a hospitalist program, markedly improved turnaround time for diagnostic testing, and an organizational commitment to making the medical center a seven-day operation by enhancing inpatient and outpatient weekend services.

The medical staff—academics and voluntary physicians—initially cooperated with the administration to achieve better inpatient throughput, but many saw these efforts as a threat to their autonomy and to established teaching programs. The 24 chairs met regularly with the administration, but few still practiced regularly and most were not intimately familiar with operational issues outside their departments. Also, the residents felt increasingly alienated from the departments and organization. In the middle of the academic year, a cross-departmental group of residents presented the administration with a petition signed by 60 percent of the residents asking the leadership to recognize a house staff union.

Dr. Pack had become medical director three months before the house staff presented their organizing petition. He was a long-time member of the academic faculty, and had worked on the quality program and throughput in the Department of Medicine. Dr. Pack was appointed as a second institutional medical director—the incumbent medical director oversaw a traditional medical director portfolio, including quality, regulatory, risk, physician discipline, chairs, and medical staff officers. The charge for Dr. Pack was to foucs on improving the operation and integration of services and alignment of employed and voluntary physicians with the medical center. Dr. Pack was asked to lead the institution's response to the house staff's organizing efforts.

Case Questions

1. How should Dr. Pack approach the chairs and medical staff leadership to improve alignment between the hospital and its physicians?
2. What are the issues raised by a house staff union proposal? What initial steps should Dr. Pack take to respond to the organizing effort?
3. What are the implications of progressively increased hospital efficiency for the employed physicians, the voluntary physicians, and the teaching programs?
4. How would you improve communication between physicians and the hospital administration?

V

ADAPTATION

A hospital is a living organism, made up of many different parts having different functions, and to the environment, to produce the desired general results. The stream of life which runs through it is constantly changing . . . Its work is never done; its equipment is never complete; it is always in need of new means of diagnosis; of new instruments and medicine; it is to try all things and hold fast to that which is good.

—*John Shaw Billings (1889)*

COMMENTARY

Adapting to external and internal pressures for and against change is a difficult challenge for the manager of a healthcare organization. The word "adaptation" suggests a view of organizational survival and growth as dependent on a specific direction of change. A closer fit between environmental demands and organizational response allows the organization to attract greater or continued resources from society.

A key paradigm here comes from marketing. In quality improvement, this is called customer-mindedness. The central idea is to find out what people want and design a product or service to meet these preferences, rather than create a product or service and convince people that they want it. Finding out what patients want and organizing to respond to those preferences is at the core of a customer-driven organization. Patient satisfaction surveys, focus groups, follow-up telephone calls after discharge, and community surveys are now widely used.

Organizations vary in their sensitivity to environmental pressures. Healthcare organizations function in complex environments, and failure to respond to pressures—such as competition, financing problems, and workforce issues—threatens their viability.

In all aspects of healthcare, large organizations are getting larger and capturing market share, although there is room in many markets for many smaller organizations to remain viable and grow. Competitors typically cross traditional lines. For example, large health systems may often contain within them an HMO, a long-term care facility, a nursing home, housing, and neighborhood health centers. Healthcare organizations compete with each other for patients, funding, and workforce.

Medical technologies are constantly changing. Effective drugs for mental illness introduced in the 1950s led to deinstitutionalization, community-based treatment, halfway houses, and an increase in homelessness and in the jail population of the mentally ill. Over 50 percent of surgery is now done in ambulatory surgery centers and doctors' offices. Hernia surgery, which once required a 20-day hospital stay, is now routinely an ambulatory procedure. Paperless electronic health records, telemetric laboratory and radiologic testing, and computer-assisted laser surgery are already common. Digital radiology tests taken in the United States are being read by radiologists in Australia or India. Keeping up with advances in informatics and diagnostic procedures is costly, and the benefits of those advances are difficult to accurately forecast.

Healthcare organizations are physically located in communities. But the communities they serve may be geographically local, regional, or even national, as increasingly consumers shop over the Internet and travel for services they believe to be higher in quality and less costly. Some patients have surgery in India or other countries, believing they receive adequate quality care at a lower cost. But many organizations are locally controlled, and require strong community relations to accomplish their purpose—for example, relations with churches may be important in making sure that low-income mothers-to-be get adequate prenatal services. Some healthcare organizations are owned by a government, with the goal of meeting the healthcare needs of nearby residents. Others serve the poor to maintain their not-for-profit tax status.

Healthcare organizations receive funding from a variety of sources, each with their own rates, regulations, and conditions. The organizations often have little influence as to what they get paid by large payers, and often can only respond by trying to increase volume.

Payer mix is an important consideration in changing what services are started, increased, decreased, or discontinued.

Healthcare organizations are often large employers. When a healthcare facility closes, the community becomes less attractive. Conversely, opening a large new facility is a boon to local union workers and firms.

Healthcare organizations respond to external pressures in a variety of ways, from pursuing acquisitions or mergers to selling or closing services and programs to investing (or not) in highly intensive capital technology to saturating (or not) local areas with satellite health centers. Appropriate response often requires specialized management staff in planning, marketing, community relations, data generation, and other areas. Healthcare organizations must constantly scan the environment to ensure that they can adequately respond to current developments and anticipate future trends.

THE READINGS

Begun and Heatwole's cycling model of strategic planning facilitates adaptation. Traditional strategic planning does not adapt well in a dynamic environment. Begun and Heatwole emphasize continuous assessment of strategies based on feedback from benchmark analysis and dialogue with key stakeholders. They suggest using multiple scenarios and making contingency plans given the uncertainty of the future.

The supplementary readings are divided among planning and marketing articles, along with the Robinson and Dratler piece on how the Catholic Healthcare West system balances mission and margin in a capital-intensive industry. These articles focus on the organizational response rather than on the environmental pressures. Christensen, Bohmer, and Kenagy argue that the innovations that will eventually turn healthcare organizations around are ready, in some cases—but they can't find backers. Berry and Bendapundi demonstrate the Mayo Clinic's organized, explicit approach to presenting customers with coherent, honest evidence of organizational abilities.

Griffith and White explain how planning and marketing departments of large health systems work. They review how planning departments (and internal consultants) analyze and forecast statistical data; provide expertise on complex technical problems; and maintain community values in planning decisions and capital investments. With regard to marketing and strategy, they explain how marketing is a broad approach to building exchange relationships and how to use evidence-based management to frame strategies. They also discuss segmentation of markets, listening approaches, and management of the strategic discussion.

Strategic Cycling Revisited

Note from James W. Begun, University of Minnesota
From the Editor: This note updates information since this article was originally published.

The core messages of "strategic cycling" remain relevant in an environment characterized by growing pressures to improve healthcare organizations in strategic ways. For example, to argue that healthcare organizations can somehow deliver care that is safe, effective, equitable, efficient, patient-centered, and timely without strategic planning—by just doing more of what they currently do—is farfetched. Strategic planning allows an organization with limited resources to prioritize problems and opportunities for change, analyze and customize potential solutions, and go after them. Strategic planning is one of the most important practices healthcare administrators can bring to their organizations.

At the same time, strategic planning processes need to be more flexible and fluid than ever, to accommodate increased competition among organizations (e.g., hospitals and urgent care centers) and to be responsive to new community and personal health needs (e.g., health promotion and prevention, palliative care, behavioral and complementary health services, chronic care, and aging services). As promoted in the article, the strategic planning process, conceptually, should be "continuous"—plans are subject to revision depending on conditions that could change at any minute in significant ways. A useful piece of advice from management consultant Tom Peters (1991, p. 555) comes to mind: "I beg each and every one of you to develop a passionate and public hatred for bureaucracy." In the same way that bureaucracies can be mind numbingly ineffective in changing times, so can strategic plans that rigidly proscribe activity several years into the future. (Some 30 percent of healthcare organizations develop strategic plans with a time horizon of five years or greater [Zuckerman, 2007].) Administrators should question and challenge their own plans in the interests of continuous improvement.

Three concepts would be added to the discussion of strategic cycling were it to be re-written today. First is the concept of the learning organization. Learning has emerged as a key purpose of planning in a dynamic marketplace. Learning requires that organizations systematically collect feedback from strategic ventures. Learning has to be incorporated into the organization's mission/vision/values, and resources have to be devoted to it. Second is the concept of evidence-based management. Far too many strategies of healthcare organizations emerge from tradition, imitation, and fad behavior (Kaissi and Begun, 2008). The thoughtful consideration of evidence and customization of strategies to a local setting, coupled with a learning posture ("we will make mistakes and we will learn from them"), are part of a healthy planning process. A third concept that has emerged as useful in the planning process is the balanced scorecard. The idea that organizational performance is multidimensional, and that elements of success need to be comprehensive rather than just financial, has become widely accepted over the past decade.

Effective healthcare organizations and their leaders will continue to plan for the future while adapting their planning processes to a dynamic environment. The strategic cycling model is a convenient and practical way to structure a flexible and fluid planning process that also promotes learning and the use of evidence in management decision-making.

References

Kaissi , A. A. and J. W. Begun. 2008. "Fads, Fashions, and Bandwagons in Healthcare Strategy." *Healthcare Management Review* 33(2): 94–102.

Peters, T. 1991. *Thriving on Chaos.* New York: HarperPerennial.

Zuckerman, A. M. 2007. *Raising the Bar: Best Practices for Healthcare Strategic Planning.* Chicago: Society for Healthcare Strategy and Market Development.

Strategic Cycling: Shaking Complacency in Healthcare Strategic Planning

Jim Begun and Kathleen B. Heatwole
From the *Journal of Healthcare Management* 44 (5), September/
October 1999

Executive Summary

As the conditions affecting business and healthcare organizations in the United States have become more turbulent and uncertain, strategic planning has decreased in popularity. Strategic planning is criticized for stifling creative responses to the new marketplace and for fostering compartmentalized organizations, adherence to outmoded strategies, tunnel vision in strategy formulation, and overemphasis on planning to the detriment of implementation.

However, effective strategic planning can be a force for mobilizing all the constituents of an organization, creating discipline in pursuit of a goal, broadening an organization's perspective, improving communication among disciplines, and motivating the organization's workforce. It is worthwhile for healthcare organizations to preserve these benefits of strategic planning, at the same time recognizing the many sources of turbulence and uncertainty in the healthcare environment.

A model of "strategic cycling" is presented to address the perceived shortcomings of traditional strategic planning in a dynamic environment. The cycling model facilitates continuous assessment of the organization's mission/values/vision and primary strategies based on feedback from benchmark analysis, shareholder impact, and progress in strategy implementation. Multiple scenarios and contingency plans are developed in recognition of the uncertain future. The model represents a compromise between abandoning strategic planning and the traditional, linear model of planning based on progress through predetermined stages to a masterpiece plan.

The popularity and significance of strategic planning reside on a pendulum in the same manner as a host of other in-favor/out-of-favor management techniques. Strategic planning is alternately hailed as the savior or denounced as the false god of organizational management. As the pendulum swings, however, much of the contemporary literature portrays planning in a negative light, as it has become fashionable to attack formal strategic planning (Gray 1986, 89; Daft and Lengel 1998, 223). Recent empirical research on the effectiveness of strategic planning is also divided; numerous studies support its efficacy, but just as many cite no relationship with organizational performance (Boyd 1991; Bruton, Oviatt, and Kallas-Bruton 1995; Powell 1992; Sinha 1990).

This article will discuss both the negative and positive features of strategic planning. The negative concerns about strategic planning are related to the dynamic environment facing organizations in general, and more recently, organizations in the healthcare industry. Discussion of the positive and negative consequences of strategic planning and the environment in which planning in healthcare organizations must take place provides a framework for the use of a strategic cycling model. This model incorporates the positive features of planning and addresses the negative consequences to guide hospitals and other complex healthcare organizations through the turbulent environment.

Potential Adverse Consequences of Strategic Planning

Many legitimate concerns about the effectiveness of strategic planning have been voiced, particularly relating to the traditional, formal, linear method. There have been situations in which formal strategic plans have been more harmful than helpful to corporate organizations, and these issues translate to the healthcare industry. Six of the major negative consequences of strategic planning follow.

1. When "planning" is initiated by an organization merely to satisfy a regulatory body's requirement for a "plan," the effort becomes meaningless. No commitment is made on the part of key leadership, and no participation is given from those in the organization who will be responsible for implementing the plan. When the planning process becomes too bureaucratic, formalized, and irrelevant, creativity can be stifled and critical opportunities overlooked (Hax and Majluf 1991; Lenz 1985; Perry, Stott, and Smallwood 1993).
2. A bureaucratic planning process focused on top-down development may lack coordination and integration with other critical dimensions of the organization. The need for strategic integration includes not only

the operational element of the organization and middle management, but other related functions such as financial resource management and information management (Hax and Majluf 1991; Henderson 1992).

3. One of the most common complaints regarding strategic planning is the lack of flexibility and responsiveness, particularly in a dynamic and rapidly changing environment. In many organizations, strategic planning has become so much of a science, with graphs, charts, statistics, and projections, that there is no accommodation for the art, intuition, and innovation that is so necessary if planning is to be effective (Luke and Begun 1994). Plans that are too rigid and detailed can inhibit flexibility and innovation (Aaker 1992; McDaniel 1997).

4. An interesting phenomenon that can be a significant negative consequence of planning is the automatic buy-in that can occur when a "masterpiece plan" is created. After creation of the masterpiece, the tendency is to try to make the plan work. Two factors are at work: (1) a fear of loss of face if plans change fosters an adherence to the plan even in situations where a change of course is clearly indicated (Mintzberg 1994); and (2) "organizations will generally tend to make changes closely related to their current strategies . . . to stay within their strategic comfort zone beyond which the organization does not wish to venture" (Shortell, Morrison, and Friedman 1992, 35).

5. Using the past to project the future is also a potential negative consequence of a formal planning process. The often-erroneous assumption that the future will follow past trends can lead to the development of flawed strategies. This emphasis on the past can lead to "the creation of strategies that are either repetitions of a largely irrelevant past or imitations of other organizations" (Wall and Wall 1995, 49). Ohmae (1982) refers to this flaw as "strategic tunnel vision," where the greater the need to broaden the vision, the more likely the tendency to narrow the focus, eliminating potentially viable options.

6. A final and deadly complaint against strategic planning is that too much attention and effort are placed on the development of the plan and strategies, and very little on implementation and monitoring. In many cases, the plan becomes the end of the process, not the spark to move the organization to change (Abell 1993; Curtis 1994).

The Positives of Good Strategic Planning

The listed adverse consequences are all legitimate complaints about the potential of strategic planning. Just as many positive consequences are associated with planning and these play a part in the success of many organizations.

Following are several positive elements that are important to preserve as a new planning model is developed.

1. Strategic planning can provide an overarching direction or roadmap for an organization. As the various constituencies of the organization develop their individual objectives, the strategic planning process provides a framework so that efforts are coordinated with organizational strategies. The strategic planning process can help ensure that the key managers understand and are working in support of common organizational objectives (Hax and Majluf 1991).

2. Organizational discipline and control are also identified as positive results associated with a strategic planning process. The previous section identified the potential problems inherent in a process that "controls"; however, in any organization, particularly in unstable dynamic situations, a mechanism should be in place that forces the organization to envision the future, to look long term, and to be vigilant of potential opportunities and threats. In volatile settings, it is important to "find patterns in what appears to be a chaotic and constantly changing environment. The leaders will be the ones who are able to see order within the chaos . . . and who know how to use it" (Primozic, Primozic, and Leben 1991, 5).

3. Strategic planning can also provide the basis for an organizational decision-making process. Strategic planning provides the information and analysis needed to evaluate situations, opportunities, and strategies. A strategic planning process that encourages participation broadens the organization's perspective by considering divergent viewpoints and interpretations of possible strategies. The planning process is a catalyst through which an organization can develop consensus among the leadership on major strategies (Birnbaum 1990).

4. Improving overall communication among the various disciplines of an organization is another positive benefit associated with a strategic planning process (Langley 1989). The process educates the organizational team on the issues and choices faced by the organization, and can direct managers to think beyond their own departmental time frames and work with the organizational timelines in a focused and coordinated manner (Perry, Stott, and Smallwood 1993).

5. Another potential benefit of a strategic planning process is its motivational influence. Workers find the knowledge that their organization constantly assesses the dynamic environment and plans strategies to ensure organizational survival reassuring. The workforce is more secure in its future knowing that the organization is planning for whatever the future brings.

Planning in a Dynamic Environment

Many business organizations in the United States have discovered that the environment is changing too rapidly for a static, reactive planning process. Instead, attention has shifted to taking advantage of temporary gains, creating new products and markets, and staking out new competitive spaces (D'Aveni 1994; Hamel and Prahalad 1994; Moore 1996). The healthcare industry is following corporate America in facing a turbulent, uncertain environment. Healthcare is transitioning from a stable, comfortable, and complacent past to a confusing present and unpredictable future. All of the key aspects of the industry are experiencing dramatic shifts. A simple continuum analysis demonstrates the turbulence of the current healthcare environment. This continuum of the "Cs" (depicted in Figure V.1) highlights the challenges facing the healthcare industry.

Traditionally, patients and physicians were the "customers" of most healthcare organizations. Now, business and industry and insurers are major customers. In fact, in many instances, the desires of the patient and physician are secondary and the insurers dictate the hospital provider.

Control

In the past, most healthcare organizations held independent control of their strategies and futures. Now, most are part of systems or alliances—or are considering strategies to merge or partner. The individual healthcare organization must give up some control of its destiny and focus planning efforts on the partnership in addition to each member.

Capitation and Cost

The current reimbursement environment is schizophrenic, with varying degrees of managed care penetration causing a shifting mix of payment types

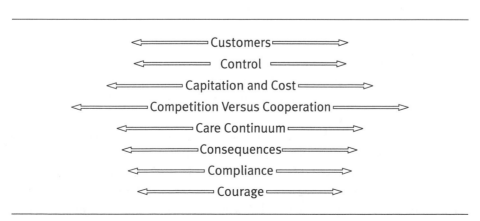

FIGURE V.1
Healthcare Continuum Shifts

from capitation to cost-based to percentage of charges. The future promises even more changes in reimbursement, and planning with future revenues and financial resources unknown will be challenging at best.

Competition Versus Cooperation

Most healthcare organizations face conflicting marketing strategies. The competitive environment has grown dramatically and organizations now face predatory attacks. At the same time, however, cooperative efforts among previous rivals are becoming commonplace.

Care Continuum

The care continuum refers to the paradigm shift from treating illness to focusing on wellness and prevention. This has been a relatively new focus for the healthcare industry. However, as the healthcare industry becomes increasingly responsible for the overall health of a defined population, the emphasis on improving health will become a primary focus.

Consequences

The "consequences" continuum acknowledges the many stakeholders that are now affected by any strategy developed by a healthcare organization. An organization's planning process must consider the consequences on other related organizations and constituencies. Equally important is the evaluation of the repercussions that strategies developed by these stakeholders will have on the healthcare organization.

Compliance

The recent increase in state and federal regulatory oversight as a means of quality control has had a dramatic effect on the healthcare industry, with increased scrutiny of the operation of healthcare delivery organizations. The public's confidence in the healthcare industry has been shaken as major accusations of fraud and abuse have been leveled at the industry. Strategies will not only need to address compliance, but also prove ethics and value.

Courage

All of these changes signal a need for healthcare leaders who have the skills to make the necessary changes—who have the vision and flexibility to lead and plan in turbulent times.

In summary, the healthcare industry is facing major changes. Changing customers, a changing product and mission, changing payment mechanisms, conflicting marketing strategies, more and different stakeholders, and a need for new leadership skills are just some of the major changes in the healthcare industry. The good news is that a dynamic and uncertain environment is not all bad. The fractious nature of the environment might prove to be the catalyst to shake the complacency from the current strategic planning process found in most healthcare organizations and encourage the development of more flexible, comprehensive models. The higher levels of tension and conflict can generate new perspectives (Stacey 1992, 39).

Strategic Cycling—A Planning Model to Shake Complacency

The previous discussion reveals that the process of strategic planning must adapt and evolve to be effective in the new healthcare environment. Although much of the current literature on strategic planning focuses on the negative qualities, the need for a process for appropriate future planning remains. In fact, most of the articles condemning strategic planning have created new terms such as strategic improvising, strategic processing, strategy application, issues management, and a wealth of other descriptive labels that still identify a thoughtful, proactive method or process to evaluate and set a course of action for an organization.

Much of the current literature on improving strategic planning focuses on a particular aspect or element of planning or addresses a specific complaint regarding a formal planning process. However, the previous discussion on the potential downsides of strategic planning and description of the environment in which healthcare organizations must chart their course indicates the need for a broader perspective. What is needed is a process that preserves the positive aspects of planning that are the "baby in the bathwater," while infusing the process with the flexibility and adaptability to not only respond to the rapidly changing environment, but to anticipate and thrive on it.

The strategic cycling model presented in Figure V.2 is a cycle or continuous process that provides a broad focus on critical issues that a healthcare organization should consider in planning strategically. The model differs from other contemporary frameworks in its emphasis on planning as a continuous feedback process rather than a set of stages that result in a relatively permanent and institutionalized plan (Ginter, Swayne, and Duncan 1998; Zuckerman 1998).

Overview of the Strategic Cycling Model

The strategic cycling model is arranged in a circular manner to avoid the linear and proscribed formal planning processes that create rigid, inflexible masterpiece plans. However, the model does not necessarily move in a clockwise manner. The arrows located in the center indicate the flexibility and responsiveness of the model, in which the process can react and adapt quickly

FIGURE V.2
Strategic
Cycling Model

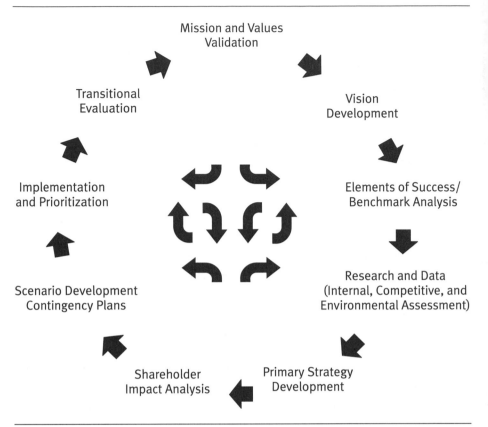

Mission and Values
Validation

Transitional
Evaluation

Vision
Development

Implementation
and Prioritization

Elements of Success/
Benchmark Analysis

Scenario Development
Contingency Plans

Research and Data
(Internal, Competitive, and
Environmental Assessment)

Shareholder
Impact Analysis

Primary Strategy
Development

to changes in the environment. For example, an ongoing assessment of the competitive environment can detect threats that cause the leadership of the organization to develop a competitive strike contingency plan; or an analysis of the effect of certain strategies on a major stakeholder can create a need to reprioritize the strategies.

The strategic cycle is a process and not a plan. It represents a moving and flowing process of analysis and evaluation to continuously monitor the environment and adapt the organization. This cyclical or process emphasis with consideration of the relationships and contingencies must be included in a strategic planning process in these transformational times. Such a perspective facilitates systems thinking—a framework for seeing interrelationships and patterns that is often presented in terms of a continuous cycle emphasizing feedback effects (Senge 1990).

The elements of the strategic cycling process provide a broad framework to structure an approach to planning. The elements are general guidelines that should be violated to preserve innovation and creativity. Without some guidelines, however, the positive features of strategic planning dissipate. The elements of the strategic cycling model are described in more detail below.

Mission and Values Validation and Vision Development

The model uses the mission, values, and vision of the organization as the foundation for the process. However, if the mission, values, and vision become too abstract or, conversely, too specific with no room for interpretation, the planning process can become a rote confirmation of an obsolete direction. Strategic cycling calls for a revalidation of the underlying foundation of the organization. Missions are often believed to be carved in stone; however, the turbulent environment can dictate a necessary adjustment or even a major change in an organization's mission, values, and vision.

Elements of Success/Benchmark Analysis

The healthcare industry is just now beginning to catch up with industrial and corporate counterparts in the compilation, analysis, and dissemination of comparative performance data. Most healthcare organizations track trends in their own performance for a variety of financial and clinical indicators, but those data alone lack relevance in a broader sense. Mandated reporting requirements on both state and federal levels are now providing healthcare leaders with a wealth of comparative data. In most cases, the benchmark data are adjusted for differences in populations with regard to age and severity of care for more valid comparisons. Hospital "report cards" are becoming widely published for both consumer and payor review. Decisions regarding which provider to use are made based on the comparative data.

As part of the planning process, organizations must evaluate their comparative position in the market and determine the elements of success by which they will evaluate their own performance. The analysis identifies "best practice" hospitals and the scores on particular indicators that can become benchmarks or targets for the planning organization. Organizations that want to remain competitive must engage in benchmarking; "avoiding these comparisons is like burying your head in the sand" (Cleverley 1989, 33). This step in the planning process identifies measurable goals and keeps the organization continuously looking for benchmarks to improve its performance in relation to other similar organizations. The benchmark analysis not only alerts the organization to potential problem areas; it provides an opportunity to correct indicators before they are published in public reports.

Research and Data Analysis: Internal, Competitor, and Environmental Assessment

This element of strategic cycling is the standard bearer of traditional planning. In the past, strategic plans collected data and performed the infamous Strengths/Weaknesses/Opportunities/Threats (SWOT) analysis. This element is still an important part of a planning process; however, rather than compiling a book of data, graphs, and trend lines that gathers dust on a shelf, the process of data assessment becomes an ongoing effort of monitoring and adjusting the organization in response to the analysis. A large amount of literature on environmental scanning, competitor analysis, and portfolio analytical tools suggests that these techniques continue to remain important in strategic planning (Drain and Godkin 1996; Ghoshal and Westney 1991). To avoid the negatives associated with this aspect of planning, focus should be placed on the use of the data and analysis to develop and implement strategies to prevent falling victim to the paralysis-by-analysis syndrome (Lenz 1985).

The means to create opportunities for product and service offerings that are not possible in the present environment and of "changing the environment to better suit the organization's goals" (Reeves 1993, 229) must also be considered. Possibilities for altering and creating new environments expand in uncertain times.

Primary Strategy Development

Although the term "strategy" in this element of strategic cycling is singular, the strategy development stage involves the development of multiple strategies. In this stage, the more scientific compilation of data and analysis combines with the less formal intuition and interpretation skills to develop workable strategies for the organization. An analysis of data and trends alone can lead to the development of erroneous strategies. The planning team must evaluate and interpret the data using experience and intuitive logic (Thomas, McDaniel, and Anderson 1991).

The coordination of the strategies among the various disciplines of the organization is a critical step in the process. This important activity solicits input and participation to avoid the problems discussed earlier in this article, where those responsible for implementation of the strategies had not been involved in nor did they believe in the validity of the strategies. Numerous anecdotal stories in the literature describe strategies that have been developed in direct conflict with other organizational directives. Clearly, one of the more important efforts involves integrating strategic development through the management team to all parts of the organization.

Shareholder Impact Analysis

Shareholders or stakeholders are "individuals, groups, or organizations who have a stake in the decisions and actions of an organization and who attempt to influence those decisions and actions" (Blair and Fottler 1998, 2). In the changing healthcare environment, shareholder impact analysis has become an even more critical aspect of strategic planning. Most healthcare organizations are now part of a system or alliance with other providers such as hospitals, physicians in PPO arrangements, and often with insurers to create a total product. Because of these vital relationships, planning becomes more complicated and the stakeholders must be considered in the planning process. In addition, the inter-relatedness among the stakeholders requires that the plans of these other individuals, groups, and organizations be considered as well. The concept of shareholder impact analysis is becoming a major focus in the planning literature. Whether called "linkage analysis" (Primozic, Primozic, and Leben 1991), "fostering generative relationships" (Lane and Maxfield 1996), or other creative terminology, the key is to evaluate relationships that can add value to the organization and to consider these potentially beneficial (or competitive) relationships in the development of organizational strategies.

Scenario Development/Contingency Plans

Scenario development and contingency planning are techniques that acknowledge that planning does not come with a crystal ball and that major assumptions can change with dramatic implications for the organization. Scenarios are "vehicles for helping people learn" (Schwartz 1991, 6). Obviously, an organization cannot anticipate all possible scenarios, nor do organizations have the time and financial resources to develop plans for all contingencies. The process of thinking about and planning for the unanticipated has the beneficial effect of moving leaders beyond their strategic comfort zone. The effort of scenario development and contingency planning leaves the organization better prepared for the unexpected. Scenario-based planning addresses one of the more serious negatives of strategic planning where only one possible "future" is considered.

Scenario-based planning can be very sophisticated, with computer models to run "what ifs," and the resulting analysis can be used to evaluate and develop possible actions in response to alternative situations that could arise (Georgantzas and Acar 1995). However, even if an organization does not have the computer or financial resources to simulate complex scenarios, a beneficial effect can be found in continuously evaluating and considering possible environmental changes or adverse conditions and thinking about the organization's options in response to these changes. This element of strategic cycling makes an organization more proactive and responsive, which will be a key factor of success in the turbulent healthcare environment.

Implementation and Prioritization

An often-cited negative consequence of strategic planning is that more effort goes into the development of a plan than into implementing it. One of the most important elements—it could be argued to be the most important element—of the strategic cycling process is the execution. Too often, the organization congratulates itself on the analysis, decisions, and creation of the plan, but rather than providing direction to a dynamic process of implementation, the "plan" is put on a shelf and forgotten. Implementation is one of the most critical aspects of the strategic planning process, but is often given little attention, which basically renders the "plan" useless.

Another important consideration in the implementation stage is the assignment of priorities. As resources are allocated to implementation of defined strategies, the allocation should be based on the strategies that have the most effect or are most critical—the top priorities for the organization. All of the key players in the organization must be committed and dedicated to the implementation of the strategies.

Transitional Evaluation

In the strategic cycling model, a continual evaluation of the implementation of the strategies completes the feedback loop. If strategies are not effective, the evaluation redirects the implementation process or redefines the strategy. Monitoring and evaluation provide for corrective action and put some control into the process. Evaluation and monitoring "make the planning effort a tangible reality rather than an academic exercise" (Birnbaum 1990, 221). In the model, the evaluation step can link back to any stage in the cycle to correct the implementation. If more data are needed, the process is flexible. If changes have taken place in the environment, then the scenario-development stage could provide possible alternative implementation efforts. Without an evaluation step, the planning process would be in serious contention to attain all of the negative results identified earlier in this article.

Conclusions

In the dynamic healthcare environment, strategic planning can be a vital and useful process to provide direction and guidance to a healthcare organization. But the possible negatives that can be associated with an ill-conceived process must be carefully considered. This article offers a strategic cycling model to broaden the planning perspective and address the potential drawbacks. The model takes into consideration the beneficial aspects of planning and focuses on a flexible, responsive, and proactive method of surviving the turbulent times. Although the current literature seems to focus on the downsides to strategic planning, a broader conceptualization of the strategic planning process provides real opportunities for healthcare organizations to face the uncertain future with confidence.

References

Aaker, D. 1992. *Developing Business Strategies.* New York: John Wiley & Sons.
Abell, D. 1993. *Managing with Dual Strategies: Mastering the Present, Preempting the Future.* New York: Free Press.

Birnbaum, W. 1990. *If Your Strategy Is So Terrific, How Come It Doesn't Work?* New York: American Management Association.

Blair, J. D., and M. D. Fottler. 1998. *Strategic Leadership for Medical Groups.* San Francisco: Jossey-Bass.

Boyd, B. 1991. "Strategic Planning and Financial Performance: A Meta-Analytic Review." *Journal of Management Studies* 28 (4): 353–74.

Bruton, G., B. Oviatt, and L. Kallas-Bruton. 1995. "Strategic Planning in Hospitals: A Review and Proposal." *Health Care Management Review* 20 (3): 16–25.

Cleverley, W. 1989. "How Boards Can Use Comparative Data in Strategic Planning." *Healthcare Executive* 4 (3): 32–33.

Curtis, K. 1994. *From Management Goal Setting to Organizational Results.* Westport, CT: Quorum.

Daft, R. L., and R. H. Lengel. 1998. *Fusion Leadership.* San Francisco: Berrett-Koehler.

D'Aveni, R. A. 1994. *Hypercompetition.* New York: Free Press.

Drain, M., and L. Godkin. 1996. "A Portfolio Approach to Strategic Hospital Analysis: Exposition and Explanation." *Health Care Management Review* 21 (4): 68–74.

Georgantzas, N., and W. Acar. 1995. *Scenario-Driven Planning: Learning to Manage Strategic Uncertainty.* Westport, CT: Quorum.

Ghoshal, S., and D. Westney. 1991. "Organizing Competitor Analysis Systems." *Strategic Management Journal* 12: 17–31.

Ginter, P. M., L. E. Swayne, and W. J. Duncan. 1998. *Strategic Management of Health Care Organizations*, 3rd edition. Malden, MA: Blackwell.

Gray, D. 1986. "Uses and Misuses of Strategic Planning." *Harvard Business Review* 64: 89–97.

Hamel, G., and C. K. Prahalad. 1994. *Competing for the Future.* Boston: Harvard Business School Press.

Hax, A., and N. Majluf. 1991. *The Strategy Concept and Process.* Englewood Cliffs, NJ: Prentice-Hall.

Henderson, J. 1992. "Aligning Business and Information Technology Domain: Strategic Planning in Hospitals." *Hospital & Health Services Administration* 37 (1): 71–87.

Lane, D., and R. Maxfield. 1996. "Strategy Under Complexity: Fostering Generative Relationships." *Long Range Planning* 29 (2): 215–31.

Langley, A. 1989. "In Search of Rationality: The Purposes Behind the Use of Formal Analysis in Organizations." *Administrative Science Quarterly* 34: 598–631.

Lenz, R. T. 1985. "Paralysis by Analysis: Is Your Planning System Becoming Too Rational?" *Long Range Planning* 18 (4): 64–72.

Luke, R., and J. Begun. 1994. "Strategy Making in Health Care Organizations." In *Health Care Management*, 3rd edition, edited by S. M. Shortell and A. D. Kaluzny, 355–91. Albany, NY: Delmar.

McDaniel, R. R., Jr. 1997. "Strategic Leadership: A View from Quantum and Chaos Theories." In *Handbook of Health Care Management*, edited by W. J. Duncan, P. M. Ginter, and L. E. Swayne, 339–67. Malden, MA: Blackwell.

Mintzberg, H. 1994. *The Rise and Fall of Strategic Planning.* New York: Free Press.

Moore, J. F. 1996. *The Death of Competition*. New York: HarperCollins.

Ohmae, K. 1982. *The Mind of the Strategist*. New York: McGraw Hill.

Perry, T., R. Stott, and W. N. Smallwood. 1993. *Real-Time Strategy*. New York: John Wiley & Sons.

Powell, T. 1992. "Research Notes and Communications—Strategic Planning as Competitive Advantage." *Strategic Management Journal* 13: 551–58.

Primozic, K., E. Primozic, and J. Leben. 1991. *Strategic Choices: Supremacy, Survival, or Sayonara*. New York: McGraw Hill.

Reeves, P. 1993. "Issues Management: The Other Side of Strategic Planning." *Hospital & Health Services Administration* 38 (2): 229–41.

Schwartz, P. 1991. *The Art of the Long View*. New York: Currency Doubleday.

Senge, P. 1990. *The Fifth Discipline*. New York: Currency Doubleday.

Shortell, S., E. Morrison, and B. Friedman. 1992. *Strategic Choices for America's Hospitals*. San Francisco: Jossey-Bass.

Sinha, D. 1990. "The Contribution of Formal Planning to Decisions." *Strategic Management Journal* 11: 479–92.

Stacey, R. 1992. *Managing the Unknowable*. San Francisco: Jossey-Bass.

Thomas, J., R. McDaniel, and R. Anderson. 1991. "Hospitals as Interpretation Systems." *Health Services Research* 25 (6): 859–80.

Wall, S., and S. Wall. 1995. *The New Strategists*. New York: Free Press.

Zuckerman, A. M. 1998. *Healthcare Strategic Planning*. Chicago: Health Administration Press.

Discussion Questions for the Required Reading

1. What is strategic planning?
2. Begun and Heatwole emphasize continuous assessment of strategies based on feedback from benchmark analysis and stakeholder impact. Why don't most healthcare organizations use this model? What would it take for these organizations to adopt the Begun and Heatwole model?
3. Who is responsible for carrying out adaptive activities for the small, mid-sized, and large non-profit healthcare organization?
4. Where does marketing fit into an organization's plans for adapting to changes in its environment?

Required Supplementary Readings

Berry, L. L. and N. Bendapundi. 2003. "Clueing in Customers." *Harvard Business Review* (February): 100–6.

Christensen, C. M., R. Bohmer, and J. Kenagy. 2000. "Will Disruptive Innovations Cure Healthcare?" *Harvard Business Review* (September–October): 102–12.

Griffith, J. R., and K. White. 2006. "Planning and Internal Consulting" and "Marketing and Strategy." In *The Well-Managed Healthcare Organization*, 6th edition. Chicago: Health Administration Press.

Robinson, J. C., and S. Dratler. 2006. "Corporate Structure and Capital Strategy at Catholic Healthcare West." *Health Affairs* 25 (1): 134–47.

Discussion Questions for Required Supplementary Readings

1. What is distinctive to the marketing approaches carried out at the Mayo Clinic?
2. The authors suggest that healthcare may be the most entrenched, change-averse industry in the United States. Why is this so? How is performance-based reimbursement changing the situation, if at all?
3. Give an example of an environmental pressure affecting large group practices, and suggest alternative ways in which the group practices can adapt to these pressures.
4. How do large hospitals raise the capital they need to adapt to change? How does Catholic Healthcare West balance mission and margin in the capital-intensive hospital industry?

Recommended Supplementary Readings

Arndt, M., and B. Bigelow. 2000. "The More Things Change, the More They Stay the Same." *Healthcare Management Review* 25 (1): 65–72.

Berkowitz, E. N. 2006. *Essentials of Healthcare Marketing*, 2nd edition. Boston: Jones and Bartlett.

Bigelow, B., and M. Arndt. 1994. "Great Expectations: An Analysis of Four Strategies." *Medical Care Review* 51 (2): 205–33.

Collins, J. C., and J. I. Porras. 1996. "Building Your Company's Vision." *Harvard Business Review* (Sept.–Oct.): 65–77.

Davenport, T. H., and J. G. Harris. 2007. *Competing on Analytics*. Boston: Harvard Business School Press.

Garvin, D. A., and M. A. Roberto. 2001. "What You Don't Know About Making Decisions." *Harvard Business Review* (Sept.): 108–16.

Griffith, J. R., and K. R. White, with P. Cahill. 2003. *Thinking Forward: Six Strategies for Highly Successful Organizations*. Chicago: Health Administration Press.

Kizer, K. W. 1998. "Healthcare, Not Hospitals: Transforming the Veterans Health Administration." In *Straight from the CEO*. New York: Simon and Schuster.

Kotter, J. P. 1995. "Leading Change: Why Transformation Efforts Fail." *Harvard Business Review* (March/April): 2–10.

Mintzberg, H. 1994. "The Fall and Rise of Strategic Planning." *Harvard Business Review* 72 (1): 107–14.

Porter, M. E., and E. O. Teisberg. 2006. *Redefining Healthcare*. Boston: Harvard Business School Press.

Reichheld F. F. 2001. "Lead for Loyalty." *Harvard Business Review* (July–Aug.): 76–84.

Rindler, M. E. 2007. *Strategic Cost Reduction*. Chicago: Health Administration Press.

Senge, P. M. 1990. *The Fifth Discipline: The Art and Practice of the Learning Organization*. New York: Doubleday Currency Publishers.

Zuckerman, A. M. 2006. "Advancing the State of the Art in Healthcare Strategic Planning." *Frontiers of Health Services Management* 23 (2): 3–15.

THE CASES

daptive capability involves organizational response to new conditions. Organizations must be innovative or proactive in responding to the pressures of competitors and regulators and to the expectations of various stakeholder groups, from customers to physicians. One indicator of adaptive capability is the presence of specialized units to carry out certain functions, such as strategic planning and marketing, that are concerned specifically with adapting rather than operations.

Strategic planning is an important managerial function. It can be conducted through a special unit, through some part of a special unit, directly by management, or by some combination of the above. Top management sees to it that information about the organization's business is gathered. Questions about the organization's mission, services, customers, competition, and strategies are addressed.

Milio (1983) reminds us that organizations have limited problemsolving capacities; they avoid uncertainty, engage in biased searches for ways of adapting, act on the basis of limited knowledge, and select alternatives on the basis of past successes.

Decisions to adapt can run counter to organizational goals and system maintenance. Even if the decisions can be shown, in hindsight, to have been technically appropriate, they may have been politically inappropriate. Managers may fail to consider the values of important stakeholders when they plan how to attain their mission and strategy. We are assuming, of course, that the healthcare organization already has a carefully worked out mission and strategy, which it constantly reassesses in terms of competitive and regulatory pressures and in terms of the preferences and expectations of stakeholders, such as physicians and nurses.

The three long case studies in this section deal with questions of partnership and alliances and with changes in product focus and delivery. How these questions are answered and what strategies are selected may have consequences that are different for specific organizations and for specific managers. In the case of "The Visiting Nurse Association (VNA) of Cleveland," the CEO, Mary Lou Stricklin, is faced with a set of choices involving new relationships with local collaborators and competitors, some of whom may be seen by certain VNA stakeholder groups as threatening the core value upon which the organization was founded and has thrived for many years. For Piney Woods Hospital, Zach Porter must address problems associated with the hospital's emergency department, considering both the perspectives of multiple stake-holders and implications for the future of the hospital. At Central Med Health System, an investment decision will impact product focus and delivery for the health system, and have broad implications for a variety of stakeholders.

The five short cases examine different issues around adaptation from multiple perspectives. The first short case study raises the basic issues from a management perspective—that of a new chief of Ob-Gyn—testing your skills at developing an organized, coherent response. Second, hospital board members provide their perspectives about a CEO's decision to sell an HMO. A physician perspective is next examined when increasing competition forces a private physician to consider a new strategic direction for her practice. The fourth short case explores the issue of disparities in care from the perspective of a hospital CEO faced with evidence that his hospital is providing disparate care. Finally, the perspective of a manager is again considered when it must be evaluated whether to fill an important position by promoting someone from within the department.

Reference

Milio, N. 1983. "Health Care Organizations and Innovation." In *Health Services Management: Readings and Commentary*, 2nd edition, edited by A. R. Kovner and D. Neuhauser, 448–64. Chicago: Health Administration Press.

Case L
The Visiting Nurse Association of Cleveland

Duncan Neuhauser

Mary Lou Stricklin, MBA, MSN, is chief executive officer of the Visiting Nurse Association of Cleveland (VNA). The home care market continues to change rapidly. Competition, the rising burden of indigent care, hospital-based home care programs, hospice, large growth of demand for home care, the explosion of specialized home care services, and the introduction of prospective payment and pay for performance for home care continue to affect this market. These rapid changes have led to a series of corporate reorganizations, and Stricklin is contemplating the next corporate transformation.

Cleveland's VNA was founded in 1902. Throughout its history, the VNA has employed professional nurses with home care experience to provide care to the residents of the greater Cleveland area, which now has a population of approximately 1.2 million. The mission and value statements for the VNA are shown in Figure V.3.

Mission
To provide compassionate, innovative, and effective community-based care that promotes health, independence, and dignity to those we serve in Northeast and Central Ohio.

Vision
- To be the leader in innovative home care.
- To be the standard for quality care.
- To be the leader in community health planning and research.

Values
- We value personal dignity, the importance of integrity, honesty, and compassion.
- We are responsive to the needs of the community and our stakeholders.
- We value quality as a measurable outcome of emerging standards of performance.
- We value education and skill development of staff and clients.

FIGURE V.3
Today's VNA
Mission
Statement

The original VNA board of trustees was largely composed of the wives of community leaders. One of the major functions those days was to provide Christmas food baskets for needy patients. By the 1990s, the board was diverse by gender, ethnicity, and professional background.

1980: About the Only Game in Town

In 1980 the core professional staff consisted of full-time salaried generalist nurses who worked out of four district offices to cover Cleveland and adjacent townships. The center office included administrative staff to coordinate several part-time social workers and physical therapists. Calls requesting care were handled by the district offices. The nurses themselves decided whether or not a patient was able to pay.

Home care aide services were also provided by the VNA under contract from another voluntary organization, the Center for Human Services. Special contracts provided care for the elderly in several apartment complexes. All services were only available during weekday working hours, and the agency was closed on weekends and holidays.

1982: Arrival of Competition

Ohio regulations made it easy to start a home care company, and more than 300 were created. The joke went that if you had a telephone and knew a nurse, you could start a home care agency. If costs could be kept down and full-pay patients selected, home care could be profitable. By 1982, competition for paying home care patients was growing. The newcomers were content to let the VNA provide home care for those who could not pay. In 1984, VNA's total income of $5 million included philanthropic gifts and endowment income of $190,000 and United Way contributions of $540,000. This allowed the VNA to provide care to all who requested it. However, the VNA needed mostly paying patients to survive.

This competitive situation led the VNA for the first time to examine the source of its patients and how the choice of home care provider was made. It turned out that 82 percent of patients came by way of hospital discharge and, of these, most came from a dozen of the area's largest hospitals. Typically a nurse, social worker, or discharge planner made the decision within the hospital. The choice of provider depended primarily on agency reputation, the ease of making a referral, and agency name recall.

Instead of being a passive receiver of telephone requests for services, the VNA decided to assign a staff nurse as contact person for each major hospital. Brochures, calendars, and small magnetized VNA symbols were distributed to promote name recognition.

The VNA organized a centralized intake service with one recognizable telephone number to make referrals easier. VNA leaders learned that one competitor was giving away transistor radios to hospital-based referrers. After some discussion, the VNA decided not to follow suit.

By 1983, prospective payments for hospital care had drastically shortened patient stay and emptied hospital beds. The hospitals were encouraging earlier discharge combined with home care. Hospitals began actively looking for new revenue-generating ventures and hospital-based home care became popular. By 1983, there was serious concern that the VNA's work would come to an end, as one hospital after another started its own home care program.

By 1984, a number of hospitals decided that running their own home care programs was not the best idea, and instead developed contracts with the VNA. The market again changed; no longer was it the individual nurse's or social worker's decision, but rather a hospital-based contract. One reason hospital contracting occurred was because hospital management was busy; the managers wanted to avoid a new program and save energy for higher-priority areas. By 1984, the VNA had contracts with eight hospitals, which accounted for about 35 percent of the VNA's patients.

Early discharge drove the demand for increasingly complex home care requiring nurses who specialized in intravenous (IV) management, pediatrics, mental health, hospice care, renal dialysis, and ostomy care, in addition to physical and occupational therapy and social work. Small suburban hospitals with paying patients and undifferentiated home care could prosper with small programs. Larger hospitals with more severely ill patients and high indigent care ratios found VNA contracting a better choice. Hospitals that started their own home care programs rarely provided home care services to nearby competing hospitals. Hospital contracts required the VNA to offer 24-hour service. Hospitals also wanted the VNA to provide additional services, so the agency started homemaker services called "Care Plus." In response to these changes, the VNA reorganized in 1989.

1990 to 2000: Prosperity for a While

Between 1990 and 2000, the single not-for-profit 501(c)(3) organization became five organizations:

- *VNA Services* encompasses the bulk of the agencies' work; within this, Medicare is the largest payer.
- *VNA Care Plus* provides home aide assistance on a private basis (cleaning, food preparation, and personal hygienic care). This is mostly paid for by the patients.
- *VNA Hospice and Palliative Care* provides care for the terminally ill at home, and also operates an inpatient unit at MetroHealth Medical Center. This is paid for largely by Medicare.
- *VNA Enterprises* is a small catch-all organization for receiving money for consulting and other services (for profit).
- *VNA Lines* provides IV solutions and other supplies needed in home care (for profit). This structure was active for several years before this market changed.

The VNA's large group of trustees was divided into a smaller group of trustees with governance responsibility and a group of overseers–loyal supporters of the VNA with no line authority, but a right to advise and contribute.

In the early 1990s, the five VNA organizations made surpluses, enough so that in 1995 the VNA could, with fundraising, move into a single new modern building in the center of the city near an expressway interchange. Two new subsidiaries, VNA Mid Ohio and House Calls, were created, but the two for-profit entities, VNA Enterprises and VNA Lines, were closed.

The current organization chart is shown in Figure V.4. See Figure V.5 for a list of services provided by the VNA components.

Over the last decade the VNA has created a group of innovative new programs in association with other organizations. Special populations served include those dealing with alcoholism, mental health problems, and AIDS,

FIGURE V.4
The Current
Visiting Nurse
Association
Organizaton
Chart

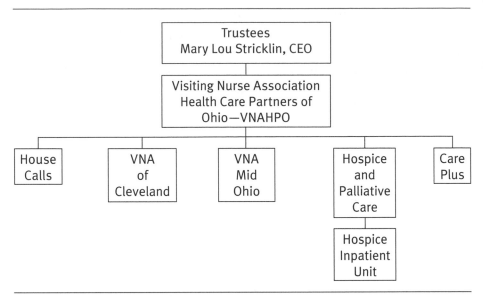

and bereaved families and elderly people living in low-income housing (see Figure V.6).

Today

The 40 separate hospitals that existed in Cleveland in 1980 evolved into three big delivery systems. One is anchored by the Cleveland Clinic Foundation, the second is based at the University Hospitals of Cleveland, and the third is the Cleveland MetroHealth Medical Center (the County Hospital). The first two have their own home care organizations. MetroHealth, which does not have its own home care service, contracts with the VNA.

By 2008 some of the five VNA components made a small surplus and others lost money. Total revenue was $55 million, and the organization was close to breaking even.

Stricklin is leading an organization that prides itself on innovative new programs. The core process of care is seen in Figure V.6. This pathway is driven by mission, vision, and values. The process of care is supported by special services, quality control, and information systems.

The activities of the core management group are shown in Figure V.7. This corporate management team provides these services to the constituent organizations, which in turn contribute funds to support the corporate staff.

Medicare, the dominant home care payer, has made several critical changes to control rising home care expenditures and monitor quality. Payment per visit has been changed to prospective payment, a fixed amount of

VNA of Cleveland
The VNA's full range of services and programs that help patients return to their optimal level of health are available in an eight-county area of Northeast Ohio.
- Medical-surgical nursing
- Maternal and infant
- Pediatrics
- Personal care
- Enterostomal care
- Older adult
- Infusion therapy
- Rehabilitation services
- Physical therapy
- Occupational therapy
- Speech-language pathology
- Social work
- Nutrition
- Behavioral health
- Mental health services
- Chemical dependency and ambulatory detox
- AIDS mental health
- Clozaril treatment
- Mental health management and support services

VNA Mid Ohio
Provides home nursing services in an area south of Cleveland

VNA Hospice and Palliative Care
VNA Hospice and Special Care are programs for patients who are terminally ill. An interdisciplinary team provides compassionate care including:
- Skilled nursing care
- Pain and symptom management
- Respite care
- 24-hour crisis support
- Social work services
- AIDS care
- Residential/nursing home care
- Home care aides
- Rehabilitation services
- Bereavement support
- Spiritual care
- Volunteer clergy, lawyers, companions, and Friendly Visitors

An in-patient hospice unit is under construction in 2008

VNA Care Plus
VNA Care Plus provides 24-hour private duty nursing and personal care. Registered nurse, licensed practical nurse, aide, or homemaker services are available for short-term rehabilitation or long-term supportive care, meal preparation, companionship, respite care, and child care.
Services include the following:
- Private duty nursing
- Personal care
- Homemaker services

House Calls
Provides physician home visits. Four physicians do this.

FIGURE V.5

Visiting Nurse Association Component Services

FIGURE V.6

1995:
The VNA
Organizaton
as a Process

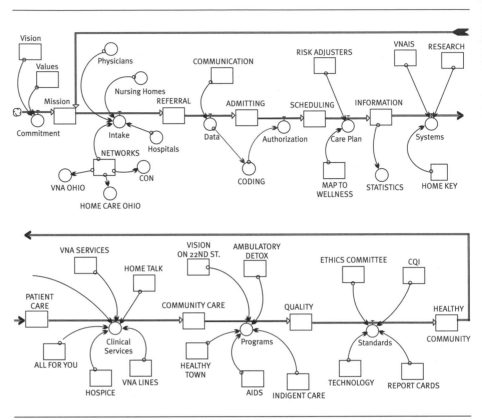

money for a predefined type of patient. This has significantly reduced the number of visits across the country. Second, a complex reporting system (OASIS) is required for each patient, put in place so that Medicare can monitor severity of illness and the outcomes of care (e.g., were activities of daily living goals met for each patient? For example, can the patient now get dressed by herself?).

Medicare fraud and abuse rules mean that unintentional reporting errors can lead to an expensive government review and harsh penalties. Complete and accurate records are essential. New privacy regulations have also required a full review of record systems to ensure compliance. Good information management has become important to the VNA. So far, the VNA has done well in this area and is recognized for it.

One consequence of these changes has been the shift of home care from a profitable small side item for a community hospital to a financially marginal business requiring substantial information management abilities and higher risk. These issues have caused many small agencies to go out of business. The VNA of Cleveland has been solicited by several small cities that have lost their local home care agencies. The VNA opened VNA Mid Ohio in one

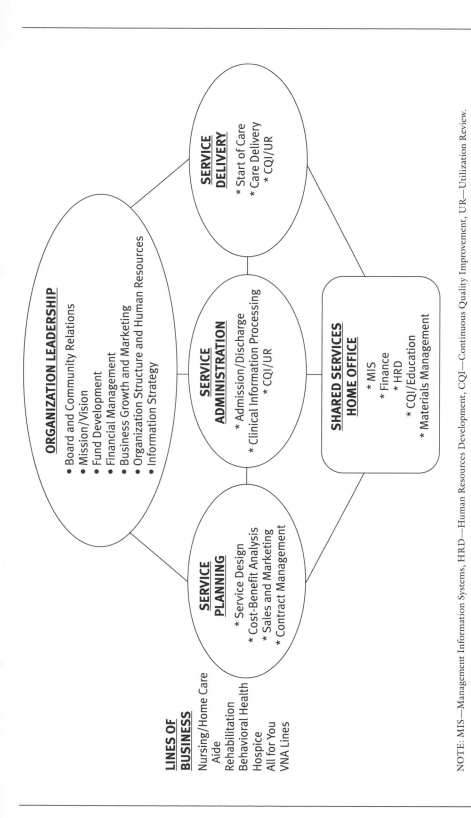

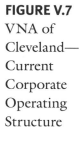

FIGURE V.7
VNA of Cleveland—Current Corporate Operating Structure

ORGANIZATION LEADERSHIP
- Board and Community Relations
- Mission/Vision
- Fund Development
- Financial Management
- Business Growth and Marketing
- Organization Structure and Human Resources
- Information Strategy

SERVICE DELIVERY
* Start of Care
* Care Delivery
* CQI/UR

SERVICE ADMINISTRATION
* Admission/Discharge
* Clinical Information Processing
* CQI/UR

SERVICE PLANNING
* Service Design
* Cost-Benefit Analysis
* Sales and Marketing
* Contract Management

SHARED SERVICES HOME OFFICE
* MIS
* Finance
* HRD
* CQI/Education
* Materials Management

LINES OF BUSINESS
Nursing/Home Care
Aide
Rehabilitation
Behavioral Health
Hospice
All for You
VNA Lines

NOTE: MIS—Management Information Systems, HRD—Human Resources Development, CQI—Continuous Quality Improvement, UR—Utilization Review.

small city with local philanthropic support. Even with this help, however, the VNA faces new business start-up costs related to such horizontal expansion.

Medicare cost control has its largest impact on traditional skilled nursing care (VNA Services). VNA Care Plus, which provides less skilled housekeeping services in the home, is paid for out the patient's pocket, and has not been affected by Medicare prospective payment.

The traditional professional nurse service of the VNA is largely dependent on Medicare funding and rules. In 2009 it is expected that pay-for-performance incentives will be implemented. The top home care agencies will get a bonus on their care outcome measures based on OASIS data, such as the percentage of patients who can dress themselves or take a bath at the end of their home care program. Medicare cutbacks are always a possibility. There is a growing shortage of professional nurses.

New technology related to home care monitoring is reducing the number of needed home visits. These monitors are expensive—$5,000 each—and are used to measure hypertension, blood sugar, and medication compliance via cell phone. The VNA has been a leader in introducing this technology. All of its machines are in use and there is a waiting list. State funding has helped in the purchase of these monitors.

In cooperation with MetroHealth Medical Center, VNA Hospice is building a dedicated inpatient unit due to open soon. The planning and building renovation has consumed time, money, and management energy.

The greater Cleveland area has competing home care agencies, but there is a need for these services in the rural and small city areas of northern Ohio. The development of Mid Ohio VNA has been steady and is meeting a need.

The All For You department provides the services of home helpers and is a private pay service. This is a competitive market and wages are not high. Because it is self-paid, patient and family satisfaction is critical. Typically care is provided to an elderly person living alone and supervised by a daughter who may be living in another state.

House Calls provides doctor and nurse practitioner home visits. There is a large need for this service for patients who are unable to leave home, but it is reimbursed on an office visit rate. The doctor can see 20 patients in an office in the same time he sees only 5 at home. This is not economically viable without special foundation grant funds. However, if these physicians could case manage such high-need, high-cost patients and share the savings from reduced hospital admissions, the revenue could be very large but risky.

Other opportunities for the VNA include providing "back office" services for other small home care agencies unable to cope with the new demands for accurate and timely information. The VNA could create a one-stop telephone site with easy access for people seeking advice about home care needs staffed by skilled people who know the complexities. Another possible opportunity could come from expanding the research center to study the data being generated and evaluate programs. Funding agencies often ask for program evaluations as part of their grants.

Stricklin is pleased with her experienced case management teams. There are many things to do, which will take time and energy.

The Future

What should the VNA's priorities be?

- Implement cost and quality control for the home care business, particularly for the Medicare part of the business, which is being squeezed for funds now and probably will be well into the future. For the first time, the VNA is getting regular national comparative performance data that can be used to measure outcomes of care and patient satisfaction.
- Expand horizontally by moving to new nearby communities in need of home care services. The VNA's current corporate headquarters structure could support such expansion. Figure V.8 shows the current grouping of activities carried out by corporate staff.
- Grow VNA Care Plus, which is not federally regulated like Medicare.
- Provide back-office services for other home care agencies unable to cope with the new demands for information.
- Start a research center to seek funding to study the data currently being collected and evaluate programs like home monitoring.

Stricklin is reviewing issues and possible other new directions for her organization.

Case Questions

1. In which direction should the VNA go?
2. How should the VNA board be brought along to agree with the change recommended?
3. How can staff morale be maintained in the face of uncertainty?
4. Who are the stakeholder groups whose expectations Stricklin must manage to succeed in implementing your recommendations?
5. What are the personal stakes involved for Stricklin in doing as you suggest? How can she maximize the upside potential and minimize the downside risks for her own career?

FIGURE V.8
Visiting Nurse
Association of
Cleveland

Innovations

Home Talk™

Through a joint venture with Telepractice in the fall of 1995, VNA introduced Home Talk, a free telephone service for patients that improves access to their VNA clinician. Patients may choose from several options, including an online library with recorded health information. Home Talk supports the clinician's assessment of a patient's health status, resulting in fewer readmissions to the hospital and unnecessary trips to the emergency room.

Ambulatory Detoxification Services

The VNA of Cleveland, MetroHealth, and Alcoholism Services of Cleveland are collaborating on an 18-month demonstration project to provide ambulatory detoxification services and chemical dependency care in home and community settings. This project is funded by a grant from the Cleveland Foundation.

Healthy Town

This program provides health promotion and disease prevention services to lower-income senior citizens and families with children at University Settlement and Collinwood Community Services Center, member organizations of the Neighborhood Centers Association. Funding is provided by the CAVS Charities and the Cleveland Foundation.

HIV/AIDS Mental Health

Through a grant from the AIDS Funding Collaborative, the VNA and the Free Clinic are collaborating to bring nursing care, social work, and consultative services to patients.

KID Connection

KID Connection nurses offer educational programs and consultation services for childcare providers. These services help daycare staff deliver high-quality care and meet state licensing requirements.

Vision on 22nd Street

To prepare students for community-based nursing, the VNA and Cleveland State University Department of Nursing formed an education-service partnership. A committee of community healthcare experts from both institutions developed new nursing curricula and began offering classes last fall. The program will educate over 200 nursing students within the next few years. Vision on 22nd Street is partially funded by the Cleveland Foundation.

Clozaril Management

Selected patients of the Mental Health program are participating in the VNA's collaborative research study, funded by Sandoz Pharmaceuticals, to evaluate the effectiveness of Clozaril, and to implement the program in other areas of the country.

Camp TLC

VNA Hospice's Bereavement Camp TLC (Together Love Continues) is an annual day-long program helping children and family members who have lost a loved one to cope with their grief. The camp is underwritten by the Bicknell Fund.

Case M
The Piney Woods Hospital Emergency Department

Julie Anstine, Kyle Dorsey, Nicholas Schmidt, Denise Hamilton, Randa Hall, and Ann Scheck McAlearney

Piney Woods Hospital (PWH) is a 575-bed not-for-profit community hospital located in the town of Piney Woods, Alabama. With a population of 50,000, Piney Woods is a growing, blue-collar community, valued for its rural scenery and easy access to outdoor activities. Piney Woods Hospital has a Level 2 designation for its emergency services, and is located 50 miles from the next nearest community hospital.

Zach Porter, the Piney Woods Hospital CEO, has dedicated a considerable amount of his time and energy to developing the acute care side of the hospital and has enjoyed positive results in this area. However, he is well aware that the emergency department (ED) presents a different story. Similar to other EDs across the country, the Piney Woods ED suffers from staff shortages, inadequate space, operational inefficiencies, and problems associated with declining reimbursement and a growing number of uninsured patients. Nursing staff are over-worked and over-stressed, evidenced by high rates of staff overtime and high turnover among nurse managers. Porter is particularly concerned about declining satisfaction scores across patient, employee, and physician populations, along with complaints about excessive ED wait times.

Assessing the Situation

Porter recognizes that problems in the ED reflect poorly upon PWH and knows he must do something. In his role as CEO, Porter realizes he has little time to dedicate to evaluating this problem, but he is not without resources. He decides that a situational assessment would be a perfect assignment for his summer resident, Gwen Roberts, who is completing her master of health administration degree.

Calling Roberts into his office, Porter outlines the "big picture" to her as follows:

- The patients are not the only ones dissatisfied. The most recent employee satisfaction survey reported a 62 percent satisfaction score (out of a possible 100 percent) for ED staff when the hospital-wide employee satisfaction score was 82 percent. The emergency physicians scored 3.3

on a 7-point scale (hospital-wide physician satisfaction was 4.6) on their satisfaction survey.

- The emergency department morale, productivity, and quality have declined over the last few years. There has been a lot of turnover in leadership, which has exacerbated the problems. In the past year, the entire hospital adopted an electronic health record system. The emergency physicians were not consulted and as a result there is a lot of ill will on their part. On Porter's latest rounds in the ED, neither staff nor physicians would look him in the eye. You could have cut the tension with a knife.

- The ED physicians' poor attitudes have burned many bridges with other physicians, both those who provide specialty coverage as well as those who serve the Piney Woods community. Hospital leadership has tried for the past 18 months to work with the ED physicians to enhance their productivity, increase chart completion rates, improve morale, and facilitate cooperation, with no success.

- The decrease in cost of physician services in FY 2007 is a result of a drop in patient satisfaction scores. The physicians receive a bonus for good patient satisfaction.

- Building a new ED is not an option at this time.

- Critical success factors for the hospital include:
  o   Maintain a high-quality workforce
  o   Improve customer service
  o   Increase quality of healthcare provided
  o   Improve financial results
  o   Expand clinical services

Starting the Analysis

Returning to her desk, Roberts feels overwhelmed, but also energized by the challenge of figuring out the ED situation. Porter has outlined a number of serious problems with the ED that clearly have broad implications for PWH overall. Fortunately, Porter's charge has also given her sufficient clout in order to request the data she needs to complete her assignment. Without further deliberation, she e-mails her request for data to the CEO's assistant, focusing on the following list of documents:

- Three-year Piney Woods Hospital comparative income statements (Figure V.9)
- Three-year Piney Woods Hospital comparative balance sheet (Figure V.10)

FIGURE V.9

Piney Woods
Hospital
Income
Statements

Years Ended September 30, 2005, 2006, and 2007
(in thousands)

	2005	2006	2007
REVENUE			
Inpatient revenue	$ 471,794	$ 510,576	$ 543,875
Hospital outpatient revenue	222,602	243,438	264,729
Behavioral health revenue	14,887	14,278	13,571
Home care revenue	31,110	29,682	34,062
Nursing home revenue	5,224	6,137	6,225
Clinic revenue	1,508	2,059	2,342
Total revenue	747,125	806,170	864,804
Deductions from revenue	(340,993)	(379,012)	(433,921)
Net patient revenue	406,132	427,158	430,883
Other operating revenue	10,968	15,083	12,804
	417,100	442,241	443,687
EXPENSE			
Nursing services	76,244	85,624	85,004
Other professional services	97,907	112,222	123,787
General services	20,227	21,815	23,016
Fiscal services	19,277	18,901	19,434
Administration services	58,927	61,319	59,965
Behavioral health expense	8,298	8,291	7,912
Home case expense	21,088	21,954	24,485
Nursing home expense	4,785	5,145	5,233
Clinic expense	3,007	3,730	3,893
Interest	4,443	2,879	3,895
Depreciation and amortization	29,297	31,460	32,789
Bad debt expense	27,930	37,685	39,788
Total operating expense	371,430	411,025	429,201
Operating margin	45,670	31,216	14,486
Non-operating revenue	16,394	14,520	16,852
Accrual for incentive bonus	(5,142)	(6,191)	(16)
Total margin	$ 56,922	$ 39,545	$ 31,322

FIGURE V.10
Piney Woods
Hospital
Balance Sheet

Years Ended September 30, 2005, 2006, and 2007
(in thousands)

	2005	2006	2007
ASSETS			
Operating cash	$ 1,574	$ 3,736	$ 32
Investments	230,150	244,152	255,239
Patient accounts receivable			
Accounts receivable, net			
of contractual adjustments	127,798	132,697	131,734
Third-party receivables	3,001	4,077	2,661
Allowance for uncollectibles	(48,648)	(49,104)	(52,734)
Net patient receivables	82,151	87,670	81,661
Intercompany receivables	38,954	33,783	51,561
Inventories	5,731	6,092	6,638
Prepaid expenses	15,584	15,547	17,674
Other current assets	4,135	6,366	5,403
Property, plant, and equipment	485,799	508,195	541,992
Construction in progress	9,388	11,697	3,396
Accumulated depreciation	(262,403)	(276,928)	(308,277)
	232,784	242,964	237,111
Bond fund	30,205	22,437	15,042
Other assets	88	38	148
Expansion fund cash and investments	31,311	33,895	38,421
Total assets	$ 672,667	$ 696,680	$ 708,930
LIABILITIES AND NET ASSETS			
Accounts payable	$ 9,688	$ 8,206	$ 9,643
Accrued payroll and withholdings	18,043	20,877	10,768
Due to third parties	7,688	8,419	8,284
Other liabilities	1,888	2,467	1,926
Bonds payable	161,171	152,071	146,059
Total liabilities	198,478	192,040	176,680
Net assets	474,189	504,640	532,248
Total liabilities and net assets	$ 672,667	$ 696,680	$ 708,930

FIGURE V.11
Piney Woods
Hospital Vital
Statistics

Years Ended September 30, 2005, 2006, and 2007 (in thousands)			
	2005	**2006**	**2007**
Patient days	150,278	150,735	142,092
Adjusted patient days	230,481	231,377	220,190
Discharges	29,220	29,902	27,917
Adjusted discharges	45,130	46,251	43,575
Home care visits	270,199	249,570	277,748
Nursing home days	38,194	38,028	37,394
Clinic visits	13,812	17,281	18,726
EMERGENCY ROOM			
Emergency room visits	54,229	55,439	57,539
Emergency room total charges	$17,405,333	$17,357,754	$16,979,267
Inpatient admissions through ED	11,495	11,864	11,289
ED RN FTEs*	48	48	49
Unit clerk FTEs	4	4	4
ER tech FTEs*	10	17	17
Left without being seen/AMA	1,030	1,497	2,301
Average turnaround time (min.)	177	247	312
Average time to be seen by physician (min.)	23	129	152
RN vacancy	4.4%	11.0%	13.0%

* In FY 2006 an observation unit was created in the ED. Eight RN FTEs were added in FY 2006 to staff this unit. ER techs increased by 8 FTEs in FY 2006 and 4 in FY 2007.

- Three-year Piney Woods Hospital vital statistics (Figure V.11)
- Three-year Piney Woods Hospital payer mix and emergency charges (Figure V.12)
- Three-year Piney Woods Hospital emergency department expense (Figure V.13)
- Physician satisfaction and employee satisfaction survey results (Figure V.14)
- Emergency department floor plan (Figure V.15)

Situational Analysis Results

Roberts's review of Porter's initial outline of the PWH problems and the documents she requested suggested a host of problems to tackle at Piney

FIGURE V.12
Piney Woods
Hospital
Payer Mix and
Emergency
Charges

Years Ended September 30, 2005, 2006, and 2007

	2005	2006	2007
INPATIENT PAYER MIX PERCENTAGES			
Commercial	21%	17%	16%
Managed care	4%	4%	5%
Medicaid	10%	11%	11%
Medicare	57%	59%	58%
Self-pay	8%	9%	10%
	100%	100%	100%
CHARGES INCURRED BY EMERGENCY PATIENTS (in thousands)			
Commercial	$ 38,007	$ 31,092	$ 30,947
Managed care	13,826	11,760	13,085
Medicaid	36,316	35,703	28,162
Medicare	46,569	41,812	51,742
Self-pay	29,734	30,759	36,361
	$ 164,452	$ 151,126	$ 160,297
EMERGENCY DEPARTMENT PAYER MIX			
Commercial	22%	21%	19%
Managed care	9%	8%	8%
Medicaid	22%	23%	18%
Medicare	29%	28%	32%
Self-pay	18%	20%	23%
	100%	100%	100%

FIGURE V.13
Piney Woods
Hospital
Emergency
Department
Expense

Years Ended September 30, 2005, 2006, and 2007
(in thousands)

	2005	2006	2007
Salaries—RN	$ 2,662	$ 2,750	$ 2,764
Salaries—other	589	838	807
Benefits	235	255	259
Administrative expense	90	107	92
Patient-related expense	456	570	616
Physician services	763	839	516
Liability insurance	428	477	538
Total	$ 5,223	$ 5,836	$ 5,592

PHYSICIAN SATISFACTION SURVEY

FIGURE V.14
Satisfaction
Survey Results

2002

	Total Hospital	ED
Physicians Surveyed	79	4
General Satisfaction	5.43	6.5

2005

	Total Hospital	ED
Physicians Surveyed	75	3
General Satisfaction	4.61	3.33

NOTE: The survey is based on a seven-point scale, 1 being negative and 7 being positive. This survey measures overall physician satisfaction concerning working relationships with the hospital.

EMPLOYEE SATISFACTION SURVEY

	Hospital	ED
2003	79	67
2005	79	78
2007	82	68

NOTE: Employee opinion survey is conducted every other year. The score represents the percentile with 1% being the lowest and 100% being the highest possible score.

Woods. Compiling her results for the CEO, Roberts focused on four particular issues: (1) satisfaction (patient, employee, and physician), (2) wait times, (3) financial, and (4) community perception. Her summarized findings are reported below:

Satisfaction

Patient

Current patient satisfaction scores at Piney Woods Hospital are among the lowest in the country. Dissatisfaction starts immediately when the patient walks through the door of the ED. Instead of being greeted, the patient must navigate his or her way to one of the three registration desks, none of which is located in plain view. After registration, the patient is not given a time estimate, but rather is told to have a seat and wait until being called back to the nursing desk. There is no additional communication with the patient until he or she is called to head through the double doors to the nurs-

FIGURE V.15
Emergency
Department
Floor Plan

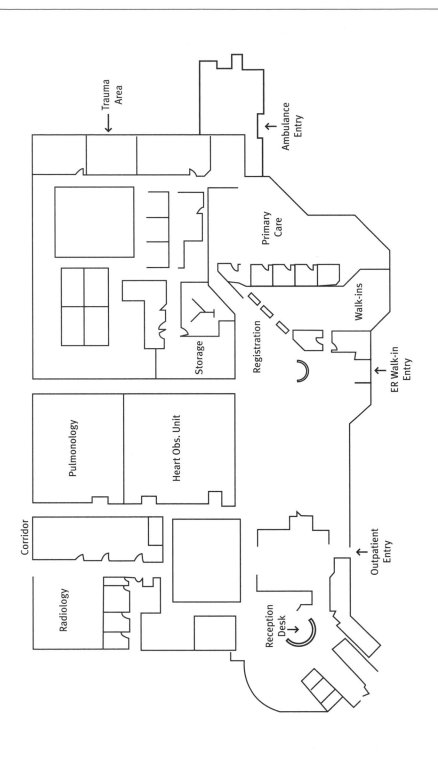

ing desk. Once again, instead of being greeted and escorted to the nursing desk, it is up to the patient to find his or her own way.

At this point, the patient is not only upset with his or her medical condition, but also with the service he or she has received. On average, it takes a patient two and one-half hours to be seen by a physician. This long wait time and lack of communication resulted in over 2,000 patients leaving without being seen or against medical advice (AMA) in the past year.

Another issue on the rise for patient satisfaction is the number of Hispanic immigrant workers now residing in the area. Most of these workers do not speak English, nor do they have health insurance. This cultural difference creates a barrier between the staff and patients.

Employee

Employee satisfaction at PWH ED increased between 2003 and 2005 but decreased to 68 percent in 2007. Work overload and poor work relationships contribute to increased stress for nurses (Institute of Medicine 2007). Stress from increased crowding is evident as PWH nurses are frustrated and tired of dealing with angry patients. In addition, the nursing schedule is inflexible and results in frequent overtime. Unfortunately, the employees at PWH do not have a consistent leader with whom to address their concerns. The lack of leadership in the ED may have been the cause for the drop in employee satisfaction after its previous increase. Satisfied employees are critical to the provision of customer service and high-quality care, so it is essential PWH leaders focus on employee satisfaction.

Physician

In 2002, physician satisfaction with the ED was 6.5 on a scale of 7, but in 2005, the survey response rate dropped, and the score declined to 3.33. The scores for the total hospital followed a similar pattern, but did not drop as sharply as those for the ED. This indicates physician dissatisfaction is a hospital-wide issue, and not just limited to the ED. Maintaining working relationships with physicians is crucial to the success of any health service institution.

The decrease in ED physician satisfaction is attributable to the high turnover in leadership. Since leadership has been inconsistent, morale, productivity, and quality have all declined in the past few years. The physicians are also upset that they were not consulted about the hospital switching to electronic health records. Since their opinions were not valued, the physicians currently do not have a good working relationship with Zach Porter, PWH CEO. Further, the contract with the physician group is set up to reward physicians on the basis of patient satisfaction, so the decline in satisfaction has cost the physicians income. Destabilization of income is disruptive to the satisfaction of any group of stakeholders. The working arrangement of the hospital with the physicians is a key area to be addressed.

Wait Times

Long wait times are another weakness of PWH's ED. The current process flow includes several points where patients endure waits. When patients arrive, they wait to be registered. Then, patients wait to be called to the nursing desk for triage. The triage process only distinguishes two levels of acuity—primary care and life-threatening trauma; as a result, most patients fall in between and wait again for a bed. After patients secure a bed they are likely to wait for nurses, physicians, and test results. Even after disposition, admitted patients may wait for inpatient beds.

Nearly 80 percent of patients' time in an ED is non-value added wait time, and longer waits correlate with lower patient satisfaction and with higher rates of patients leaving without being seen (Advisory Board Company 2004; Crane 2007; Institute of Medicine 2007). As shown in Table V.1, PWH's experience is similar to that reported in the literature. From 2005 to 2007, PWH's average time to see a physician increased over 500 percent and average turnaround time increased 76 percent; as expected, patient satisfaction is low and the number of patients who left without being seen or against medical advice increased 124 percent. Since improving customer service and quality of care are critical success factors for the hospital, PWH's ED must reduce wait times.

Financial

The hospital has obviously been in a downturn over the past three years. Year-to-year bottom lines have been declining, leaving fewer resources available for updating and expanding the current services. Surprisingly, analysis of ED performance shows this department is not significantly draining on the hospital. There are other places the hospital should be more concerned about when evaluating overall financial performance.

For example, growth of expenses in "other professional services" has been quite large. The increase in these costs accounted for 82 percent of the

TABLE V.1 Status of Emergency Department Visits	**2005**	**2006**	**2007**	**'05–'07**
Visits	54,229	55,439	57,539	6.1%
Left w/o being seen/AMA	1,030	1,497	2,301	123.4%
% left w/o being seen/AMA	1.9%	2.7%	4.0%	
Average turnaround time (min.)	177	247	312	76.3%
Average time to physician (min.)	23	129	152	560.9%

total margin decline from 2005 to 2006. There may be revenue associated with these costs, but they do not appear to adequately offset the costs. Also, there has been an enormous amount of growth in the home care business. This rapid expansion, 633 percent growth from 2005 to 2006, may have flown under the radar of the business office, which could be struggling to collect. Lack of management attention might lead to high expenses in the business office, preventing it from covering costs. These two issues alone are more financially alarming than the situation in the ED.

The most immediate financial problem presented by the ED is the influx of self-pay patients, particularly the uninsured. These individuals seem to be causing a large amount of stress on the staff. Lack of attention to the special requirements of billing and collecting from self-pay patients makes the situation more burdensome than need be. Appropriate and proactive collection methods could assuage this.

Community Perception

Little information was available regarding the current state of the PWH brand. However, the state of the ED has significantly damaged the brand of the hospital, whether there is an official brand strategy or not. The patrons—patients and their families—of PWH form perceptions about the hospital based on the care and satisfaction they receive while there. They pass along these perceptions to their friends by word of mouth. Every institution, private or public, for-profit or non-profit, has an image and associated set of values. PWH needs to actively improve that image and those perceptions by managing the brand. Managing the ED brand and the hospital's brand are not mutually exclusive.

What's Next?

Porter appreciated Roberts's detailed review of the Piney Woods situation, and decided he needed some concrete suggestions about what to do next. In particular, he wanted solutions to address the four issues Roberts outlined.

Case Questions

1. What could be done at Piney Woods Hospital to reduce ED wait times?
2. What steps could be taken to improve the patient payer mix?
3. How could PWH improve patient satisfaction scores?
4. What could be done to improve employee satisfaction?
5. How could physician satisfaction issues be addressed?
6. What could be done to improve community perceptions about PWH?

References

Advisory Board Company. 2004. "Accelerating Emergency Department Through-put: Reducing Bottlenecks in the ED." In *The Throughput-Focused Hospital.* Washington, DC: Advisory Board Company.

Crane, J. 2007. "Redesigning Your Front End and Transforming Patient Care." Institute of Healthcare Improvement. [Online document; accessed 4/4/09.] http://www.ihi.org/IHI/Topics/Flow/EmergencyDepartment/Emerging Content/PresentationsIHIEDCommunityOct07.htm.

Institute of Medicine. 2007. "The Emergency Care Workforce." In *Hospital-Based Emergency Care: At the Breaking Point.* Washington, DC: National Academies Press.

Case N
An Investment Decision at
Central Med Health System

Emily Allinder, Jason Dopoulos, Breanne Pfotenhauer, David Reisman, Erick Vidmar, Jason Waibel, and Ann Scheck McAlearney

Background

Central Med Health System (CMHS) was created on January 1, 1996, with the mission of "providing expert healthcare to the people of North Central Iowa." The non-profit organization is comprised of two general, acute care hospitals, Central Med Hospital and Shelty Hospital, with a combined total of 395 beds. The service area consists of a six-county region in North Central Iowa: Rich, Crawford, Ashville, Morris, Huron, and Knowell counties. Central Med is the largest provider of healthcare services between the cities of Cletan and Flagship. The health system provides a complete range of primary care and specialty practices. Central Med Hospital offers a Level II trauma center and a Level II perinatal department. Other featured services include cardiac care, comprehensive neurological services, cancer care, behavioral health, maternity services, sports medicine, surgical services, pediatric therapy services, speech therapy services, industrial health and safety services, home care, and hospice care.

All services and business units are driven by the mission, vision, and values of Central Med. Central Med's vision is to provide "expert care close to home." The organization seeks to be the provider of choice for residents of North Central Iowa and strives to dissuade residents from traveling to Cletan or Flagship for care. The core values as stated by Central Med include:

- *Quality*: We will be known for excellence in all that we do.
- *Customer service*: We will work to fulfill the individual needs of every patient, family member, and visitor.
- *Innovation*: We will continually strive to develop and work with the latest processes available in every department.
- *Teamwork*: Our staff will work together to provide our patients with the best care possible.

Financial Status

CMHS is a financially stable organization. Operating margins have been consistent with similar BBB–bond rated organizations over the past three years and currently stand at 3 percent. A $12 million endowment provides consistent investment returns, which contributed to a total margin of 8 percent last fiscal year. CMHS maintains a prudent balance sheet with a debt to capitalization ratio of 25 percent. Days cash on hand has averaged 225 over the last three years, and the current ratio was 2.5 last year, demonstrating the facility's ability to cover its operating expenses. CMHS has historically used debt to finance capital projects, but due to evaporation of liquidity in the municipal bond markets, the system decided to fund certain projects with cash from operations.

The Problem

Like other non-profit healthcare providers, CMHS struggles to enhance patient care with limited financial and capital resources. Investments in new clinical programs are evaluated carefully to ensure that patients have access to the appropriate new programs and services. CMHS strives to balance the need to invest in the clinical programs that are most important to its patient population with the need to remain financially viable.

CMHS leadership is currently faced with a difficult decision. The system has $13 million to invest in a clinical expansion project, and stakeholders throughout the organization have varying ideas about which program is most deserving of the new capital investment. While certain members of the leadership team want to invest in an expanded radiation oncology program, others are interested in bolstering heart services by enhancing the interventional cardiology program.

Option 1: Radiation Oncology

According to the American Cancer Society, the *Journal of Oncology Management*, the Health Care Advisory Board, and other expert sources, there is a

TABLE V.2
Current Market
Share—
Radiation
Oncology

	Total 2007 Radiation Oncology Pts.	Central Med 2007 Radiation Oncology Pts.	Central Med 2007 Radiation Oncology Market Share
Ashville	138	50	36.2%
Crawford	135	61	45.2%
Huron	189	15	7.9%
Knowell	163	24	14.7%
Morris	68	3	4.4%
Rich	419	327	78%
Total	1,112	480	43.2%

Projected Market Share—Radiation Oncology

	2007	Year 1	Year 2	Year 3	Year 4	Year 5
Conservative (43%–51%)	43.2%	43.3%	45.2%	47.2%	49.2%	51.1%

20 to 25 percent increase projected in the number of newly diagnosed cancer cases in the next ten years. In addition to newly diagnosed cases, the five-year relative survival rate has increased significantly as a result of newer technologies and treatments. As people live longer, the demand for cancer services will grow. Table V.2 provides additional information about projected demand for radiation oncology services, and Box V.1 describes the perspective of a nurse executive interested in expanding this program at CMHS.

Dr. Moh, the only radiation oncologist at Central Med Health System, sees up to 70 patients a day, which is 40 percent more patients than the average radiation oncologist. The facilities are cramped and the schedule is tight, but somehow he is able to complete the day's work. Perhaps it is the friendly culture of CMHS that keeps the staff content with current operations, but Dr. Moh believes something needs to be done differently in order to continue to provide high-quality care.

Every radiation oncology department in the country needs two components, a board-certified radiation oncologist and the essential equipment to create a treatment plan. Central Med has both of these components, but there is growing concern regarding the need for additional equipment to accommodate treatment plans. Linear accelerators are traditionally used to program a patient's treatment plan and can be accessed for each appointment. Central Med currently has two machines and averages between 40 and 50 patients per day.

BOX V.1
A Nurse Executive's Argument for Building a New Radiation Oncology Facility

Isabelle Gonzalez had served as the chief nursing officer at CMHS for 20 years. She had worked in several different departments, and was well respected and admired by her colleagues and superiors. She was known for her solid work ethic and unwavering dedication to the success of CMHS and to the provision of excellent patient care services.

Isabelle felt that building a new facility to house the radiation oncology department and its equipment was the best option. She noted that the existing facilities were "old, inefficient, cramped, and not patient friendly." She was concerned that Central Med could lose a considerable amount of market share if the health system did not remain on the leading edge of cancer care. "Cancer patients are very sick and require a high intensity and frequency of care," Isabelle stated. "We have a duty to our patients to provide comprehensive cancer services close to their homes. Besides, radiation oncology is a growing service line that contributes significantly to our operating margin."

The literature recommends that one machine treat 30 to 35 patients per day; therefore, it is important that CMHS has two machines running. Technical difficulties are a problem because CMHS's linear accelerators are unmatched. This means that if one machine goes down, the patient plan for that machine cannot be transferred to the other machine. This results in wasted time and resources.

In addition to these operational challenges, Dr. Moh is concerned that CMHS is vulnerable to competitors who might want to enter the radiation oncology market in CMHS's primary service areas. Such competition would be difficult to withstand with CMHS's current facilities. Dr. Moh knows he needs to act quickly to secure the future success of the program.

Option 2: Interventional Cardiology

Although the cardiology program has been quite successful for CMHS, further investment in the interventional cardiology segment of the department is desperately needed. Current industry trends favor interventional cardiology procedures over traditional open heart operations. Expert industry organizations predict that this trend will continue. CMHS needs to make a significant investment in its interventional cardiology program if it wants to retain and expand market share in this specialty. Additional data about interventional

TABLE V.3
Current Market
Share—
Interventional
Cardiology

	Total 2007 Interventional Cardiology Pts.	Central Med 2007 Interventional Cardiology Pts.	Central Med 2007 Interventional Cardiology Market Share
Ashville	276	75	27.2%
Crawford	270	92	34.1%
Huron	378	23	6.1%
Knowell	326	36	11%
Morris	136	5	3.7%
Rich	838	491	58.6%
Total	2,224	722	32.5%

Projected Market Share—Interventional Cardiology

	2007	Year 1	Year 2	Year 3	Year 4	Year 5
Conservative (32%–52%)	32.5%	39.7%	43.2%	46.8%	49.9%	52.3%

cardiology are provided in Table V.3, and the perspective of a board member interested in expanding the program is provided in Box V.2.

As the number of patients requiring specialized cardiology care continues to increase throughout the service area, CMHS has been struggling to expand its service offerings to this patient population. New cholesterol lowering and antihypertensive medications introduced over the last ten years have resulted in significantly extended life spans for cardiology patients. However, Americans leading more sedentary lifestyles and eating high-fat diets have contributed to a larger number of patients requiring specialized cardiac care. At the same time, a large competing health system in the area has recently invested in a significant expansion of its cardiovascular service line. Dr. Peak, an interventional cardiologist and CMHS's director of cardiology, knows that in order to ensure the future success of the cardiology division, he needs to secure additional financial support from hospital leadership.

The cardiology program at CMHS has overcome significant challenges in the past. Several years ago the division faced a need for more cardiac surgeons and operating rooms to handle the increased number of coronary artery bypass graft procedures. The solution to the problem was to remodel the cardiac operating rooms and recruit several highly qualified physicians. The program has since become one of the more profitable units at CMHS and a model that other divisions within the hospital hope to emulate.

BOX V.2
A Board Member's Argument for Expanding the Interventional Cardiology Program

An influential hospital board member, Brandon Gerner, argued that CMHS should invest the $13 million in an expanded interventional cardiology program. Gerner felt the radiation oncology program was not headed in a positive direction. In his opinion, the program should be discontinued and the money should be allocated to the interventional cardiology program, which would produce higher margins for the institution. "Let's beef up our interventional cardiology program," stated Gerner. "The future impact of radiation oncology has been drastically overestimated and the need for interventional cardiology will continue to grow as the population continues to age. Furthermore, favorable reimbursement for interventional cardiology procedures is likely to continue in the future, making this a sound financial decision for the organization."

Advances in treatment options for cardiology patients have focused on minimally invasive interventional procedures that are more comfortable for patients and have significantly reduced recovery times. In fact, the number of minimally invasive interventional cardiology procedures performed at CMHS has nearly doubled in the last few years. These procedures are completed in specially designed treatment areas where sophisticated imaging equipment is used to guide small catheters and instruments through patients' cardiovascular systems. The single interventional cardiology suite at CMHS is no longer adequate to serve this expanding clinical need. Dr. Peak knows that in order to retain market share in this competitive environment, CMHS needs to invest significant capital in the creation of additional interventional cardiology treatment areas.

Implications of the Investment Decision

Given Central Med's location, the health system is continually concerned about its ability to retain market share and avoid losing patients to hospitals in Cletan or Flagship. While the financial stability and reputation of CMHS are enviable, the hospital has been unwilling to expand beyond the North Central Iowa region. Further, Central Med's clear mission and strong organizational culture have made affiliation options such as alliances or other cooperative arrangements with competitors virtually impossible to consider. As a result, any CMHS investment will be pursued on its own.

In previous discussions about investment options, hospital leadership has raised alternative uses for the $13 million at CMHS. However, the board has rejected other alternatives and has narrowed the options to the two currently on the table. They are unwilling to further explore avenues that might make the two options jointly possible. Even though an exclusive investment in radiation oncology will threaten the success of the interventional cardiology program, and vice versa, the board wants to force a decision between the two, and it wants the decision made now.

Case Questions

1. What are the pros and cons of each alternative investment? Does the radiation oncology project or the enhanced interventional cardiology program better align with Central Med's mission and vision? Why?
2. Whom does Central Med serve? At what cost?
3. Who are the stakeholders at Central Med who will be affected by this decision? Which stakeholders should be included in discussions leading to a decision about which alternative investment to pursue?
4. What time sequence would you propose for the planning process around this investment?
5. What additional information would you need to make a solid business decision? Are there non-financial data you should consider?
6. What would be implications for the alternative service that is not selected for investment? What might happen to volume and market share for that service?
7. If the two alternatives were not mutually exclusive, what types of financing strategies would you propose to permit investment in both options?

Short Case 21
New Chief of Ob-Gyn: The Next Three Years

Anthony R. Kovner

Since Dr. Mikhail has taken over as chief of Ob-Gyn at North Heights Medical Center in New York City, the following have occurred: a slight increase in deliveries; a significant expansion of primary care centers and number of visits; a large increase in the number of abortions done; a large increase in research grants received; improvement in facilities; and an improvement in patient service. However, patient revenues have decreased slightly because of improvements in health for premature births (preemies), and use of the preemie nursery has decreased significantly. North Heights serves a low-income, diverse population and is a large hospital and health system with a $200 million budget.

The following discussion has occurred among a group of consultants brought together by Dr. Bright, the medical director.

Dr. Strong: The service needs to increase its share of the market. St. Brennan's Hospital represents a threat in this regard and Washington Hospital represents an opportunity.

Dr. Light: There is a leakage in primary care away from North Heights. Hire an outreach worker to find out the reasons for the leakage and do something about it.

Dr. Bright: Dr. Mikhail should increase marketing efforts, including advertising.

Dr. Quick: Dr. Mikhail should continue with the present strategy. Deliveries are down in the Bronx, and market share is slowly increasing.

Dr. Rough: Dr. Mikhail should reduce the number of full-time staff and produce the same number of deliveries with a smaller budget.

Dr. Clever: Dr. Mikhail should alter his research strategy and seek grants aimed at interventions that will increase the number of deliveries.

Case Questions

1. What are the key facts in the situation?
2. What are the problems and issues?
3. What should Dr. Mikhail do, and why?

Short Case 22
To Sell or Not to Sell

Anthony R. Kovner

Clark Medical Center in New York City is losing $2 million a year on sales of $750 million. Clark Hospital serves a low-income, diverse population and is located in an old facility. Besides owning a hospital, the Medical Center owns HelpYou, a Medicaid HMO with over 250,000 patients. HelpYou contributes its surplus of $2 million per year to Clark Medical Center, which meets the Medical Center's deficit.

Sam Hayes, Clark's CEO, has determined that the best way to save the hospital is to sell the HMO and believes that Clark can get up to $200 million for it. Sam has convinced all but two members of the executive committee that "this is the way to go." The two unconvinced board members are Luke Reacher and Harry Smith, who have the following conversation about the prospective sale at Joe's Pub:

Luke: I'm not against selling, but the HMO is worth $300 million and I would only sell if Sam told us in advance how much of the money is "net" and what he would use it for.

Harry: I think we should sell the hospital and invest in the HMO. The hospital continues to lose money. Why do we pay Sam $1 million a year anyway?

Luke: Shouldn't we at least review the experience of other hospitals that have sold their HMOs?

Harry: Sam says we're unique.

Luke: The next question is, What should we and what can we do about the situation as board members? The hospital board has already agreed to sell the HMO if we can get $200 million.

Harry: No one will offer us that. What if they offer us $100 million?

Luke: What worries me is that Sam will take the $100 million to pay off underfunded reserves for malpractice and the nurses' pension plan. This may be up to half of the $100 million.

Case Questions

1. If selling the HMO is such a bad idea, why are the hospital CEO and the board in favor of the sale?
2. What is the hospital likely to do with the proceeds of the sale?
3. What are the choices available to Luke and Harry?
4. What do you recommend that Luke and Harry do now, and why?
5. List barriers to implementing your recommendations and how Clark Medical Center and its board can overcome them.

Short Case 23
A New Look?

Ann Scheck McAlearney and Sarah M. Roesch

Dr. Elinor Cooke is a renowned cosmetic surgeon, highly dedicated to healing and restoring well-being for those affected by aesthetic issues. She believes that her line of work builds the confidence and self-esteem of those who seek her services. Dr. Cooke received her medical degree from Case Western Reserve University and then completed four years of residency and two additional years of residency in plastic surgery at the Ohio State University Hospitals. Dr. Cooke's current practice, North City Aesthetic and Plastic Surgery, Inc., affiliated with Northside Community Hospital, is located in a suburb of Cleveland on a beautiful wooded lot next to Lake Erie. In addition to Dr. Cooke, there is one other doctor affiliated with North City, Dr. Ryan Thomas, who specializes in men's reconstructive surgery. The practice also employs two nurses and an office manager. The practice enjoys an excellent reputation and is known for its compassionate approach to care.

While North City Aesthetic and Plastic Surgery is considered one of the premier practices in the Midwest market area, Dr. Cooke is concerned about some of the changes she has observed in the field of plastic surgery. When she started her practice in the early 1980s, cosmetic surgery was a relatively new field. Plastic surgery was available for those affected by disfigurement, but not readily available for those who wanted to fix something just because they didn't like their appearance. Over the years, Hollywood, new techniques, and new trends sparked tremendous growth in the cosmetic surgery industry, and with this growth, the profile of a typical cosmetic surgery practice changed. Whereas patients used to be amazed that a tummy tuck, breast augmentation, facelift, or rhinoplasty were possible, now the average patient tends to want more than surgery alone.

Another trend Dr. Cooke has observed is the increasing level of competition for aesthetic surgery services. She is aware of the expanding availability of surgical procedures through ambulatory surgery centers, but a recent invitation to a Botox party event provided evidence of a new competitive threat—even if the quality of care provided might be suspect. Dr. Cooke's North City practice has managed to grow based on patients' word-of-mouth recommendations and other physicians' referrals rather than through advertising. Yet given local and regional competition for well-paying patients, Dr. Cooke knows that she must develop her own strategy to ensure that her practice can survive and thrive into the future. The practice's prosperity is important to Dr. Cooke and she is continually looking for ways to grow her practice's business.

Dr. Cooke, who also has a bachelor's degree in business, is a problem solver by nature. In considering the new trends in the aesthetic surgery area, Dr. Cooke senses that she has a choice to make. Abdominoplasty (tummy tuck) is the most popular form of surgery that she performs. After surgery, the patient often has trouble with activities such as moving from a sitting to a standing position, walking, and caring for the post-operative drains. Dr. Cooke has often thought it would be nice to have a 24-hour care alternative for post-operative patients.

One particularly intriguing option is to develop a "hideaway" for her aesthetic surgery clients where they can relax and recover after their procedures. She knows that her patients desire complete confidentiality at all times, and that they also want a high degree of professional and personal attention—before, during, and after the procedures. Creating a hideaway would allow Dr. Cooke to provide top-notch medical care in a spa-like atmosphere, and enable her staff to offer professional and personal attention to the healing patients during the days following surgery. Further, given her knowledge of the important connections between individuals' minds and their bodies, she is certain that a relaxing atmosphere would enhance the healing process while offering a safe place for her demanding clientele to recover. Moreover, there is no such facility in the Cleveland area and she feels that this would definitely give her practice an edge over other practices. She also feels that her building's scenic locale would be perfect for this type of post-operative hideaway.

While Dr. Cooke suspects that this hideaway concept would have considerable appeal to her well-heeled patients, she knows that potential patients are not the only individuals she would need to consider in developing a new approach for her North City practice. When she shared her idea with Dr. Thomas, he was less than enthusiastic. Dr. Thomas reminded her that they were surgeons, not innkeepers. He noted that the overhead costs associated with such a practice change would be high, and he was particularly worried about management of the facility. Dr. Thomas also brought up the issue of insurance liability. Then he mentioned that he had heard that St. Clare's, another community hospital, is also looking into opening a similar type of facility not too far away.

Dr. Cooke, discouraged, yet not defeated, understands Dr. Thomas's concerns. As the lease is soon up on the building for her current practice, Dr. Cooke knows she will need to make any decision about changing the direction of her practice quickly so that she can take action. The possibility of a facility opening at St. Clare's motivates Dr. Cooke to further investigate her idea. She believes the wooded lot with lake views that her practice occupies would be an ideal location for a recovery retreat. And she feels that Dr. Thomas's male patients would also benefit from a discreet hideaway to recover.

Case Questions

1. What are the pros and cons of changing the focus of Dr. Cooke's practice?
2. What would you predict would be the reactions of the various stakeholders to Dr. Cooke's new business concept (e.g., patients, referring physicians, Northside Community Hospital, her professional colleagues).
3. What would you recommend for Dr. Cooke?

Short Case 24
Disparities in Care at Southern Regional Health System

Ann Scheck McAlearney

Tim Hank leaned back in his chair and closed his eyes. While he had been afraid the reports might have bad news, he now had to figure out what to do with this new information. Flipping through the first binder on his desk, reporting results of the recent Robert Wood Johnson Foundation–sponsored assessment of the cardiovascular care provided by his organization, he was increasingly concerned. Southern Regional Health System was based in Jackson, Mississippi, an area known for a highly diverse population and high poverty rates. Black and Hispanic residents in the area were about three times more likely to live in poverty than were whites. Unemployment was also a big problem that affected whites and nonwhites differently—in the Jackson area, black residents were two and a half times more likely to be unemployed and Hispanics over twice as likely to be unemployed as white residents. Beyond poverty and employment differences, though, was the issue of different care given to different patients. This issue of disparities in care was receiving increasing national attention, but Hank had thought the care they provided at Southern Regional was "color blind." Given the health system's mission of providing "excellent quality of care for all," he assumed that the care was equitably delivered across patients and patient populations.

Apparently, this was not the case. This first report showed that there were indeed disparities in the care provided by Southern Regional. Data on heart care had been collected by race and ethnicity for the past year, and these baseline data showed differences. For instance, using the four core measures for heart failure that the Centers for Medicare & Medicaid Services currently collects and reports, only 41 percent of patients were receiving all recommended heart failure care, and the numbers were worse based on race and ethnicity. The analysis showed that while 68 percent of whites received all recommended care, the comparable number among non-whites was 27 percent. For one measure—the percentage of heart failure patients receiving discharge instructions—only 65 percent of Hispanic patients received the information, compared to 85 percent of non-Hispanic patients. Also troubling Hank was the fact that none of these measures were close to 100 percent—this certainly wasn't the type of care he'd want offered to his own family. Yet he truly didn't understand how his hospital could be providing such disparate care.

The second binder on his desk offered little information to ease his concern. This report, the "Assessment of Organizational Readiness to

Change" for Southern Regional Health System, showed that few individuals in his hospital were aware of the nation-wide problem of disparities in care, and even fewer were aware that such an issue might be problematic within their own hospital. Now he had the data for Southern Regional that showed significant gaps in care provided to African American and Latino patients relative to white patients, but the accompanying readiness-to-change evaluation showed a strong tendency among hospital employees and physicians to resist any proposed changes and instead "go with the flow." Hank knew that his ability to bring the issue of disparate care to the forefront of hospital concerns and successfully make strides to reduce these disparities would be a legacy he would love to leave. Yet he didn't know how he could possibly begin to address this issue at Southern Regional Health System.

Case Questions

1. What should Hank do with the information contained in these reports?
2. What reactions would you predict he might receive from various hospital stakeholders, such as other executives, physicians, board members, or the community?
3. What can Hank do to raise the level of urgency at Southern Regional Health System to address the issue of disparities in care?
4. What are the constraints he will face?

Short Case 25
Annual Performance Evaluation:
Can You Coach Kindness?

Ann Scheck McAlearney

Bob Carter, RN, has been working at New Hope Hospital for six years, ever since he finished nursing school. He has always planned to become a manager at some time in his career, and it seems that the opportunity might soon be available. As a floor nurse Carter has earned the respect of his peers, never taking "no" for an answer and, in many cases, saving patients' lives because of solid clinical instincts. At this point Carter has been working for two years as a case manager in the Clinical Case Management Department, participating in case management and discharge planning within the hospital. Carter is considering applying for a promotion to manager of discharge planning to fill a newly vacated position in the Clinical Case Management Department, and he is looking forward to his upcoming performance review with the director of clinical case management as an opportunity to discuss this possible promotion.

Sally Valen is the vice president of clinical operations, and the Clinical Case Management Department is one of her areas of responsibility. She is particularly concerned about the role of this department in ensuring appropriate discharge planning for all patients, especially in light of the new attention focused on discharge planning through the Centers for Medicare & Medicaid Services (CMS) Core Measures Program.

You are the director of clinical case management, and eager to fill the vacant manager of discharge planning position. You know that any manager in the department will require a strong clinical background, but you are also aware that this individual must have the ability to work well with others in process improvement activities needed to strengthen discharge planning and clinical case management services throughout the hospital.

In reviewing Carter's file before his performance evaluation, you are reminded of several issues that might affect your decision about his promotion. First, you are aware that Carter's attitude toward social workers within the department has been less than collegial. Your observations of his work style would indicate that he feels superior to the social workers, but you have not discussed this directly with him. Second, you are somewhat concerned about Carter's potential management style. While he has yet to be tested as a manager, you have seen him verbally reprimand other nurses in front of other employees, and this has frustrated some of his co-workers. On the positive side, though, you know that Carter has excellent clinical instincts. Further, while he may seem to have a superior attitude in interactions with some of his co-workers, his interactions with patients have been consistently outstanding. His ability to help patients manage challenging health issues and take responsibility for their care post-discharge has been noted several times in his file.

Your reflections about Carter's possible promotion have left you confused. You have several considerations:

Case Questions

1. What is the relative importance of clinical competence and patient focus over one's ability to work as a member of a clinical team in this department?
2. Do you want Carter to be a manager in your department?
3. What should you tell Carter to help him improve and develop his managerial skills regardless of your recommendation for him to apply for the manager position?

4. Based on your recommendation about Carter's possible promotion, what do you do now to help him succeed in a managerial role, or how do you encourage his professional development within New Hope so that he does not leave for a different job?

ACCOUNTABILITY

Let's not be too hasty; speed is a dangerous thing.
Untimely measures bring repentance.
Certainly, and unhappily, many things are wrong in the Colony.
But is there anything human without some fault?
And after all, you see, we do move forward.
—*C. P. Cavafy*

COMMENTARY

Organizations receive resources from society based on the acceptability of their products or services to their users and purchasers. If health services are perceived as acceptable, the organization providing them is meeting the expectations of purchasers, employers, or patients, all of whom have an interest in organizational performance. Of course, expectation levels can be changed—for example, by communicating to patients or employees what the organization is promising them in terms of performance in return for their patronage or willingness to work.

According to Pointer and Orlikoff (2002), the boards of trustees (directors) of healthcare organizations have five functions: formulating the organization's vision and key goals and ensuring that strategy is aligned with vision and goals; ensuring high levels of management performance; ensuring high-quality care; ensuring financial health; and ensuring the board's effectiveness and efficiency. The CEO is the board's agent, on site.

Primary accountability in health services organizations is shifting away from focusing on physicians, who presumably know best which services patients should receive and how, to customers or potential customers, based on a trajectory of the patient. For an example of the context for building organizational supports for change, see Figure VI.1, which is taken from the Report of the Committee on Quality of the Institute of Medicine, *Crossing the Quality Chasm* (2001).

Healthcare is increasingly purchased wholesale, rather than retail, by purchasers or their agents, who pay providers for specified benefits at specified amounts. Agents for wholesale purchasers exchange increases in patient volume for price discounts. The exchange works when customers are satisfied with quality and service, and have a number of providers to choose from.

Healthcare managers are concerned with production costs on the one hand and customer preferences on the other, a situation that American business organizations have faced for years. Two factors are vital in applying the concept of accountability: (1) a specification of organizational performance that is mutually agreed upon in advance by stakeholders and (2) the capability of managers to control the resources and behavior necessary to achieve such specified performance objectives.

FIGURE VI.1
Making Change
Possible

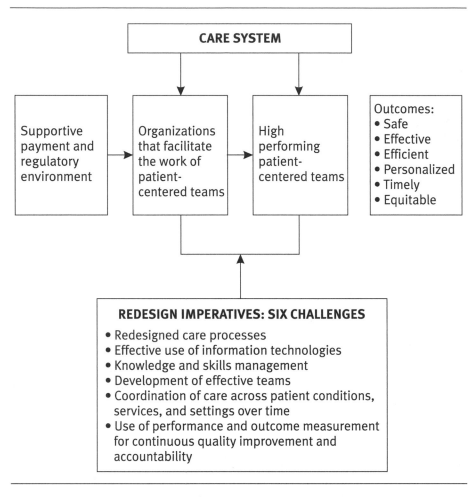

SOURCE: Committee on Quality, Institute of Medicine (2001).

Expectations of Organizational Performance

Stakeholders assess levels of organizational performance in a variety of ways. Increasingly, organizations are using "balanced scorecards" as strategic management systems. As posited by Kaplan and Norton (1996), the measures come from four perspectives: (1) financial, such as return on investment; (2) customer service; (3) internal business processes, such as the hospital readmission rate for the same illnesses; and (4) learning and growth, keyed to employees' morale and suggestions. This framework can easily be adapted to the expectations for performance on the part of stakeholder groups such as physicians or consumers. For example, physicians are concerned that the hospital makes a sufficient surplus to finance capital equipment, while consumers want a high level of customer service, as manifested in a same-day appointment system for ambulatory care.

To meet consumer expectations for service, managers can undertake marketing studies to find out what patients say they like and do not like about the organization's services. And physicians can be regularly surveyed for likes and dislikes. Using information from those surveys, managers can take steps to improve the situation. They can set up special units to advocate for patients or physicians. They can designate individuals in the marketing department or community advocacy department, for example, to advocate for patients or physicians. Managers can reorganize work so that fewer people provide more services for each patient or physician. Managers can reevaluate organizational routines regularly in terms of impact on patient outcomes or convenience of physicians. Special units or committees can be organized for quality improvement.

The manager can tour the facility regularly; talk with physicians, nurses, and patients; and observe how services can be improved and made more convenient. The manager can make it easier for patients or physicians to complain by establishing a hotline to her office or to that of another manager. The manager can analyze patient and physician complaints, review their resolution and follow-up, and talk to complainants personally. The manager can let patients and physicians know what service levels they should expect and what behavior is expected from them. Similar sets of activities can be conducted to improve employee perceptions and employer accountability.

The manager can report regularly as well to other stakeholders—such as purchasers and employee representatives—on performance, plans, and problems. Members of such constituencies can be included on policymaking and advisory committees. Management information systems can be developed for planning and evaluating services; information should include population served, population using various services, quantities of services, cost of service, quality of service, and patient satisfaction. Summaries of reports of regulators and accreditors can be shared with constituent groups. Organizational goals and performance can be analyzed, as can information on trends in turnover, overtime, and absenteeism; fundraising; profitability; and new capital equipment.

The process of decision making can be examined and improved, either as a process, given certain ends, or as a structure, such as considering whether constituent groups who are affected by organizational policy are included. By making itself more formally accountable, the leadership incurs substantial costs in terms of management time spent on the process, dollars spent on information systems upgrades, and conflict raised by differences about present and future direction. But the leadership may also reap substantial benefits: plans that are more acceptable to constituents, and therefore more feasible to implement; greater commitment from key clinicians to organizational goals; and a sharper focus on the organization's mission so that goal attainment is more easily obtained and justified to employees and customers.

Stakeholder Claims on the Organization

Organizational performance can be improved (or negatively affected) by governmental legislation, regulation, and the media. For example, pay-for-performance legislation at the federal or state level can reduce the use of certain procedures and their associated problems. One example of this is the Omnibus Budget Reconciliation Act enacted by Congress in 1987, which was, at least in part, responsible for a decline in the use of physical and chemical restraints and rates of urinary incontinence and catheterization. In New York State, the government publishes a consumer's guide to Medicaid managed care in New York City, ranking health plans according to the quality of care provided to children and adults and according to patient satisfaction with access and service. Such guides are also available to the public in magazines, such as *Consumer Reports*, and over the Internet.

Managers may have less control over accountability than they do over control systems, organizational design, professional integration, or organizational adaptation, because they lack influence over external groups that have their own expectations and interests regarding organizational and managerial performance. And health services is particularly challenging for managers because of the difficulties in specifying organizational performance in measurable terms and in isolating the contribution of a delivery system to an improvement in health status for a community or a population. These difficulties make it hard for organizational leadership, internal stakeholders, and external groups to reach agreements as they seek to influence each other's expectations and behavior.

Managers can, however, successfully affect stakeholder expectations. The Mayo Clinic has succeeded in this regard. According to Berry and Bendapudi (2003), Mayo manages a set of visual and experiential clues so that stakeholders recognize that care is organized around patient needs rather than around doctors' schedules or hospital processes. The Mayo workforce is hired because they embrace the organization's values. These values are emphasized through training and reinforced in the workplace.

To encourage collaboration among professionals, physicians at Mayo are paid salaries; sophisticated internal paging, telephone, and videoconferencing are used; and electronic medical records have been implemented. The facilities are designed to relieve stress, offer a place of refuge, create positive distraction, convey caring and respect, symbolize competence, minimize crowding, facilitate way finding, and accommodate families (Berry and Bendapudi 2003).

Managers can ensure that key stakeholders are identified and that their expectations and satisfaction levels are regularly measured. For objectivity in this regard, measurement should usually be done by external organizations explicitly organized for this purpose, such as Consumers Union, which publishes *Consumer Reports* magazine.

References

Berry, L. L., and N. Bendapudi. 2003. "Clueing in Customers." *Harvard Business Review* 81 (2): 100–04.

Institute of Medicine, Committee on Quality. 2001. *Crossing the Quality Chasm: A New Health System for the 21st Century.* Washington, DC: National Academies Press.

Kaplan, R. S., and D. P. Norton. 1996. "Using the Balanced Scorecard as a Strategic Management System." *Harvard Business Review* 74 (1): 75–85.

Pointer, D. D., and J. E. Orlikoff. 2002. *Getting to Great: Principles of Health Care Organization Governance.* San Francisco: Jossey-Bass.

THE READINGS

The required reading for Part VI, Accountability, is "Transparency—'Deal or No Deal?'" by Sandy Lutz. Lutz suggests that "as employers push more cost sharing to workers, hospitals and health systems will have to construct a pricing structure that is meaningful to consumers." Providers will have to "know the market, know what their own prices mean, consider the customer, and reengineer business processes around the patient rather than around the billing side of the business."

Transparency—"Deal or No Deal?"

Sandy Lutz
From *Frontiers of Health Services Management* 23 (3): 13–23, Spring 2007

Summary

In the United States, transparency is becoming an ideal worthy of Mom and apple pie, like quality in healthcare. Physicians, payers, hospitals, business associations, and organizations representing patients have all chimed in expressing support. At the local, state, and national levels a variety of transparency initiatives are under way.

How will transparency affect the healthcare industry? Transparency could profoundly change today's balance of power, for it is about information, and information is power. As employers push more cost sharing to workers, hospitals and health systems will have to construct a pricing structure that is meaningful to consumers.

What are providers to do? To be successful with this new demand, providers should make sure they are making quality information as well as pricing information available to consumers. They will have to know the market, know what their own prices mean, consider the customer, and reengineer business processes around the patient rather than around the billing side of business.

The winds of change are blowing in the health industry with President Bush, payers, employers, and consumer groups clamoring for increased transparency. Transparency could provide a window into quality and pricing information, and that is a scary thought for most providers.

Could transparency commoditize medical services? Will it turn health-care into a version of the game show "Deal or No Deal?" "Here is the price: Deal or no deal?" Well, yes and no.

Transparency is here to stay. Trends often ripple slowly through healthcare—we are still waiting for online adjudication to kick in—so some may be tempted to wait until this one runs its course before jumping on board. Not a good idea. As Victor Hugo, the author of *Les Miserables,* once wrote, "there is nothing more powerful than an idea whose time has come." One may feel "les miserables" about the prospect of pricing transparency, but it is an idea whose time has come. And long after "Deal or No Deal" has left the air, the healthcare industry will be operating in a far more transparent environment.

In fact, the only thing more powerful than an idea whose time has come is an idea force-fed by government. That is where we are with transparency today. The government, from the president on down, is on the transparency band-wagon. On a website devoted to transparency, the U.S. Department of Health and Human Services defines the term through "four interconnected corner-stones," one of which is to "measure and publish prices" (USDHHS 2006).

The United States is not the only place where transparency is seeping into the healthcare lexicon. The issue came up prominently in Pricewater-houseCoopers' global research for *HealthCast 2020: Creating a Sustainable Health System.* More than 80 percent of survey respondents globally identi-fied transparency in quality and pricing as important for a sustainable health system. Respondents included nearly 600 executives from health systems, government agencies, health plans, employers, and pharmaceutical compa-nies in 27 countries (PricewaterhouseCoopers 2005).

In the United States, transparency is becoming an ideal worthy of Mom and apple pie, like quality in healthcare. Who could oppose it? Physicians, pay-ers, hospitals, business associations, and organizations representing patients have all chimed in expressing support. At the local, state, and national levels, a variety of transparency initiatives are under way. Unfortunately, they are not coordinated. This suggests the possibility of multiple proofs of concept, which is a long way from the government's vision of "four interconnected cornerstones." What is more, each group has its own list of imperatives for, and obstacles to, progress on transparency.

This article will examine how transparency will affect the healthcare industry and provide recommendations for providers.

Information Is Power: Transparency Diffuses That Power

Transparency could profoundly affect today's balance of power in the indus-try. Transparency is about information, and information is power. Healthcare is an information business, and power lies with the organizations or individuals who hold the information and control its flow.

While providers often complain about the power wielded by payers, hospitals and physicians really are the undisputed rulers of information, both clinical and financial. Nearly all information starts with them—how care is delivered, how much it costs, and who should get what types of treatment. What is more, providers are the most highly trusted sources of information. Physicians were the most trusted professionals and hospitals were among the most trusted industries in recent polls by Harris Interactive (Harris Interactive 2006; Taylor and Leitman 2006).

The fact is that consumers today scour the Internet for information when they are diagnosed with cancer or diabetes or heart disease. What do they do with all of that information? Typically, they will print it out, take it to their doctor and ask, "Gee, what do you think?" A patient can have a world of online information at his or her fingertips, but it all leads to the same end: What does the most trusted adviser think about it? Close behind physicians in the hierarchy of trust are the nurses and other clinicians who treat patients in hospitals. PricewaterhouseCoopers' *HealthCast 2020* survey (2005) asked which healthcare stakeholder had been the most successful at communicating with consumers in the recent past. The clear answer was nurses.

How does transparency change these relationships and positions of trust? It could change the source and flow of information from providers to payers. Medicare and numerous private insurers are starting to publish prices online. That is a first step to becoming the knowledge broker on pricing information for patients, for employers, and for other providers. Once payers become a trusted source of pricing information, they will not have to take much of a leap to become the trusted source of other health information. Why ask the doctor about whether you need that surgery when the payer has better knowledge of pricing and outcomes? Is the back surgeon really the right person to ask about whether you need back surgery? This shift in trusted source is one possible result.

Many of the numbers presented as medical prices have been generated by providers themselves via charges. While most healthcare insiders acknowledge the worthlessness of charges in today's market, they are still hardwired to the reimbursement system. Many health plans continue to pay hospitals based on a discount off charges for inpatient and outpatient services.

Transparency and Pricing

Charges Are Becoming Surrogate Prices, but the Dollar Sign May Be the Only Thing the Two Have in Common

Charges, costs, prices, and payments: They are similar but different definitions of the expense incurred in providing a medical service and how providers are compensated for that expense.

Prices are what insurers, the government, and individuals must pay for the healthcare services they receive. Costs are the resources required for the health system to provide the healthcare services—what the service costs the hospital. Charges may be the most difficult and controversial concept in the current debate. Charges are a standard healthcare finance measure used for analytical and statistical purposes. Setting charges for medical services is complex and varies by hospital. Hospitals can use a variety of sources to establish a charge rate, including publicly available charge data, competitor pricing, insurance plan fee schedules (reimbursement), and the hospital's own cost information (The Lewin Group 2005). Decades ago, charges were primarily used to set prices; today, charges are essentially meaningless to the patient.

Unlike in other industries, prices have not been part of healthcare. Ever since the third-party payer system was invented in the 1930s to shield patients from catastrophic bills, little attention has been paid to prices. Reimbursement and negotiation more appropriately define financial transactions in the industry. Because negotiations are proprietary, prices generally have not been made public. As the healthcare market moves toward transparency, the industry is trying to construct a pricing structure that may or may not be meaningful to consumers.

The costs, payments, prices, and charges can all be different amounts, yet are all blurred together in the taxonomy of transparency. By nearly everyone's estimation, charges have grown out of line in respect to costs. According to at least one study, the ratio of costs to charges has grown from 1.1 to 2.6 over the past 25 years (Tompkins, Altman, and Eilat 2006). Another recent study found that hospital charges increased annually at an aggregate average rate of 7 percent. The most common reason for increasing hospital charges cited by the hospitals was overall cost inflation (The Lewin Group 2005).

Of these four terms—costs, payments, prices, and charges—the logical hierarchy would be that costs are the lowest amount and charges are the highest. After all, grocers mark up their costs and post the amount that they are charging. To those in the industry this seems logical, but consumers are rightfully confused. Sometimes items and services are priced below cost. All consumers want to know is what they personally are responsible for paying. Accordingly, when a health plan publishes a price for hip replacement surgery, a consumer assumes that is what he or she is going to have to pay.

Employers Are Increasingly Pushing More Cost Sharing onto Workers, Creating More Demand for Pricing

For the past three decades, consumer out of pocket spending for healthcare has been dropping steadily as a share of overall spending. Only about 13 percent of all health spending today is out of pocket (Smith et al. 2006), compared to about a third in the 1970s. For that reason, consumers have largely been shielded from the full magnitude of healthcare cost increases.

No more. All forms of cost sharing are up: copayments, deductibles, and premiums. When employers were asked in a PricewaterhouseCoopers' survey (PricewaterhouseCoopers Health Research Institute 2005) if cost sharing would lower their costs, 15 percent said yes, by a great deal. Another 63 percent said yes, somewhat. Clearly, consumers are bearing a bigger share of healthcare costs than in the recent past.

Consumer-driven health plans are the most flexible benefit design in terms of cost sharing. Workers pay the first thousand dollars or more in health expenses out of a health savings account (HSA), giving them exposure to cost that they may never have seen before. It is an eye-opener for many consumers, who increasingly will ask what they are getting for their money.

Pricing Should Serve a Purpose Beyond Curiosity

A great deal of media interest has surrounded healthcare pricing disclosure, but providers need to focus on what kinds of pricing the market really wants. Ironically, Medicare and other payers are beginning to publish hospital charges and prices while the larger demand is for prices of physician and outpatient services. Most nonelderly consumers will spend money on these charges, either out of pocket or out of their HSAs. Workers in consumer-directed health plans are more likely to scrutinize the bills of physicians and outpatient providers. As Figure VI.2 shows, nearly half of the insurance premium goes to pay for physicians and outpatient services. Only a small amount—18 percent—goes toward inpatient care.

This does not mean the heat is off hospitals. They compete for patients in outpatient services as well. That is why some have focused their pricing strategies around outpatient services.

A hospital's chief customer is not the patient but the physician, who may bear the brunt of pricing inquiries from consumers, particularly those navigating consumer-driven health plans. Answering detailed questions about prices, after all, is not among the things that physicians' offices are equipped to do.

Lack of Demand for Hospital Prices Can Be Deceptive

Some hospital executives are saying that they are not concerned about price-shopping consumers because so little of their revenues come from them. With 90 percent of reimbursement coming directly from the government and private insurers, hospitals may not have time to worry about the small share that is coming from individuals.

The hearts and minds of pricing-shopping consumers already may have moved beyond considering hospitals for certain procedures. Ambulatory surgery centers now outnumber hospitals, a significant shift in the delivery

FIGURE VI.2
Estimated
Breakdown
of Insurance
Premiums,
2005

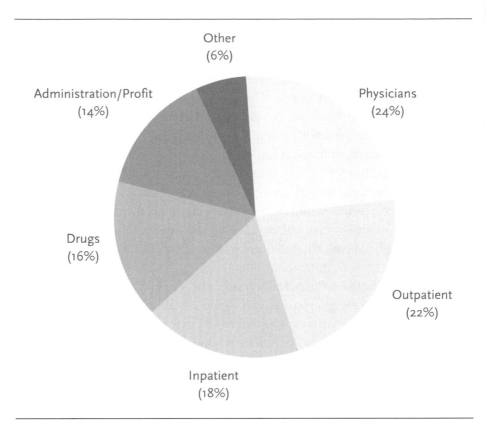

SOURCE: PricewaterhouseCoopers. 2006. "The Factors Fueling Rising Healthcare Costs." Prepared for America's Health Insurance Plans. New York: PricewaterhouseCoopers LLP.

system. Clearly, consumers and physicians are choosing the convenience of ambulatory surgery centers over hospitals. Could consumer readiness be a factor in this shift? Certainly, those who are brought in on a stretcher are not going to ask prices. Those who can walk in on their own may, and they may choose to go somewhere else.

The Way Forward

What can providers do? Operating in a more price-transparent environment requires new thinking and strategy. Here are some recommendations:

Don't Be Left Standing with Only Prices Out There

Prices have little meaning without quality. Price is only one dimension of the value consumers seek through transparency. Once pricing information is available, quality components should be added to offer patients financially quantitative as well as outcome-oriented qualitative perspectives prior to making healthcare choices.

Spectrum Health, one of the first hospitals in the country to voluntarily report clinical outcomes, has implemented both components, but in reverse order. The hospital started with a quality report card on its website and then started publishing prices on 1,000 procedures, mainly outpatient procedures, organized by CPT code. The system includes links to insurance company websites to make it easy for patients to figure out copayments and deductibles (PricewaterhouseCoopers Health Research Institute 2006).

Public access and scrutiny of this information is likely to improve the overall quality in the healthcare marketplace while keeping prices consistent, unlike the current climate in which drastic variations of price can be found for the exact same procedure.

Scan the Market

Work with the state hospital associations, physicians, and insurance companies to implement pricing transparency. Some states, such as California, Wisconsin, and, soon, Minnesota, require that providers release pricing information for many of the most common medical procedures. In Wisconsin, the WHA Information Center, a subsidiary of the Wisconsin Hospital Association, posts charges for approximately 60 types of inpatient procedures on its website (www.whainfocenter.com). New Hampshire has a similar website (www. nhpricepoint.org).

When communicating this issue, it will sound better if providers, payers, and regulators work together. By creating an environment that fosters relationships between the payers, the government can assist in this team approach toward price transparency.

Healthcare executives often argue that current hospital pricing is generally neither understandable nor relevant to most consumers, nor is it understood even by many industry professionals. What is paramount to consumers today is predictability and reasonableness of their actual out-of-pocket costs—without or after insurance payments.

Healthcare is not the only industry in which pricing does not correlate directly to costs. Some products are loss leaders. Junk mail subsidizes first-class mail, business travelers subsidize leisure travelers, and, in healthcare, insured patients subsidize those in government programs and the uninsured.

Private-pay patients pay as much as one-third more than Medicare and Medicaid patients for the same service. Because Medicare and Medicaid are government programs, they set payment and hospitals take it. Private patients must pay more, as shown in Table VI.1.

Private health insurance often provides a cross-subsidy for patients with no insurance or ability to pay and patients with government-sponsored insurance that may not cover the full cost of care for beneficiaries.

TABLE VI.1
Cost-Payment
Percentages

	1997	1998	1999	2000	2001	2002	2003	2004
Medicare	103.7%	101.9%	100.0%	99.1%	98.4%	97.9%	95.3%	91.9%
Medicaid	96.0%	96.6%	95.7%	94.5%	95.8%	96.1%	92.3%	89.9%
Private Payer	117.5%	115.8%	115.1%	115.7%	116.5%	119.0%	122.3%	128.9%

SOURCE: The Lewin Group. 2006. *AHA Chartbook*, Analysis of American Hospital Association Annual Survey data (Includes Medicaid Disproportionate Share Payments). Falls Church, VA: The Lewin Group.

In the auto insurance industry, the cost of the uninsured is transparent; it is called "uninsured motorist coverage." In the healthcare industry, that cost is less transparent but is a real cost nonetheless and one that providers are obliged to communicate.

Know What Your Prices Mean

Analyze current charge structure and integrate market-driven cost pricing. Analysis of the current charge methodology is a viable corrective response to charges that have grown out of line. However, a complete overhaul of a hospital's charge description master (CDM) is difficult. Not surprisingly, such an overhaul is also rare, according to a Lewin Study that found that the most common reason hospitals increased their charges was to account for inflation (The Lewin Group 2005).

Hospital systems today are challenging historical CDM rate-setting strategies, moving from rate optimization to more defensible cost-based pricing and stringent market rate comparisons. Other progressive institutions are working with payers to ensure a defensible pricing strategy. For example, one solution is to realign payer reimbursement for inpatient services to cover costs while providing concessions on more profitable and competitive outpatient services. Another solution is to work with payers to reduce charges in exchange for a payer realigning discounts off those charges to arrive at some level of payment neutrality. Finally, some providers are looking at fixed-rate reimbursement on all services, virtually eliminating the dependence on CDM based pricing.

Some hospitals have continued to use charges for self-payers, which has raised the hackles of patient advocacy groups. That strategy is quickly transitioning out as health systems move to more market-driven pricing for the uninsured. Often, this pricing is comparable to the discounts offered managed-care payers.

Prices charged to the uninsured also should be evaluated in light of recent state legislation. In Minnesota, prices for the uninsured must be equal to the rate paid by the commercial insurer that generated the most revenue in the prior year. In other jurisdictions, hospitals are charging uninsured patients the average price negotiated by the three largest managed-care plans. Rates offered to the uninsured should be adjusted based on a formula that incorporates managed care or Medicare rates, and should be applicable to all uninsured patients who do not qualify for charity care. For example, North Mississippi Medical Center saw that its discounts for managed care were in the 10 percent to 30 percent range. Therefore, it structured the discount for the uninsured at about 20 percent, with an additional discount for those paying in cash (The Lewin Group 2005).

Consider the Customer

Be ready for patients asking about their financial obligation. Hospitals need to think about how patients are receiving pricing information when they inquire. When "mystery shoppers" for the California HealthCare Foundation called about pricing information in 2005, they were sent to admitting departments, financial counselors, billing offices, and cashier's offices. The foundation found that pricing information was given inconsistently, which creates doubts about how reliable it was (PricewaterhouseCoopers Health Research Institute 2006). This underscores other research by PricewaterhouseCoopers' Health Research Institute around the readiness of hospitals for empowered consumers. When asked whether hospitals were ready for empowered consumers, 25 percent of healthcare leaders in 2005 said they agreed or strongly agreed, down from 38 percent in 1999 (DelPo 2005).

Hospitals that are experiencing a noticeable increase in patient requests for pricing information should begin to document those requests. By tracking the number and types of requests, hospitals can direct resources to improve the process and prepare to meet the demand generated by the vast new offerings of consumer-driven or high-deductible health plans. One hospital chief financial officer noted: "We participated in a study with the American Hospital Association and did not warn our employees, where 'patients' would call in with questions about pricing and charity care. We did a good job in responding, but out of this we are now trying to come up with a standard response. We now have a sheet that explains our pricing and that the amount is only an estimate based upon prior patient experience. In addition, we share our charity care and discount policy" (PricewaterhouseCoopers 2005).

When quoting the price range, providers should clearly define the service, assess personal patient data, apply insurance coverage, and document the quote. In addition, the business office should also maintain statistics on patient requests, so hospitals can gather useful information about market needs and continually improve their processes for responding.

Reengineer Billing to Focus on Front End Rather than Back End

The Healthcare Financial Management Association's Patient Friendly Billing effort (www.patientfriendlybilling.org) has focused on how to reengineer business processes around the patient. As depicted in Figure VI.3, this means turning the billing process on its head. By focusing more on the front end rather than the back end, hospitals can be better prepared for pricing transparency.

One solution is to establish a central pricing office to provide timely verbal quotes for care based on insurance coverage and the charity care policy. A central pricing office can act as a communications conduit between physicians, payers, the hospital, and patients as it relates to insured and uninsured pricing. As was so aptly illustrated in the California HealthCare Foundation's "mystery shopper" study (DelPo 2005), most hospitals do not have a good process in place to communicate prices to patients who call.

Prior to service, financial counselors can build an estimated out-of-pocket price range based on physician directives to accurately identify the procedure, provide personalized patient information to anticipate risks and assess proper time allowance, and explain the applicability of actual insurance coverage. This process can also enhance charity care identification and shorten the revenue cycle by informing patients about their financial responsibility up front rather than after services are delivered. Access to useful data for the insured and uninsured prior to choosing healthcare services empowers the patients and improves the prospect of collection by the hospital.

FIGURE VI.3
Focus Business Processes Around Patients

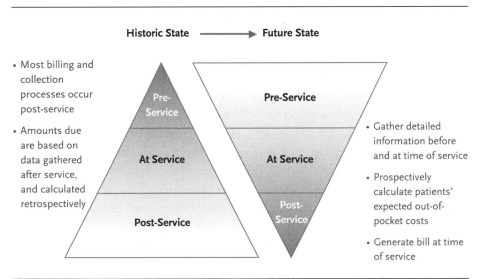

Reprinted by permission of Patient Friendly Billing® Project of the Healthcare Financial Management Association.

Expect the Unexpected

The law of unintended consequences is strong in healthcare, so it would be wise to think about how the journey to transparency could take some unintended turns. Some scenarios:

- As price and quality information expands, consumers may migrate toward the highest-quality providers and health plans. In a market-driven economy, high-quality products in demand often raise their prices. However, a patient looking for the best cardiac surgeon or the best orthopedic implant likely may be paying only a portion of the overall cost. This runs counter to the theory behind price elasticity. As the price of a luxury car climbs, fewer drivers can afford it. As the price of an elite surgeon or implant climbs, the patient is likely paying the same deductible or copayment. The excess cost would be borne by the health plan or employer. Such a scenario could increase overall health spending.
- In many industries, pricing is tied to demand. Airline seats are cheaper on routes with fewer passengers. Movie theaters charge less during the day. Providers and health plans may soon begin experimenting with pricing along time dimensions, which adds another layer of complexity for providers.
- Widespread knowledge of pricing could lead to a trend in retailing known as "death in the middle" (Reibstein 2006). Consumers seeking high-end or low-cost goods squeeze retailers in the middle. In the same way, price-hunting consumers may seek care in inexpensive retail clinics, which they pay out of pocket, and high-end luxury hospitals, where costs are largely paid after the deductible is satisfied. Such a consumer-directed trend could squeeze community hospitals, which would be left with the bread-and-butter business of medicine.

References

DelPo, A. (ed.). 2005. "Price Check: The Mystery of Hospital Pricing." White Paper by the California HealthCare Foundation. [Online article; created 12/05.] http://www.allhealth.org/briefingmaterials/PriceCheckMysteryHospital-Pricing-12.pdf.

Harris Interactive. 2006. "Doctors and Teachers Most Trusted Among 22 Occupations and Professions." [Press release; created 8/8/06.] Rochester, NY: Harris Interactive.

The Lewin Group. 2006. "Analysis of American Hospital Association Annual Survey Data (Includes Medicaid Disproportionate Share Payments)." *AHA Chartbook*. Falls Church, VA: The Lewin Group.

———. 2005."A Study of Hospital Charge Practices and Their Relationship to Hospital Costs, Prepared for TheMedicare Payment Advisory Commission." [Presented at the Healthcare Financial Management Association's 2006 Spring Summit.] Falls Church, VA: The Lewin Group.

PricewaterhouseCoopers. 2005. *HealthCast 2020: Creating a Sustainable Health System.* New York: PricewaterhouseCoopers LLP.

PricewaterhouseCoopers' Health Research Institute. 2005. "Take Care of Yourself: Employers Embrace Consumerism to Control Healthcare Costs." New York: PricewaterhouseCoopers LLP.

———. 2006. "My Brother's Keeper: Growing Expectations Confront Hospitals on Community Benefits and Charity Care." New York: PricewaterhouseCoopers LLP.

Reibstein, D. 2006. "Death in the Middle: Why Consumers Seek Value at the Top and Bottom of Markets." Knowledge@Wharton. [Online article; created 5/10/06.] http://knowledge.wharton.upenn.edu/article.cfm?articleid=1477.

Smith, C., C. Cowan, S. Heffler, and A. Catlin. 2006. "National Health Spending in 2004: Recent Slowdown Led by Prescription Drug Spending." *Health Affairs* 25 (1): 186–96.

Taylor, H., and R. Leitman. 2006. "Survey on Trust in Different Industries Finds Reasonably High Trust in Pharmaceuticals, Less Trust in Biotech and High Distrust of Health Insurance and Managed Care." *Health Care News.* Rochester, NY: Harris Interactive, Sept. 18.

Tompkins, C. P., S. H. Altman, and E. Eilat 2006. "The Precarious Pricing System for Hospital Services." *Health Affairs* 25 (1): 45–56.

U.S. Department of Health and Human Services. 2006. [Online article; retrieved 11/6/06.] www.hhs.gov/transparency.

Discussion Questions

1. How serious and extensive are the transparency problems Lutz refers to in the American healthcare system?
2. If they are serious and extensive, why hasn't more been done by healthcare organizations to satisfactorily meet consumer and patient expectations for transparency?
3. What are the opportunities and constraints facing managers seeking to improve transparency in healthcare organizations?
4. How should patients and consumers and their advocates be involved in improving the transparency of healthcare organizations?
5. How do incentives under which healthcare organizations operate impact transparency?

Required Supplementary Readings

Batalden, P., J. J. Mohr, E. C. Nelson, S. K. Plume, G. R. Baker, J. W. Wasson, P. K. Stolz, M. E. Splaine, and J. J. Wisniewski. 1997. "Continually

Improving the Health and Value of Health Care for a Population of Patients: The Panel Management Process." *Quality Management in Health Care* 5 (3): 41–51.

Herzlinger, R. E. 2002. "Let's Put Consumers in Charge of Health Care." *Harvard Business Review* 80 (7): 44–55.

Weil, P., and R. Harmata. 2002. "Rekindling the Flame: Routine Practices that Promote Hospital Community Leadership." *Journal of Healthcare Management* 47 (2): 98–110.

Young, D., D. Barrett, J. W. Kenagy, D. C. Pinakiewicz, and S. M. McCarthy. 2001. "Value-Based Partnering in Health Care: A Framework for Analysis." *Journal of Healthcare Management* 6 (2): 112–33.

Discussion Questions on the Required Supplementary Readings

1. How realistic is population-based health to the management of primary care practice?
2. What are the pros and cons of Herzlinger's approach to consumer sovereignty in healthcare?
3. What strategies should hospitals consider in managing relationships with other community organizations?
4. How should non-profit boards and CEOs be accountable to the communities their healthcare organizations serve?

Recommended Supplementary Readings

Anderson, G., and J. R. Knickman. 2001. "Changing the Chronic Care System to Meet People's Needs." *Health Affairs* 20 (6): 146–60.

Berry, L. L., and N. Bendapundi. 2003. "Clueing in Customers." *Harvard Business Review* (February): 100–106.

Berry, L. L., and K. D. Seltman. 2008. *Management Lessons from Mayo Clinic.* New York: McGraw-Hill.

Evans, R. G. 1995. "Healthy Populations or Healthy Institutions: The Dilemma of Health Care Management." *Journal of Health Administration Education* 13 (3): 453–72.

Institute of Medicine. 2001. *Crossing the Quality Chasm.* Washington, DC: National Academies Press.

McAlearney, A. S. 2003. *Population Health Management: Strategies to Improve Outcomes.* Chicago: Health Administration Press.

Neuhauser, D. 2003. "The Coming Third Health Care Revolution: Personal Empowerment." *Quality Management in Health Care* 12 (3): 171–84.

Leape, L. L., and D. M. Berwick. 2005. "Five Years After To Err Is Human: What Have We Learned?" *Journal of the American Medical Association* 293 (19): 2384–90.

Lindenauer, P. K., D. Remus, S. Roman, M. B. Rotherberg, E. M. Benjamin, A. Ma, and D. W. Brazler. 2007. "Public Reporting and Pay for Performance in Hospital Quality Improvement." *New England Journal of Medicine* 356 (5): 486–96.

Nolan, T., and D. M. Berwick. 2006. "All-or-None Measurement Raises the Bar on Performance." *Journal of the American Medical Association* 295 (10): 1168–70.

Porter, M. E., and E. O. Teisberg. 2004. "Redefining Competition in Health Care." *Harvard Business Review* (June): 65–76.

Schroeder, S. A. 2005. "What to Do with a Patient Who Smokes." *Journal of the American Medical Association* 294 (4): 482–87.

Studer, Q. 2003. *Hardwiring Excellence.* Gulf Breeze, FL: Fire Starter Publishing.

Walshe, K. 2001. "Nursing Home Regulation: Lessons Learned for Reform." *Health Affairs* 20 (6): 128–44.

Weiner, B. J., J. A. Alexander, and H. S. Zuckerman. 2000. "Strategies for Effective Management Participation in Community Health Partnerships." *Health Care Management Review* 25 (3): 48–66.

THE CASES

Accumulating evidence suggests that a significant amount of medical care resources are misallocated relative to the general health needs of Americans. At a time when nutrition, health education, and even literacy among low-income groups is relatively neglected, there are too many hospital beds, too much surgery, and too few medical specialists available to low-income patients. Who is accountable? What are the consequences to the manager of pursuing organizational accountability?

When a patient reports his experience, such as in "Letter to the CEO" below, how is the manager to know whether the patient's complaints are justified? When the manager knows complaints *are* justified, what can she do to resolve them satisfactorily? It takes time to complain, and patient expectations regarding remediation may be low. To what extent should the manager make it easier for patients to voice their responses to care, or help develop and share organizational goals that will limit and focus patient and consumer expectations?

Obviously, if services are being provided satisfactorily, management need not get involved. This is seldom the case, however, because of scarce resources and high patient expectations. Quality and service will not usually improve significantly unless leadership gets involved in the process. Management should have responsibilities for improving quality and service, and physicians and nurses should be accountable to top management for performance.

Of course, in some organizations, physicians and nurses are formally accountable for patient care only to their peers and to patients. Often, however, the manager notices something wrong or patients complain to her. The manager can respond directly to certain problems, such as uncleanliness, lack of information systems, or lack of interpreters. Other problems, such as physician or nurse rudeness, malpractice, and lack of physician visits to patients, can be referred to departmental chiefs or nursing management. The manager can communicate with patients by survey or interview to find out how they perceive services and how services can be improved.

As a rule, patients do not wish to get involved with organizational functioning. They want things to run smoothly. Patients expect to be treated equitably compared to other patients. They expect not to be harmed by physicians, nurses, and others. For many patients, time is valuable, and they expect it to not be wasted. Patients want to be relieved of pain. They expect appropriate access to care, and some want explanations of their problems and the treatment options open to them with probable related costs and benefits. Patients wish to be treated with dignity and with respect for their privacy. They wish to pay a fair price. How patients feel about the care they receive varies by factors such as demographic and provider characteristics, patient condition, and services offered.

Managers expect patients to return to the facility for services, to complain if they feel they are not properly treated, to make decisions about their own healthcare, to expect only the possible from providers (e.g., certain illnesses are not curable, sufficient staff are not always available), to respect the rights of other patients and providers, and to respect the facility's equipment and supplies.

These expectations seem reasonable. Why then don't those who work in healthcare organizations behave as patients expect, and vice versa? First, there is the lack of formal accountability of physicians, notably when they are not employees of the organization. Or hospital trustees may only pay lip service to improving quality, rather than backing management initiatives that are resisted by physicians. Consumers may lack price or consumer information to make informed choices, or insurance plans may limit their choice of providers. When providers are paid primarily based on their costs, they may lack an incentive to be efficient. When physicians are paid fees for service, there may be an incentive to provide extra services rather than spend extra time with patients. When physicians are paid on salary or by capitation, they may have a tendency to see fewer patients in the office. Physicians and patients are human beings, as are managers, and all have their own failings and strengths.

When service breaks down, what options are open to patients and consumers? Patients may take or threaten to take their business elsewhere. They may complain to the departmental chief, a manager, or a member of the board of trustees. Letters, such as the "Letter to the CEO" in Case Study O, are few and far between, especially in that detail. Patients may form organizations (as in chronic care facilities) to advocate for their rights. Patients can sue to recover costs from a provider's malpractice insurer. Patients can lead healthier lives, so they are less dependent on the healthcare system, or they can raise their threshold tolerance for pain and discomfort. Consumers can control organizational performance by obtaining positions on governing boards and reporting to their constituencies. Government regulatory agencies, national accrediting agencies, and large purchasers can represent consumers and patients in holding providers accountable for meeting minimally adequate standards of care.

Managers are paid to help the organization attain goals and to obtain a level of resources and productivity necessary for system maintenance (which is what Don Wherry, CEO of Brendan Hospital, is attempting to do in the case study "Whose Hospital?"). But there are many stakeholders in healthcare organizations, including trustees, managers, physicians, other health professionals, non-professionals, patients, other payers, accreditors, and regulators. Vendors and volunteers also have a stake in organizational performance.

We believe accountability is blurred unless some mutual agreement is specified among stakeholders on mission, goals, satisfactory ways of measuring goal attainment, and ways to change organizational goals. Some of the consequences when such specification does not occur are shown in "Whose Hospital?"

An alternative to formal accountability is mutual adjustment. Rather than establishing goals, interest groups confront each decision on its merits and its effects upon them. Should a hospital purchase or lease a CT scanner, provide services to the chronically ill, or purchase several physician practices? If a significant minority of the ruling coalition objects to a new policy direction, the new direction may be stymied until consensus can be achieved.

To whom is the healthcare organization accountable? How is it accountable? How can its level of performance be ascertained by those who wish to hold it accountable, or by those who are concerned with demonstrating that it *is* accountable? Lutz's article describes the increasing importance of transparency in healthcare and its impact on the availability of information and the power derived from that information.

The cases in Part VI deal with the concept of accountability from different perspectives. First, the long case, "Letter to the CEO," is written from a patient's point of view (but can be considered as well from the perspective of prospective patients and taxpayers). "Whose Hospital?" is written from the manager's point of view, and involves trustee and physician stakeholders. The third long case, "What Happens when Patients Cannot Pay?" raises the issues of access, reimbursement, and the hospital's obligation to provide services to the uninsured. The six short cases continue to consider different perspectives about accountability and management. Short case 26, "The Conflicted HMO Manager," describes the conflicts of interest between the manager and the organization, while "The Great Mosaic" raises the issue of the management of diversity in a nursing home. The short case "No Parity in Behavioral Health Coverage" presents the issue of differential coverage from the perspective of a physician. The short case "Ergonomics in Practice" considers the needs of employees in a healthcare setting. The short case "What's in a Name?" raises the consumer perspective about hospital donations. Finally, the short case "Patient Satisfaction in an Inner-City Hospital" describes issues associated with patient satisfaction from the perspective of both physicians and administrators.

Case O
Letter to the CEO

Anonymous
From *Quality Management in Health Care* 14 (4): 219–33, 2005
Copyright Lippincott Williams & Wilkins, Inc. Used with permission.

Dear Chief Executive Officer:
The Perceptions of a Recently Discharged Patient

Editor's Note The following material represents a report based on the actual hospital experience of a health professional and his wife, who also is a health professional. They are well qualified to make the assessments set forth in this report. Quality Management in Health Care *is treating this as a quality management case study, and, to preserve the authors' confidentiality, is omitting their names and that of the hospital.*

Foreword

Dear CEO,

Attached is a description of my recent experience at your hospital. I and my wife share this with you because we are committed to improving the delivery of health care services in hospitals. We believe that our perceptions reflect problems in the system of care and are in no way meant to reflect upon individuals.

We hope you will find the perceptions useful.

We have many professional colleagues and many friends who work at your hospital. We plan to continue to get our health care there. In fact, I expect to have another operation there 3 months from now.

We shall be happy to discuss any aspect of care with you or your staff, and do whatever we can to improve care. We plan to share this document with my physicians and with your Director of Nursing.

Sincerely,
Patient and Spouse

Perceptions of a Hospital Experience

Operation: Cardiac Arterial Bypass Graft (CABG) October 2004
Operative Report:

I. Semi-urgent coronary bypass grafting employing aortosaphenous bypass grafts to the first and second circumflex marginal coronary artery.

II. Anastomosis of the right internal mammary artery (skeletonized) to the right coronary artery.

III. Anastomosis of the left internal mammary artery (as a pedicule) to the left anterior descending coronary artery (2 venous and 2 arterial grafts)

The heart was returned to the pericardial cavity.

The heart spontaneously defibrillated in a few minutes.

The procedure was tolerated well and the patient was discharged from the operating room in good general condition.

This is our story of a common surgical procedure that saves lives every day, but is painful and stressful for patients and their families. The heart has spiritual meaning—our "heartfelt" thanks; "I love you with all my heart." We also know that we cannot live without our hearts. Knowing that my heart would stop beating for a large part of the surgery brought with it the special fear of truly being on the brink of death or of coming back (or not coming back from the dead). My wife and I were both terrified.

I underwent cardiac catheterization at an urban medical center in the Fall. The surgical plan at that time included insertion of a stent. However, the physician found a 70% blockage of the main anterior artery and similar damage to the posterior vessel. He said, "In 2004, in this city, a stent is not an option." The bypass graft had to wait until Plavix, the drug I took in anticipation of the stent, had passed out of my system. This circumstance was similar to that experienced by former President Clinton earlier in the year. The cardiologist required that I be given heparin, and kept under continuous hospital monitoring until a quadruple bypass could be performed 6 days later.

The quadruple bypass graft was performed by an outstanding surgeon, who typically performs more than 300 each year. Four days later I was sent home with plans for rehabilitation therapy to begin in 3 weeks. As I write this account 5 weeks after surgery, I am up and about and feeling much healthier, with more energy than before the surgery. So we could conclude that nothing went wrong. But, can we be so sure? True enough, the attending physicians provided excellent technical care and were also admirably comforting. The nurses were extremely pleasant and, for the most part, efficient. Nevertheless, we observed numerous errors or potential errors (near misses) in the way that ancillary staff, nurses, and even some physicians failed in or neglected their responsibilities, both medical and humane. There were system failures, largely in the provision of nonclinical, so-called hotel services. Opportunities were lost for staff to teach and provide emotional support, and that seriously marred the entire hospital experience. We have organized this narrative on the following themes.

Errors and potential errors

1. *Potential infections:* I never observed any physician, nurse, or staff member wash hands before approaching us, nor were we told that they had washed elsewhere.

2. *Fire hazards:* At least 8 gurneys, in addition to wheelchairs and linen carts, clogged the hallway outside my room, in violation of state regulations and JCAHO standards.

3. *Medication error:* Late one afternoon, a physician prescribed Cipro to be administered twice daily. A nurse gave me the first dose that evening. The next day she brought only 1 dose.

   Only on the third day she did follow orders and deliver morning and evening doses.

4. *Potential medication error:* The evening nurse came to say goodnight on one of the presurgery nights because she said she had nothing else to do for me. Only after my spouse asked about prescribed bedtime medications did the nurse leave to check, and returned to say, "Oh, I see he does have medications and I didn't see that in the computer." My spouse asked why these medications were not found in the computer.

   The nurse replied, "Oh, I guess they *are* listed for 10:00 PM. I'll get them for you." That same night, Proscar, one of my drugs, was missing from the medication drawer. The same nurse finally had to get Proscar from the pharmacy and brought it to me at 11:30 PM.

5. *Potential unnoticed cardiac event:* Another nurse left my heart monitor disconnected for 40 minutes prior to my transfer to another unit, explaining that he needed to have me ready for the transport crew. (Disconnecting a monitor takes about 3 seconds.)

6. *Potential blood clot:* At one point, the registered nurse failed to notice that the heparin intravenous bag was empty. My wife had to call him, and it took him more than 15 minutes to replace the fluid.

7. *Allergic reaction to tape:* I broke out in a skin rash from tape used during the cardiac catheterization. My wife told a physician resident, who ordered silver nitrate. On the evening before surgery, my wife told the surgical resident about the tape allergy, recommending that he not use the same tape during surgery. The resident said that the allergy was not recorded in the chart and asked us to find out from the catheterization laboratory what kind of tape they had used.

   But that was an impossible assignment for a patient or spouse. My wife asked that at least a yellow self-stick be put on the chart to note the tape problem. The resident told us to remember to tell the surgeons about it in the morning.

   As our anxiety about the surgery mounted, my wife called a nurse acquaintance on the hospital staff. She finally was able to learn the name of the offending tape (Dermaclear) and placed a large warning on the chart.

8. *Informed consent:* The same surgical resident asked me to sign a consent form that did not specify any surgical procedure. He said that he would fill it in afterwards.

9. *Potential delayed recovery.* Three days after surgery, I was too tired to speak to the physical therapist (PT) who visited with instructions. The PT called my wife at home and asked her to be available the next day to help persuade me to participate in therapy. They set a time for the meeting; my wife arrived on time, but the PT failed to appear at all that day.

10. *Potential dental problems:* I occupied 2 private rooms in sequence during my stay. Neither had a toothbrush, floss, or toothpaste. There was a mouthwash of some sort—but not the kind that studies have shown works as well as dental floss in preventing gum problems.

System failures

Absence of follow-up

1. A cardiology fellow, who worked me up in preadmission testing, promised to attend the cardiac catheterization but never showed up.

2. The evening before surgery, the anesthesia resident was unable to confirm that the attending anesthesiologist would be present throughout the cardiac surgery and would be handling only 1 patient. The resident's reaction to my inquiries suggested that she considered them bizarre. She said she would find out, but never returned with an answer. Once again, my wife called someone she knew, who verified that the anesthesiologist would be handling only my case.

Poor communication

1. Immediately after the catheterization and prior to surgery, the cardiologist called my wife to report that I would have to be monitored and remain in the hospital until surgery. He had already told me the same thing. But when I arrived in the postcatheterization unit, a nurse congratulated me on going home that day. Similarly, a patient facilitator for the catheterization service left a message for my wife that she could take me home in a few hours.

2. I and the entire unit had no phone service for several hours one day. On another day, my extension number, untypically, did not match the room number. So my callers ended up disturbing another patient.

3. No one explained how to get a newspaper. My wife or a physician friend brought one each morning by 8:00 AM. Only days later did we learn that a newspaper deliverer came to the floor each morning.

4. We could not get TV service for several hours in one of the rooms. The TV service's phone was continually busy.

5. No one told us what personal clothing and supplies to bring to the hospital either for the catheterization or for the surgery.

6. No one informed us how we could make use of helpful volunteers, social services, or pastoral counseling. We never saw a nutritionist, who could have explained the presurgery diet, which seemed low on salt, or the desirable posthospital diet.

7. No one explained how to work the electric bed. It may surprise readers, but my wife, a nurse, did not know either (but being a public health nurse she soon figured it out).

8. When my wife was asked to leave the recovery room following her brief visit with me, the nurse offered a phone number for checking on my condition during the night. Confident that she had a contact with a registered nurse (RN), my wife left the hospital. But when she called the number a few hours later she got the main switchboard operator who reported on my condition, secondhand.

Insensitivity to patients

1. At 10:30 PM, the night before the surgery, several nurses were laughing and talking outside of my room for one half hour, until I requested quiet.

2. On at least 2 occasions, nurses spoke loudly over the speaker in my room, in search of a nurse who was not there.

3. The waiting area of the cardiac catheterization laboratory was in the corner of a crowded, cold hallway, with only 1 chair for me. My wife had to stand. There was no privacy for me in a patient gown. Hospital staff passed regularly through this hallway, threading between us and the laboratory equipment that cluttered the hall.

Environment and housekeeping

1. My private room featured a broken chair, dirty windows, and inadequate light for reading. The nurse sent for a reading lamp, which arrived the next day, broken. The lamp was never fixed or replaced. On several occasions, full waste baskets were not emptied. The bathroom towels were thin and worn.

2. Environment: The room temperature in one of my rooms was consistently either too hot or too cold.

3. Unnecessary moves: The postangiogram unit was closed from Saturday noon to Monday morning, forcing my transfer to another floor—up one crowded elevator, down another.

4. When I arrived in the new unit, there was no holder for my cardiac monitor, and I had to carry it in my hand for several hours.

5. Missing belongings: When transferred from one unit to another, my belongings were not transferred with me. It took several requests and phone calls to retrieve them.

Food service

The food was consistently tasteless, sometimes delivered late (after 10:00 AM one morning) and, one evening, to the wrong room. We were never told that we could bring in take-out food (at least prior to surgery, we did anyway). On one occasion, my wife saw a dietary manager in the visitor cafeteria and told him that my food had been found in another unit and that it was cold. He advised her to call the dietary department and ask the nutritionist to provide a new meal. When my wife called, the woman who answered the phone said rudely, "We don't have a nutritionist here. He should never have told you that." She finally agreed to send up a new meal.

Lost opportunities (to provide comfort, improve health, and/or improve safety)

1. No one gave us information or any educational materials about cardiac disease, risks affecting the course of disease after discharge, or behavior that might keep me healthy. By flipping the TV channels, we saw that the hospital has some educational videos on various topics, including meditation.
2. The cardiac surgery house staff (which sometimes included a nurse practitioner) usually visited in groups of 5 or more, but never introduced themselves by name or professional title. They spoke in murmurs, mainly to each other. They actually stood away from me, as if I had a communicable disease. They never provided emotional support or taught us anything about my illness or approaches to preventing future cardiac problems.
3. Only nurse friends, who visited me, offered emotional support or asked about our feelings and fears. Only 1 hospital aide offered hope, a hug, and kind words before surgery. My wife asked for a visiting nurse following discharge. The hospital nurse declined. She then asked for physical therapy at home and one of the nurses said that a PT would be arranged, but it never was.

Discussion

According to a physician friend, I am incredibly lucky that I was diagnosed and treated as quickly as I was. Another physician told us "of people with my problem 10% die each year." For probably saving my life we are grateful to talented and caring physicians and nurses. Our internist is the real hero for following up on my vague and not very serious symptoms. We are grateful that we have adequate insurance and live in the United States, where I had to wait only 1 week to get the echocardiogram that began my course of care. We were fully paid by our employer during my recovery and my wife's care for me in the hospital.

Fortunately for us, we had the financial resources to go back and forth to the hospital, fly in our children, and buy whatever I wanted, from take-out food to TV and phone. We worry about people who do not have our resources, notably health insurance, or who do not speak English, have no primary care physicians who care about them, and whose spouses cannot manage to arrange good patient care.

There were many wonderful RNs and aides who cared for me. One of the RNs got me up to the chair, got me to use the nebulizer, and arranged for me to have a bed bath. That is ordinary nursing care in some hospitals, but we saw it as especially kind.

Nothing we encountered resulted in poor outcomes, but there were too many near misses, and we suspect similar mishaps occur at almost all hospitals.

The near misses usually are not reported and therefore do not inspire changes in hospital routines. Hospital managers and others can claim that our negative experiences were minor (some would say petty—like the non-functioning TV) and blame a lack of adequate funding. The managers might make a similar claim about the "lost" opportunities we noted, saying "There is a nursing shortage." This is not the place to discuss revenues and expenses, except to note that the hospital charged more than $68,000 for this 11-day stay, not including physician fees.

We believe that many of the problems we have identified result not from inadequate resources, but rather from insufficient focus on patients and a lack of accountability for performance at the patient level of care. If our experience is typical, it has important implications for hospital administrators and for the training of patient care managers.

Case Questions

1. How do you feel about the level of patient care given in this medical center? How do you think other patients feel? The doctors? The managers?
2. What are some of the problems with patient care in this hospital? What are the most important problems that the manager can do something about?

3. What are the causes of these problems?
4. As the hospital CEO, what would you do, if you had received this memorandum?
5. How would you have solved the problems to which the memorandum refers?
6. What organizational factors would constrain implementation of your recommended solutions?
7. How would you, as the CEO, overcome these constraints?

Case P
Whose Hospital?

Anthony R. Kovner

Tony DeFalco, a 42-year-old electrical engineer, and president of the board of trustees of Brendan Hospital in Lockhart, East State, wondered what he had done wrong. Why had this happened to him again? What should he do now? The trustees had voted, at first 10 to 6 and then unanimously, to fire Don Wherry, the new chief executive officer. Brendan Hospital had hired Wherry, who had been DeFalco's personal choice from more than 200 candidates, just 18 months before. DeFalco had told the trustees that he shared the burdens of managing Brendan Hospital with Wherry, that there was no way of dissociating Wherry's decisions from his own decisions. So in a way, DeFalco pondered, the board should have fired him, too.

Tony DeFalco had lived in Lockhart all his life, and he loved the town, commuting one-and-a-half hours each day to his office at National Electric. Lockhart was one of the poorest towns in the poorest county in central East State, with a population of about 50,000, of which 30 percent were Italian, 25 percent Puerto Rican, and 10 percent Jewish. The leading industries in town were lumber, auto parts manufacturing, and agriculture.

On June 7, 1979, Joe Black, president of the Brendan Hospital medical staff, had called Tony DeFalco, telling him that some doctors and nurses had met over the weekend and that they were going to hold a mass meeting at the hospital to discuss charges against CEO Wherry. DeFalco had called Wherry immediately in Montreal, Canada, where Wherry was giving a lecture to healthcare administration faculty about the relationship between the chief executive officer and the board of trustees. Wherry was as shocked as DeFalco had been and returned immediately to Lockhart. That night DeFalco and Wherry went to a hospital foundation meeting near where the mass meeting was being held in the hospital cafeteria.

DeFalco and Wherry had been planning the foundation meeting for several months. It had been scheduled and rescheduled so that all eight of the prominent townspeople could attend. The key reasons behind forming the foundation were to enlist the energies of community leaders in hospital fundraising, thereby freeing the hospital board for more effective policymaking, and to shield hospital donations from the state rate-setting authority. Brendan Hospital had held a successful first annual horse show the previous fall, netting $10,000 and creating goodwill for the hospital, largely through the efforts of DeFalco and two dedicated physicians who owned the stable and dedicated the show and all proceeds to the hospital. Because this was an important meeting, and because they had not been invited to attend the mass meeting, DeFalco and Wherry decided to attend the foundation meeting. There, they elicited a great deal of verbal support for the foundation, and for DeFalco's leadership. The community leaders were familiar with the problems of employee discontent in their own businesses and with the political maneuverings of former Brendan medical staffs. It would all calm down, no doubt. The wife of the town's leading industrialist said she appreciated DeFalco's frankness in sharing the hospital's problems with them.

But, of course, everything was not yet calm. The mass meeting was held and a petition signed to get rid of Wherry. The petition was signed by half the medical staff and by half the employees as well. A leadership committee of four doctors and nurses demanded Wherry's immediate resignation, and it was rumored that if the board didn't vote Wherry out, the committee wanted the board's resignation as well. Brendan Hospital was being site-visited for Joint Commission accreditation that Thursday and Friday. A board meeting was held on Wednesday afternoon, before the site visit. After much discussion, a decision emerged to meet with the staff and employee representatives on the following Monday. The accreditation site visit somehow went smoothly.

The four doctor and nurse representatives met with the board on Monday afternoon, stating that they could not speak for the others. They delivered the petition to DeFalco, who read it to the trustees. The petition stated that the undersigned demanded Wherry's resignation because he was "incompetent, devious, lacked leadership, had shown unprofessional conduct, and had committed negligent acts." The representatives would not discuss the matter at that time. They had been delegated only to deliver the petition. Thus, DeFalco scheduled another board meeting for the following Wednesday afternoon to hear all the charges by all the accusers and to allow Wherry to confront his accusers, 13 days after the mass meeting of June 8.

The meeting of June 22 was attended by eight physicians, 18 registered nurses, 5 department heads, a laboratory supervisor, one dietary aide, and the medical staff secretary. (For an organization chart of Brendan Hospital

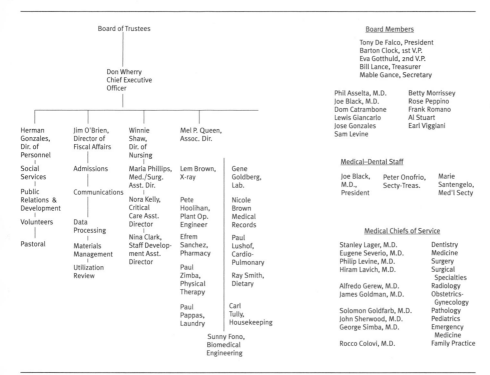

FIGURE VI.4

Brendan Hospital Organizations Chart, Board of Trustees

see Figure VI.4.) All but one of the 18 hospital trustees were in attendance, including Wherry, who was a member of the board. The meeting was held in the tasteful new boardroom of Brendan Hospital, complete with oak tables and plush burgundy carpeting. The committee's presentation is summarized as follows.

The Accusers' Charges

Perrocchio: The most important thing we have to discuss today is patient care. That's why all of us are here. Many of us are not here because we have a personal gripe, but because we want to do what's best for the patient.

Tully (department head): Mr. Wherry humiliated and intimidated three department heads: Mr. O'Brien, Mrs. Williamson, and Mr. Queen.

Pappas (department head): There is a bad morale problem in the laundry.

Patrocelli (supervisor): Laboratory morale is low. There are too many people in other departments and not enough personnel in our department. Companies who deliver to us have put us on COD.

Fong (department head): Mr. Wherry humiliated Mr. Queen.

Frew: There has been a problem in staffing new areas of the hospital. We were told that these would be adequately staffed. I realize they haven't opened yet.

Tontellino: Several months ago a nursing survey was sent around by Mr. Wherry, and we all sent in our responses. We have received no response from Mr. Wherry about the survey.

Carter (RN): We need more help on the floors.

Greenberg: Insensitivity is the problem. The administrator, as you can see from all the comments made so far, is insensitive to the people who work in the hospital.

Santengelo (medical staff secretary): The director of volunteers' salary should have been explained to the rest of us. Employees should continue to get the Christmas bonuses. It means a lot to many of them. Mr. Wherry has created a whole lot of unnecessary paperwork. I don't feel he heard what we were telling him.

Lafrance (RN): There has been a lack of communication between administration and employees. Mr. Wherry actually has asked people to give him the solution to a problem they presented to him.

Shaw (RN and former director of nursing): Mr. Wherry used four-letter words in his office with me. He called one of our attending physicians a . . .

Levari (RN): When there was a bomb scare, Mr. Wherry came to the hospital and stayed for 20 minutes. Then he left before the police came, which I definitely think was wrong.

Leon (RN): It took Mr. Wherry ten months to call a meeting with the head nurses. Problems in nursing have to be solved around here by the nursing department.

Kelly (RN and assistant director): The problem has been lack of communication. I was humiliated when I presented a memo to Mr. Wherry about increases in operating room expenses. He said he couldn't understand what was in the memo, although it was right in front of him. His whole manner was rude.

Phillips (RN and assistant director): When the state inspector came on one of her inspections, she said that Mr. Wherry should be dumped.

Santengelo: He told Dr. Burns one thing and me another when we needed extra help in my office.

Bernstein (RN): Mr. Wherry was evasive and showed a lack of concern. He asked me for my suggestions. I told him to put an ad in the paper to get more help, and it was in the next day. Nurses were not present at administrative meetings.

Brown (department head): Mr. Wherry said Dr. Black would also have to sign an X-ray equipment request for $100,000. That is poor leadership.

Ferrari (RN): I didn't like the tone of his response when I called him at home to ask about treating a Jehovah's Witness in the emergency room.

When we call Mr. Queen, the associate administrator, we nurses never experience that kind of problem.

Lashof (department head): I felt intimidated by Mr. Wherry. The hospital has a morale problem that interferes with patient care.

Brown (department head): He said to me, "If you can't handle the problem [we were having in X-ray], I'll find someone who can."

Charlotte (RN): I've had a problem with my insurance and the personnel department still hasn't gotten back to me for three weeks now. I am divorced and I have a little girl, and it's really creating a hardship for me. I don't understand why Mr. Gonzales, the personnel director, hasn't gotten back to me. I've called him about it many times.

Lafrance: Mr. Wherry sounded upset and annoyed when I called him at home about the electrical fire in maternity.

Gerew: The problem is communication. Mr. Wherry promised something and he didn't deliver. I have been working here for three years trying to develop a first-class radiology department. How can we cut costs and improve service in the outpatient department? I asked for help from fiscal affairs and I didn't get any.

Lavich: The family no longer has any confidence in its father. There was a unanimous vote of no confidence for Mr. Wherry in my department.

Greenberg: Mr. Wherry has a repressive style. There has been a tremendous turnover of personnel in the nursing department since he became the administrator.

Mendez: There is poor morale at the hospital. The nurses are upset. Mr. Wherry used derogatory language concerning foreign medical graduates. This was in the student administrative resident's report on what to do about the emergency room. Let's remove what is causing the problem.

Black (president of the medical staff): Department heads should be on board committees. No one came around and told department heads that they were appreciated. People at Shop-N-Bag make more money than nurses. Our medical people want to be appreciated, too.

Frew: Tony DeFalco, the board president, is seen as being in Mr. Wherry's pocket. There must be accountability for the situation that arose. I have no personal grievance. Accountability starts at the top.

Black: Dr. Fanchini was behind a good deal of what I was doing. A lot of critical things have happened, making for a crisis situation. Dr. Simba was hired to head up the emergency room, without adequate participation of the medical staff. Dr. Fanchini resigned as a board member. Dr. Burns resigned as president of the medical staff because of his personal problems. Mr. Wherry said that Dr. Severio was not really a cardiologist. The radiologists at Clarksville Hospital asked for emergency privileges. What made the medical staff unhappy was when Mr. Wherry said we weren't going to get a CT scanner and when he said that there were no problems in nursing morale. At the meeting of the medical executive committee held this Monday night, June 20, the committee reaffirmed our lack of support for Mr. Wherry, giving him a vote of no confidence by a vote of ten for the motion, one against, and one abstaining.

Listening to the doctors and nurses, DeFalco felt as if he was a spectator watching a Greek tragedy. The committee representatives left the boardroom. DeFalco remembered when the board had met in the old private dining room only two years before, voting to dismiss the previous administrator of 22 years, Phil Drew, because Drew allegedly hadn't kept up with the times, some doctors said he had sexually harassed several of the nurses, and the hospital wasn't doing well financially. Drew had been a good man, and Tony DeFalco had promised himself that he would do everything in his power to prevent this from happening again.

Wherry's Defense

"First I'd like to go through the state of the hospital, as it was when I got here," Wherry began nervously. And yet DeFalco thought Wherry seemed perfectly assured of himself, confident in the rightness of his cause. That was probably one of the things the doctors held against him. Don had attended Princeton undergraduate and Harvard Business School, and had worked for a government regulatory agency in hospital cost containment before taking the Brendan job.

Wherry: There was bad leadership in the nursing department and in several other departments, a lack of medical staff leadership, and few competent department heads. Nursing is a difficult occupation. Morale is always a problem in this department. These are young people with children; they are working evenings, nights, and weekends; and the work is physically, emotionally, and administratively demanding. The doctors at this hospital are like doctors in other hospitals like Brendan, fearful of anything that threatens to affect their livelihood or freedom. I can understand that. But there is a small, embittered group with axes to grind against me. [For a list of 1978 Brendan Hospital goals and accomplishments, see Table VI.2. For 1979 Brendan Hospital goals, see Table VI.3.]

I have been busy with the finances of the hospital and in improving external relationships with the Latinos, state officials, and other

1978 Goals	1978 Accomplishments
1. Stablize hospital finances	• $75,000 surplus • Improved Medicaid and Blue Cross reimbursement • Expenditures reduced in line with lower than expected occupancy
2. Increase fundraising	• Modernization fund pledges on target • Successful first annual horse show
3. Improve hospital morale	• Regular employee-administration meetings • Regular publication of *Brendan News*
4. Improve quality of nursing care	• High patient evaluations in survey • New director of nursing recruited
5. Organize department of emergency medicine	• Department organized and Dr. George Simba recruited as chief
6. Establish effective management information and control system	• Implemented auditors' recommendation • Evaluating new data processing alternatives
7. Increase communication with Spanish-speaking community	• Several meetings held with Hispanic leaders • Increased Hispanic staff in patient areas, including social services
8. Increase accountability of medical departments for quality assurance	• Board resolution requiring annual reports • Joint conference committee and trustee seminar for better communication between medical staff and trustees
9. Increase community participation in long-range planning	• Four community members added to long-range planning committee • Wide distribution of annual report with attendance encouraged at annual meeting
10. On schedule, on budget, fully accredited new wing	• New wing scheduled to open in April 1979 • Building is roughly within budget and on schedule

TABLE VI.2
Brendan Hospital 1978 Goals and Accomplishments (from 1978 Annual Report)

TABLE VI.3

1979 Brendan
Hospital Goals
(from 1978
Annual Report)

1. Stabilize hospital finances and improve cash flow
2. Improve board, administration, and medical staff communication
3. Increase hospital involvement of Spanish-speaking community
4. Fill administrative vacancies and recruit needed medical staff
5. Increase pediatric and obstetrical inpatient occupancy
6. Accomplish complete availability of new wing by April and obtain full hospital accreditation
7. Establish quality assurance programs for all professional departments
8. Establish productivity and efficiency goals for all hospital departments
9. Develop an operational long-range plan, including time and dollar estimates for new programs
10. Continue to contain increases in hospital costs

groups. Mel Queen, the associate administrator, has been busy with the new construction and the move into our new $5 million wing.

We've had a new director of nursing on board for five weeks now, and I wish that everyone would have just given her a chance. Dr. Burns's resignation as president of the medical staff didn't help me any, and I have had a director of personnel, Gonzales, with acute personal problems, which has been a problem for me, too. Next, it's quite unusual for someone to have to defend himself on the spot to a list of specific charges that I have been waiting for these past 13 days and just now have been made aware of. I think the way this whole thing has been handled by the doctor and nurse ringleaders is disgraceful. The charges they have made are largely not true and could not be proven even if they were true. Even if the charges are true to a substantial extent, there is still not sufficient reason for your discharging me, certainly not suddenly as they are demanding you to.

The doctors are out to get me because I'm doing the job you've been paying me to do, what I'm evaluated on, and for which I received a very good evaluation and a big raise at the end of last year, presumably because I was doing a good job. [For Wherry's evaluation, see Appendix VI.1; for DeFalco's raise letter, see Appendix VI.2.] Certainly none of you have told me to stop doing what I have been doing to assure quality, contain costs, and improve service. During the past year I gathered information for the medical staff on a new reappointment worksheet so that reappointments aren't made on a rubber stamp process every two years. I pointed out the problems that the low inpatient census in pediatrics would create in retaining the beds in the years to come. I obtained model rules and regulations for the medical staff and shared these with the president, Dr. Black. I questioned the effectiveness of the tissue committee, which hasn't been meeting, and when it has met, whose minutes are perfunctory. I questioned the performance of the audit committee after our delegated status under PSRO was placed in question by a visiting physician, Dr. Lordi. I suggested we explore mandated physician donations to the hospital, as was passed and implemented two years ago by another East State hospital. When patients made complaints about doctors I took these up with the respective chiefs of departments. I investigated the assertion by a lab technician that tests were being reported and not done by the laboratory. I questioned and had to renegotiate remuneration of pathologists and radiologists, all with knowledge of the president of the board, Mr. DeFalco, and I have done nothing without involving the medical executive committee.

I have been involved in the lengthy and frustrating process of getting support from other hospitals for a CT scanner and in justifying financial feasibility of the CT scanner at this hospital. I have suggested ways to recruit needed physicians into Lockhart and have shared with the staff other approaches used by East State hospitals, such as a guaranteed income for the first year. I followed up a trustee's question about the appropriateness of fetal monitoring with the chief of obstetrics and gynecology, and worked out a satisfactory response to poor ophthalmology coverage in the emergency room with the chief of ophthalmology. I became involved in trying to convince one of our three pathologists not to resign because of a run-in with the chief of pathology. I have to get after physicians who do not indicate final diagnosis or complete their charts on time, because this delays needed cash flow for the hospital. I suggested that the hospital develop a model program for providing day hospital and other care to the elderly and chronically ill, and sought the cooperation of State University in designing a research protocol to measure the need for such services. This action was resented by several members of the staff, although we have not gone ahead with the State research program pending staff approval, and, if they disapprove, I said we would not go ahead with it.

I initiated a study of how we can prevent malpractice at the hospital, conveyed board disapproval of radiology equipment, which we had scheduled to buy but couldn't afford because other radiology equipment broke down in an unforeseen way. There are several very difficult physicians on the medical executive committee who have never gotten along with any administrator or with other physicians. I am the one who has to discuss with the surgeons and the radiologists ways to decrease costs in their units when these costs are way above the state medians and we have to reduce them or face financial penalties.

As far as nursing goes, here is a list of what I have done: I have met with all shifts, with head nurses, with supervisors, and regularly with the director and assistant directors. I hired a new director and fired an old assistant director whom the nurses said showed favoritism, lied to them, and overpromised. This was opposed, by the way, by Dr. Fanchini, former director of obstetrics and gynecology. I hired an expert nursing consultant to help us develop appropriate goals and ways of meeting these goals. I was in the process of obtaining the services of an operations research consultant, at no cost to the hospital, to help us with our scheduling problems. We implemented a study done by an administrative resident on improved staffing and scheduling. I pointed out all the problems of authoritarian leadership, lack of adequate quality assurance programs, and lack of appropriate scheduling and budgeting to the previous nursing director, which is why she had to be demoted. Mrs. Shaw always tried to do her best, but she lacked the proper education and skills. I obtained 15 additional approved nursing positions, including one additional full-time RN in in-service and an additional $80,000 for in-service, from the state rate-setters, something that no one has been able to do at this hospital for the past eight years. Our expenditures in nursing are already above the state median. I obtained a staffing plan from another hospital for the director of nursing and influenced her to distribute a questionnaire to all nurses to better find out their feelings and ideas.

I could go through each of the charges made by the people assembled here, but it won't really prove anything. Yes, I did call a doctor a . . . in my office. Yes, I did leave the hospital after the bomb scare before the police came, but only after I was convinced that it was a scare. I had a meeting to go to in Urban City, and I called one hour later to see that everything was all right. I think it is significant that none of the department heads supposedly humiliated by me showed up at this meeting. You have asked me to resign, but I'm not going to resign. That would not solve the hospital's problems. Firing me will not solve the bad nursing morale here or the doctor distrust. It will show the doctors and nurses and the community who runs this hospital. Is it the board of trustees or some doctors and nurses (the nurses are mainly being used by the doctors)? Whose head will these doctors be asking for the next time they want to get rid of somebody? The bond issue set for next month that could refinance our debt on the new wing will not go through if you fire me. And we shall have a $355,000 payment to make in August, which will be difficult to meet.

"Does anybody have any questions?" DeFalco asked the other trustees. There were a few questions, but nothing significant, no major contradictions of anything Wherry had said. A vote was taken to clear Wherry of the charges without rebuttal, and this passed 7 in favor, 5 against, with 4 abstentions. Then the trustees asked Wherry to leave the room and told him that they would make a decision.

That evening, after dinner with his wife and teenagers, DeFalco watched a baseball game on television. He couldn't get his mind off that Friday night board meeting, the vote 10 to 6 against Wherry, and the ultimate unanimous vote to dismiss him with two months' severance. During the previous week, DeFalco had made it his business to discuss the Don Wherry situation with the other 16 trustees (Wherry and he made 18). As best as he could recollect, the following was the essence of their comments to him.

Board Comments

Clock (age 55, life insurance salesman, first vice president of the board, former mayor, and DeFalco's long-time confidant): I have been one of Don Wherry's strongest supporters since he got here and before he got here. I was a member of the search committee that selected Don, as you remember. I still like Don personally, really I do, but it has become obvious to me, at least, that Don can no longer manage the hospital. Whether Don is right or wrong, the docs don't like him. [Wherry told DeFalco that Clock sold a lot of life insurance to a lot of doctors.] Don's biggest mistakes have been in not firing Mel Queen, the associate administrator, who never has supported him properly, and Winnie Shaw, the ex-director of nursing, whom he should never have kept around and I told him so.

Gotthuld (age 50, second vice president of the hospital board, president of the board of Preston College, and wife of a beer distributor): I have been spending one or two weeks out of every month in Vermont, you know, George, where we bought a distributorship, and last year Sam and I spent six months on a luxury liner trip around the world. So I really don't know what's going on that well. As chairman of the executive committee, I know we gave Don a good evaluation and if he isn't acting properly as chief executive officer, then at least part of the fault is ours. I see no reason to fire Don abruptly because of these alleged charges.

Lance (age 45, president of a local lumber company, treasurer of the hospital, and chairman of the buildings and grounds committee): I have always been one of Don Wherry's closest friends, although he may not admit it now. I think Don could do an excellent job managing a university hospital, but that he definitely cannot do the job here at Brendan and that we should get rid of him now. Don might care more than anyone else, certainly more than I do, about the welfare of the hospital employees, but Don just hasn't communicated that to them.

Gonce (65 years old, RN, secretary of the hospital, recently returned for the board meeting from University Hospital in Urban City where she was recovering from a heart attack): Tony, you know I fought bitterly against Don Wherry's coming to Brendan in the first place, voted then for Mel Queen, the associate administrator, to do the job, and I vote for him now to do a better job than Don Wherry. Don should be working for the government somewhere, not in a small town. Mel Queen will make an excellent administrator of Brendan Hospital. We should have given it to him in the first place.

Giancarlo (age 60, president of a local canning firm, newly elected to the board in January): I don't know much about the facts of the situation, Tony; I like Don Wherry personally, but obviously the doctors and many of the employees are unhappy with him. They must be listened to. It doesn't seem that anything they are complaining about is new or isolated.

Gonzales (age 40, secondary school teacher, was one of Don Wherry's strongest supporters): I see what Don has done to meet with all the Latino leaders without any crisis, to hear out our problems and respond to us. Don has reorganized and improved services in the emergency room, hired a Spanish-speaking social work assistant, increased the number of minority supervisors. I am not that impressed, really, by these charges. There's no meat to them. I think this is just a bunch of doctors trying to get rid of Don as they got rid of Mr. Drew, the last CEO, and I do not think the board should bow down to them this time.

Peppino (age 34, senior bank vice president): Knowing Don Wherry as I do, I can understand a lot of the charges and sympathize with those making the complaints. Don Wherry is cold and authoritative, and if he knows so much, maybe that isn't what the job needs anyway. Mel Queen can run the hospital perfectly well, I'm convinced of that. And if the doctors are going to stop admitting patients as they threaten to do, they must feel very strongly about Don Wherry. It's important to calm the doctors down and get on with business as usual, and the sooner the better. Don Wherry will have no problem finding a job somewhere else. Maybe he was going to leave Lockhart anyway after a few more years.

Black (age 45, president of the medical staff): We have to get rid of this guy. He's nothing but trouble. I tried to work with him, but the guys don't like him. Maybe it's because he went to Princeton or something. He gives the guys this feeling that he feels superior to us. He's the big-time administrator and we're the lowly doctors. We'd much prefer Mel

Queen running the hospital. We don't have to put up with this Wherry guy, and now's the time to get rid of him.

Romano (age 50, president of a lumber company, newly elected to the board in January): I feel the way Lew Giancarlo does. I never thought being elected to this board would involve all these problems, and I'm certainly spending more time on this darn hospital than I would like to be spending. It's a tough thing for this Wherry guy. I like Don personally, but I really think we're going to have more problems with him than without him.

Levine (age 45, attorney, newly elected to the board in January): I think this is disgraceful what we're doing to Don. I don't like the way the whole thing was done, even if Don has made mistakes. You don't treat an employee this way, certainly not the chief executive officer. But I don't think that Don has handled it right, either. He should have gone to the mass meeting and defended himself. He should have organized people to speak on his behalf. That's the advice I would have given Don as a lawyer. And I think it's a darn shame this has to happen. It doesn't have to happen, really, if someone would only stand up and fight for Don and his cause. I'm doing the best that I can, but I've only been on the board a short time, and I feel I'm therefore limited in what I can do.

Morrissey (age 47, housewife): Don and his wife Sue are personal friends of mine, but I can't let that get in the way of making the right decision for the hospital. Don is certainly a brilliant guy who cares about people and doesn't want to see the patient or the consumer taken advantage of. He wants to do all the right things and he has done a lot of the right things. The hospital is a safer, warmer, financially sounder place than it was when Don took over. I'm certainly going to vote for Don. I'm sorry, but I don't feel I know enough to be really energetic about this.

Viggiani (age 60, owner of a large real estate firm and chairman of the county Democratic Party): I think it's a terrible thing what they're doing to Don. It's just like with the other guy, Phil Drew. This guy has always been there when we needed him. He works night and day. If anything's the matter, then it must be our fault because this guy has been doing what we've been telling him to do. He hasn't done anything without telling the doctors and us first. I think it's a disgrace.

Asselta (age 70, general practitioner): The staff just doesn't like him. I like Don Wherry. I know he's been trying to do the right thing. I've tried to help Don, after I made sure of him, every way I can. You know my wife has been very sick and I haven't been able to attend to hospital affairs lately as I would like. I guess I'll go along with the majority, either way.

Goldman (age 61, chief of ob-gyn, newly elected to the board in January): I don't think the man knows how to manage the hospital, asking the employees to come up with the solutions to their own problems. That's bad management. Our group is against him.

Catrambone (age 50, director of a large funeral home): Tony, I'm only sorry I won't be at the meeting to speak for Don. There's a right and a wrong, and I can tell the difference. Ask yourself who is right and who is wrong and you've got to vote for Don Wherry. I happen to think he's a pretty fair manager to boot. I wish you would count my vote. Since my open heart surgery, I've got to be in Rochester, Minnesota, for my annual heart examination.

Stuart (age 41, senior vice president of the same bank of which Mrs. Peppino is assistant vice president.) [Don Wherry had told DeFalco that Stuart and Peppino were against him because he gave all the bank business, per finance committee recommendation, to a competing bank.]: I don't like Don Wherry. I never have. I served with him on the personnel committee and we were usually in disagreement. Don always made me feel somehow that I was ignorant, that he felt himself superior to me. This is not how he should have acted. And I'm sure a lot of the employees feel the same way about Don that I do.

APPENDIX VI.1		Rating 1–5 (1 is high, 5 is low)	
Summary of CEO Evaluation (November 25, 1978)		Self	Avg. Trustee
I. Goal Achievement			
1. Stabilize hospital finances		1	2.7
2. Increase fundraising		3	3.6
3. Improve hospital morale		3	4.9
4. Improve quality of nursing care		1	3.7
5. Organize emergency room department		1	2.9
6. Establish an effective management information and control system		2	2.1
7. Maintain on-schedule, on-budget west wing building program		3	2.3
8. Establish plan for utilization of west wing and integration with total hospital operations		3	2.1
9. Increase communications with the growing Spanish-speaking community		1	3.1
10. Increase accountability of medical departments for quality assurance		1	3.1
11. Prepare to obtain three-year hospital accreditation upon completion of west wing		3	1.9

12. Increase community participation in hospital long-range planning	1	2.2

CEO Remarks:
1. CEO is goal-oriented.
2. He needs to spend yet more time developing consensus and persuading key stakeholders and earning their respect.

Trustee Remarks:
1. Many of these "specifics" are difficult for an outside director to judge.
2. I think CEO's contributions are acceptable except in items 3 and 4, where they should have been significantly greater.
3. Morale is a question.
4. CEO is doing a fine job for Brendan.
5. CEO's capability is great for achieving all goals. Sometimes his motives are not understood, and some obstacles are not of his doing.
6. The answers to some of these questions are based more on perceptions than actual knowledge.

President's Remarks:
   I agree that the CEO is goal-oriented. He has attained goals we have given him about as well as anyone could reasonably expect.

II. System Maintenance	2	3.5

CEO Remarks:
1. Given what the CEO was hired to do, a certain amount of distrust is inevitable.
2. The CEO tries diligently to establish regular and continuing dialogue with all key hospital groups and individuals.

Trustee Remarks:
1. Greatest weaknesses in this category are in maintaining adequate commitment of employees to organizational goals and developing adequate trust between management and medical staff.
2. The board is not made aware of exactly the number of employees needed and the department that has this need. There seems to be a feeling of unrest among the

(*continued on next page*)

administrative staff (department heads). Trust between management and medical staff is currently very poor.

3. CEO's capabilities are limitless, but I feel he has developed a schism between himself and the medical staff.
4. Small areas of difference need to be cleared by better communication and understanding of mutual problems. Main problem area is with doctor contracts.
5. I suspect that the only positive factor in the above list would be "maintaining adequate administrative and control systems."

President's Remarks:

1. Our "hospital system" has undoubtedly provided sufficient patient care of adequate quality at reasonable cost. I therefore believe the trustee evaluation to be too low in this area.
2. A mistrust of the administration by the medical staff does exist. I am also apprehensive about the "team play" of the administrative staff. We must address these problems in 1979.

III. Relationships with Important External Publics	1	2.1

CEO Remarks:

The hospital had done well with licensing, regulatory, and reimbursement agencies, and with other provider agencies during 1978. The CEO speaks frequently to consumer organizations and volunteer groups as well and has been well received.

Trustee Remarks:

1. The CEO had done an especially good job with third-party payers.
2. This is definitely the CEO's strongest area.
3. Excellent record.

President's remarks:

I am pleased with the CEO's accomplishments in this area.

IV. Management Roles		
1. Interpersonal	3	3.6
2. Informational	1	2.4
3. Decisional	1	2.8

APPENDIX VI.1

(*continued*)

CEO's Remarks:

The CEO is intelligent and quick. He works long hours and is subject to constant pressures. He cannot possibly talk at length continuously with 18 trustees, 40 key doctors, 20 department heads, and other key personnel outside the hospital. He must try harder to be cheerful, quiet, friendly, and low-key.

Trustee Remarks:

1. I think the CEO has done a good job in 1978, especially in view of what he walked into.
2. The CEO has weakness in providing motivation, also in recognizing disturbances of uneasiness within the hospital personnel, and in dealing with incompetent or unproductive personnel.
3. The CEO seems to be seeking many changes. His method for achieving this isn't always productive. The CEO has great potential but doesn't seem to implement it well.
4. I'm not too sure if CEO is handling personnel adequately. Morale has not improved within the hospital.
5. The CEO has done and is doing an outstanding job. I am proud to work with him and would give him even higher marks if possible.
6. The CEO is excellent on a one-to-one basis. He handles groups well. He is anxious to please and to get cooperation.

President's Remarks:

1. Changes in staff personnel in 1978 have hampered the efficiency and effectiveness of this group. When stability of this group occurs, provided the right group has been chosen, improvement in hospital management will be most evident.
2. The dissemination of information is exceptional.
3. I have confidence in the decisions that are being made. I am not sure about their method of implementation.

V. President's Summary

1. Areas of evaluation:
   The CEO has exceeded my expectations. In sum total, I am extremely pleased with his accomplishments.

(*continued on next page*)

2. Strengths:
   Planning, establishing priorities, dealing with regulatory agencies, understanding and articulating hospital organization, financial management, intelligence, creativity, ability to negotiate, potential, sincerity, and directness.

3. Weakness:
   Impatience and aloofness (coldness).

4. Uncertainties:
   Evaluation of personnel, evaluation of situations, employee motivation, and non-peer and subordinate relationships.

5. Recommendations:
   Attempt to gain trust and respect of medical staff.
   Improve trust and respect of employees in presence of others.
   Refrain from reprimanding employees in presence of others.
   Work toward having assistant responsible for day-to-day operation of hospital.
   Continue to attempt to improve morale.
   Improve patience; realize that few people can match intelligence quotient.
   Continue to develop administrative staff.

6. Conclusion:
   The CEO has performed well in 1978. He has acceptably attained his goals. As a new manager, he has been severely tested by the board of trustees, medical staff, and employees and has withstood their challenge. I believe his inherent intelligence will allow him to correct any and all identifiable deficiencies.

   The CEO's self-evaluation was extremely accurate. It is comforting to know that he has the ability to correctly assess his strengths and weaknesses.

   The following elements will be necessary for his continued success:
   a. Constructive advice and support by board of trustees
   b. Trust of medical staff
   c. Melding of administrative staff into stable, competent, and qualified team with common objectives

APPENDIX VI.2
Letter from
Tony DeFalco
to Don Wherry
on January 10,
1979

Personal and Confidential

Mr. Don Wherry   January 10, 1979
Brendan Hospital
Lockhart, East State

Dear Don,

The Board of Trustees of Brendan Hospital, on January 8, 1979, unanimously approved a 10 percent increase in your annual salary along with a $500 increase in automobile allowance for 1979. The above increases will result in a per annum salary of $57,750 and an automobile allowance of $2,300. Your receipt of this letter provides you with the authority to make the stipulated adjustments effective January 1, 1979.

Our board believes that you have done an outstanding job as our chief executive officer and hopes that the above increases have fairly rewarded your effort.

Very truly yours,

Tony DeFalco, President
Brendan Hospital, Board of Trustees

Case Questions

1. How do you feel about what happened to Don Wherry?
2. Do you feel the board was justified in acting as it did?
3. What could Wherry have done to prevent being fired? What could the board have done to have prevented this? Should the medical board have acted any differently?
4. Should Wherry have resigned as the board wished him to?
5. Whose hospital is Brendan Hospital? What are the consequences of this being the case, for consumers, patients, managers, physicians, and trustees?

Case Q
What Happens When Patients Cannot Pay?

Ann Scheck McAlearney and Paula H. Song

Susan Lawler, CEO of Sunrise Memorial Hospital, leaned back in her chair to reflect on the topic just debated at this morning's board meeting. She was delighted that the hospital was financially stable, but, as echoed in the comments of several board members during the meeting, she thought the not-for-profit hospital should be doing more for its community. While each year the hospital reported that it had provided a substantial level of uncompensated care, given the morning's discussion, it seemed clear that now was a good time to revisit this issue.

As Lawler knew, a hospital's report of its uncompensated care level consists of both charity care and bad debt. While charity care is care provided to individuals for which the hospital does not ever expect to be paid, bad debt represents care for which the hospital bills and reasonably expects to be paid, but ultimately is unable to collect. Charity care visits do not appear as an expense on the hospital's financial statements. Rather, the dollar value of charity care is included in a note to the financial statements. In contrast, the revenue and expense associated with visits characterized as bad debt appear on the hospital's income statements.

For Sunrise, as at all hospitals, reporting uncompensated care using these two categories has several implications. With respect to bad debt, the most salient issue is how aggressively the hospital pursues payments. Lawler was comfortable with this area, and aware that the hospital would never be accused of overly aggressive collections practices as had been reported by several other hospitals in an adjacent state. However, with respect to charity care, she was less convinced. The current charity care policy was based on family income level. But Lawler wondered whether this policy was designed as a marketing tool to protect Sunrise Memorial's tax-exempt status, rather than a tool to appropriately decide who should receive charity care.

Lawler was particularly concerned that the hospital may be missing opportunities to help patients and the community with their healthcare needs. While she knew the Sunrise emergency department (ED) was legally obligated to stabilize all patients who presented there for care regardless of ability to pay (i.e., under the legal restrictions associated with the Emergency Medical Treatment and Active Labor Act), she also knew there were no plans or policies in place to help those patients when they were discharged from the ED. Further, she knew that if these patients did not have another place to go for care (i.e., a "medical home"), they would be at risk for several downstream problems, such as repeat ED visits or declining health, if they chose not to pursue recommended follow-up care. While there was a federally qualified health center (FQHC) not too far from Sunrise, no effort had been made to establish any relationships with the FQHC, and Lawler wondered whether this was even possible.

A Charity Care Challenge

Not long after the board meeting, Lawler learned of the case of Jeremy Spring, a patient who had arrived at the Sunrise ED complaining of severe pain in his arm. After being processed through triage, Spring was admitted for treatment of myocardial infarction (a heart attack). He ended up staying at Sunrise for a full week due to the need to both treat his acute condition and manage several complications associated with his chronic heart disease. After Spring was stabilized, a Sunrise case manager, Anneliese Campbell, asked him about his insurance status and discovered he had no coverage. Upon further investigation Campbell determined that Spring's income level was around 250 percent of the federal poverty level, thus slightly too high for him to qualify for the hospital's free care program.

Campbell raised this issue with her supervisor, Owen Williams, and they agreed that Spring's situation was indeed complicated. While the patient did not qualify for the hospital's charity care program, they were concerned that the costs associated with Spring's stay might create an insurmountable financial burden for him. Further, Spring's condition upon arrival at Sunrise indicated that he had not received appropriate primary care for some time, and, as a result, had a number of comorbid conditions that contributed to his ill health and long hospital stay. Campbell also pointed out that the hospital's doctors had already expressed concern about Spring's future well-being. While Spring clearly needed both short-term follow-up and long-term monitoring, his past history provided no evidence that he would adhere to a recommended treatment plan because of both limited financial means and no "medical home," or place where they could refer him for care within the community.

Williams and Campbell scheduled a meeting with the hospital's chief financial officer (CFO), Kelly Brady, to raise their concerns. Brady was aware of the hospital's charity care policy, but felt her hands were tied in this situation. She advised Williams and Campbell to "do what they could" to help Spring make the transition back to the community, and pointed out that the local FQHC might be an appropriate place to refer Spring for ongoing care.

Now What?

While Lawler supported her CFO, she was not comfortable with the decision that had been made. In particular, she was unconvinced that discharging a low-income patient with a referral slip to go to the local FQHC was sufficient.

She knew that the most likely next chapter of Spring's story would be another expensive visit to the Sunrise ED, and, potentially, another hospital stay. Given Sunrise's financial condition, she sensed there was an opportunity to address the case of Spring and other patients with similar situations, but she was unsure how or where to start.

Case Questions

1. What issues are raised in this case for Lawler to address?
2. What are the options for Sunrise with respect to treating patients who cannot pay for care?
3. What key stakeholders would be involved (both internal and external) in revising the Sunrise charity care policy?
4. What steps would you take to learn more about the options available to Sunrise Memorial Hospital with respect to treating its low-income patients?
5. What would you recommend that Lawler do to better help patients who cannot pay?
6. What might change if Sunrise were a for-profit hospital?

Short Case 26
The Conflicted HMO Manager

Anthony R. Kovner

Bill Brown had built up University Hospital's HMO over the past ten years so that now it had 100,000 members. His boss, Jim Edgar, had decided to sell the insurance part of the business (retaining the medical groups) because University wasn't in the insurance business. Brown was asked to recruit some bidders, one of whom, Liberty National, Edgar came to prefer because of its financial strength and excellent reputation. In the process of working with Liberty National, Brown learned that it wanted to hire him, after the sale, to be the president of its regional HMO activities. Brown told Edgar what was likely to happen in this regard. The deal was subsequently approved by Brown's board (of the HMO) and by Edgar's board (of the hospital). Two years after the sale, Brown works for Liberty and is making $5 million a year, while University is losing $5 million a year. Joe Kelly, University's new CEO, figures out that the contract that Brown negotiated for University was highly favorable to Liberty and now University can't get out of it for another nine years.

Case Questions

1. Did Brown act unethically? If so, how? What should Brown have done? Why didn't he do it?
2. Did Edgar act competently? If not, what should he have done differently? Why didn't he do it?
3. What should the University CEO, Joe Kelly, do now?

Short Case 27
The Great Mosaic:
Multiculturalism at Seaview Nursing Home

James Castiglione and Anthony R. Kovner

Alice O'Connor is the new director of the Seaview Nursing Home (SNH), a large investor-owned facility in Far West City, which provides services to 98 ethnic groups speaking 68 different languages. Most of the top management jobs at SNH are held by white females. Although Far West City has a 23 percent Latino population, Latinos hold only 6 percent of the higher level management positions at SNH. SNH has an affirmative action program and, as a result, staff members at lower levels come from a wide range of backgrounds. Twelve percent of SNH employees are classified as minorities.

According to O'Connor's predecessor, Una Light, SNH has had an exemplary affirmative action program, promoting diversity awareness, hiring more minority staff at lower-level positions, and being responsive to the health needs of the minority populations served by the nursing home.

SNH has a diversity awareness training program that has been offered 14 times over the last two years. The need for this program has been assessed through internal surveys and interviews of all staff. The purpose of these meetings is to increase the level of awareness and sensitivity of the staff of SNH as service providers; to promote awareness within the organization and increase the level of informed cross-cultural interactions among staff; and to expose potential problems and keep them from increasing in severity.

Only 8 percent of students who graduated last year from local accredited schools of nursing or healthcare administration were minorities. Latinos accounted for only 3 percent of graduates.

As part of becoming familiar with the organization, O'Connor has had conversations with each of SNH's middle managers. Anna Gonzales, who is

Latino, feels that given the large minority population in the area, SNH is not doing enough to grant power to minority groups. She would like to be considered for the position of deputy director, currently occupied by a 60-year-old white female. Jim Leone, another of the middle managers, points out that white men have not occupied positions of power at SNH for the last 20 years, and that positions should be allocated strictly on the basis of merit.

Case Questions

1. Do you feel SNH has been doing an adequate job in managing diversity?
2. What, if anything, do you think the new director should do differently?
3. How useful is the concept of "minorities" in managing diversity?

Short Case 28
No Parity in Behavioral Health Coverage

Ann Scheck McAlearney

Dr. Elizabeth Rosendale was concerned. As medical director of a community health center (CHC) located in downtown Miami, many of her patients suffered from mental and behavioral health problems. Yet she was continually amazed by the difficulty she had obtaining appropriate medications and treatments for her patients. Many of the patients who came to the CHC for help with their behavioral health problems had insurance coverage, but these insurance plans never seemed to cover the types of treatments and medications necessary to address the issues bringing her patients to the clinic. Rosendale was getting increasingly frustrated by the limits placed on her by restrictive insurance policies.

Most recently, a new patient had arrived who needed treatment for depression. Rosendale was able to get the required medications covered by insurance, but the policy had a limit on the number of visits the patient could have with a mental health provider. Rosendale knew the medications would be less effective if her patient could not be regularly seen by a therapist, and she also knew that it was likely that the side effects from the medication would make her patient less likely to continue with the medications without regular oversight by a mental health provider.

Rosendale had built a good relationship with a local therapist, Dr. Gayle Orman, but this therapist was complaining that too many of her patients were unable to pay enough money for their therapy to justify continuing treatments.

Case Questions

1. What can Rosendale do?
2. With whom could she work to begin to address these problems?

Short Case 29
Ergonomics in Practice

J. Mac Crawford and Ann Scheck McAlearney

Riverlea Rehabilitation Hospital's administrators had recently begun to notice high levels of absenteeism, workers' compensation claims, and time off from work associated with back and other injuries suffered by their workers. Staff were prone to injuries when patients lost their balance while being moved—especially when staff were required to use their own bodies to prevent patient falls. Patients, in turn, could be injured when staff were unable to secure the patients due to the overwhelming physical load or because of preexisting injuries or deficits in staff members' physical strength. Tim Montana, the administrative director, had heard that the new system of patient-lifting devices planned for installation at Riverlea Hospital could effectively reduce both the number of workers' injuries and associated workers' compensation claims and absenteeism rates, but the new system was expensive. Montana believed the lift system's cost would be worth the benefits, but he wanted to make sure.

The new lift system had been designed so that patients could be placed in a harness and moved from a bed to a chair, the bathroom, or anywhere else in the room. It was meant to be used consistently, and consistent use was apparently associated with reduced risk of injury to both staff and patients.

In order to prove that the new lift system helped address the problems associated with the musculoskeletal injuries reported by Riverlea nursing staff, Montana enlisted a team of researchers from the local School of Public Health. Montana wanted to be able to provide quantifiable evidence that the new system had made a positive impact at Riverlea.

During Montana's meeting with the research team, Dr. Jason Terry, the lead environmental health services researcher, explained that the best approach to evaluating the impact of the lift system would be to undertake a longitudinal study of the health of Riverlea personnel. As Terry explained, the research team could first collect baseline information using existing injury data, then supplement these data by collecting new information about work practices, shifts, and musculoskeletal symptoms among the target workers.

After installation of the new lift system hospital-wide, the researchers could collect follow-up data to assess the system's efficacy.

Montana convinced the rest of Riverlea's administrative team that a research study was justified, and approved the budget request to support the investigation. Baseline data were collected before the lift system was installed, and plans for the follow-up assessment were made. However, Montana observed the implementation and initial use of the lift system at Riverlea and was concerned about the process. He and his team had seen evidence that many staff members were using the devices incorrectly, were using them intermittently, or were not using them at all. Well aware that improper use of the system would bias any research data collection process, Montana decided to ask the engineering department to check whether the lift system was operating as planned. After a week of study, the engineering personnel reported to Montana that the lifts themselves were functioning properly, so that was not the problem.

Montana next asked individual staff members for their opinions about the lift system. After only a handful of conversations, Montana realized that there were plenty of opinions about the lift system, and most of these were negative. Staff appeared unconvinced about the value of the lift system, and instead were delighted to tell Montana stories about how they had managed to "work around" the system to lift their patients in the "usual way." Montana still believed that the lift system could have a positive impact at Riverlea, but he knew that current use patterns were inconsistent and inappropriate. He knew he had to do something to intervene, but he didn't know where to start.

Case Questions

1. What options does Montana now have to convince staff to use the new lift system consistently and properly?
2. Are there appropriate metrics and goals by which to evaluate the success of the lift system implementation? What metrics should be used to meet what goals? And what is an appropriate timeline for meeting those goals?
3. What would be an appropriate role for a research team evaluating the impact of a new lift system?
4. Who should be accountable for correct adoption and use of the new lift system?
5. For a different organization considering installing a new lift system, what type of process would you propose to build staff support and buy-in for the system? Who would be the relevant stakeholders to include in planning for the new lift system's introduction?

Short Case 30
What's in a Name?

Ann Scheck McAlearney and Sarah M. Roesch

Donna Taylor was on her way to the mall to pick up an item donated to the carnival silent auction benefiting her daughter's school. In her head, she was going over the last-minute list of things she had to do to get ready for that night's carnival. Taylor really didn't have anything to worry about, because she was a master planner of fundraisers and community service events. Ten years ago, Taylor had worked in the insurance industry, but left to stay home with her kids after her third child. Taylor enjoyed staying home with her children, but soon realized she needed more responsibilities than monitoring her children's nap schedules and play dates to make her feel useful. As a result, Taylor became active in the community through volunteerism, and participated in many service projects offered by the Junior League, YWCA Women's Board, and Children's Hospital Auxiliary. Taylor also participated in various capital campaigns and was a natural fundraiser. Taylor was an organized, creative, and capable volunteer who quickly climbed the volunteer hierarchy and became a leader of these organizations. As her three daughters each entered school, she also became active in their school's PTA, and this involvement had led to her current run to the mall to pick up a donated auction item.

Taylor sprinted into the mall to gather her item and let out a deep sigh as she passed the Ashley and Mitch store. Taylor's oldest daughter, Stella, was in the sixth grade and just getting interested in fashion. A pair of Ashley and Mitch jeans was at the top of Stella's birthday list. Taylor shook her head at the large poster in Ashley and Mitch's window. Taylor was no prude, but she didn't quite agree with the photo of three scantily clothed teenage models. Ashley and Mitch was infamous for its risqué promotional material and sexual imagery enticing pre-teens and teens to buy its clothing. She did not think it was appropriate to entice teenage consumers with this type of marketing. However, it certainly seemed to work, since most pre-teens she knew were very interested in Ashley and Mitch's clothing. Taylor personally believed this type of advertising was sleazy and demeaning to young people. Even though she was able to shrug her shoulders at the poster with a mental note that, "it's only clothes," she knew her daughter would not be getting those jeans for her birthday.

Taylor hurried to pick up her donation. Back in the car, she again went over her mental list for the fundraiser, and decided she had everything covered. She was just beginning to relax when the news came on the radio. The reporter was relating a story about the local Children's Hospital renaming its emergency room "The Ashley and Mitch Emergency Department and Trauma Center" in exchange for a $10 million donation. With this new information, Taylor was struck by the realization that maybe this wasn't "only clothes." Taylor thought back to several middle-of-the-night trips to Children's Hospital and how thankful she was that her children had such a good place to go in an emergency situation. She also thought about the hours she spent volunteering at Children's Hospital, pushing a book cart and delivering books to patients. Taylor knew what $10 million could do for a children's hospital. Yet to name an emergency room after a company with a reputation for relying on sexual image marketing to target pre-teens and teens? She wasn't convinced. As the mother of three pre-teen girls, Taylor knew how insecurities about image can damage self-esteem. She was confused about the apparent inconsistency with Ashley and Mitch's message and Children's Hospital's mission of "protection and caring for children." As she approached the school for the carnival fund-raiser, Taylor's confusion had changed to anger at Children's Hospital for deciding to associate with a company notorious for egregious advertising.

Arriving at the school, the first person Taylor ran into was her fundraising co-chair, Meg Flynn. After telling Flynn about the new partnership between Ashley and Mitch and Children's Hospital, she was amazed that Flynn appeared ambivalent. Flynn's first response was to ask, "Why would Children's turn down such a large donation? They would be crazy to turn down that kind of money for all it could do to improve healthcare for children." Further, Flynn argued, despite the advertising, the consumer is the one with the true power. "No one is forced to buy Ashley and Mitch clothing. People can choose to look away." Flynn also suggested that maybe Ashley and Mitch owes something to the consumer, and *should* give back to children. Since it makes millions of dollars each year selling its inappropriate clothing, giving back some money to help children makes a lot of sense. While Taylor saw Flynn's points, she didn't think she could actually look the other way. Even though she knew how hard it is to raise money and realized that $10 million is a sizeable donation, Taylor thought Ashley and Mitch should donate the money, but not get naming rights. She remained unconvinced that this was a good trend for an industry focused on health and well-being.

Case Questions

1. What are the pros and cons for Children's Hospital in accepting the donation from Ashley and Mitch in exchange for naming rights?
2. Are there alternatives, such as a donation without naming rights, that you might propose?

3. Given the sentiments among community members, are there steps the hospital should take to work with the community to establish donation guidelines, or are such decisions only relevant to the hospital itself?
4. Should guidelines be established about which companies or industries should be allowed to donate money?

Short Case 31
Patient Satisfaction in an Inner-City Hospital

Claudia Caine and Anthony R. Kovner

Lutheran Medical Center is a 400-bed, inner-city, community teaching hospital located in Southwest Brooklyn. It is also one of only two Level I trauma centers in the borough of Brooklyn. There are three major competing hospitals within five miles of the hospital and this competition continually challenges the hospital's efforts to grow and gain market share. Lutheran's community is made up mainly of immigrants and blue-collar wage earners. The payer mix is 75 percent Medicare and Medicaid. Recent efforts, therefore, have focused on reaching out to the neighboring community of Bay Ridge where the population is dense, better insured, and facing the closure of its only hospital (one of the aforementioned three hospitals).

With low New York State reimbursement rates, the high cost of New York healthcare (wages, malpractice, benefits, etc.), the hospital must keep 90 percent of its beds filled in order to break even. Lutheran is already known as a low-cost provider, so growth is its only real option.

Most hospital administrators know that having a hospital routinely filled at over 85 percent creates many challenges. Safety, quality of care, and patient satisfaction must be emphasized more than at hospitals at lower, more comfortable occupancy rates.

In response to its primary objective (i.e., growth and maintenance of high census while still improving quality of care, safety, and patient satisfaction levels), the hospital embarked upon an effort to dramatically improve its emergency department (ED). Generally known to be the "front door" to the community, over 70 percent of Lutheran's admissions come from the ED. Lutheran's thinking about the ED is that if it works beautifully, patient satisfaction will go up, first impressions will be positive, quality of care and patient safety will be improved, and more and more residents of the community, and beyond, will choose the hospital for care.

The hospital did three main things to address the goal of becoming the ED of choice in Brooklyn:

1. Replaced the leadership of the ED.
2. Expanded the ED's space by 60 percent and modernized it.
3. Redesigned all ED systems and processes.

The specific measurable goals for this redesign project were to:

1. increase the percentage of patients reporting being "satisfied" or "very satisfied" from 52 percent to 70 percent;
2. increase visits from 147 per day to 175 per day;
3. have a provider see every patient within 30 minutes of arrival in the ED;
4. have fewer than 2 percent of patients return to the ED for a second visit within 48 hours of their first visit; and
5. hire 100 percent ED-trained physicians in the ED.

The project began in 2002 and was completed in 2006. The first step was to replace the leadership. The leaders, at that time, were reluctant to change and were not familiar with national best practice models in emergency department care. Also, 80 percent of the physicians were non-ED-trained. Replacing the chairman and the vice president of nursing for the ED took one year to accomplish. Turning over the staff to have 100 percent ED-trained physicians took three and a half years.

Next, in 2005, the hospital formed an ED Process Redesign Task Force. Previous leadership had attempted a redesign in 2002, but it failed. A major lesson learned was that redesign and "overhaul" are impossible without the right leadership in place.

This effort was led by the hospital chief operating officer and the new chairman of the ED. The other members of the team included the chief nursing officer, the vice president of nursing for the ED, the nurse manager for the ED, the ED educator, and the VP of operations responsible for the ED.

There were seven main results of the process redesign:

1. A care team model for the ED was created, allowing small groupings of patients to be treated by a team that included MD, RN, and aide.
2. A position called ED patient navigator was created. This person was available to communicate with referring physicians about their patients and serve as a case manager for ED patients.
3. The role of the ED nursing care coordinator/charge nurse was redefined to be the daily "director" of movement, operations, and oversight of the entire ED.
4. The traditional nursing triage model was replaced with a combined triage/fast-track model. Physician assistants (PAs) replaced nurses at

triage and triaged, treated, and released (when appropriate), or triaged and moved patients to the main ED when appropriate.

5. All ED staff were given portable internal zone phones to increase communications and reduce the noise level.
6. Paper charts were replaced with a fully automated medical record and tracking system.
7. Bedside registration was implemented, so patients go directly from triage to an ED bed without stopping to be registered.

Within 18 months of introducing the process redesign team, the following occurred:

- Patient visits went from 147 per day to 172 per day.
- The average door-to-provider (MD or PA) time went from 90 minutes to 30 minutes.
- 100 percent of MDs were ED-trained.
- Two percent of patients needed to return to the ED within 48 hours of their initial visit.
- ED patient satisfaction went from 52 percent to 66 percent (still 4 percentage points short of the goal).

Clearly the team was disappointed by the lack of progress in patient satisfaction, but they were not confused by it. The reason was that as patient volume increased, the number of available hospital beds remained fixed, so patients waited longer as more time was needed to move patients from the ED to a hospital bed. Because the hospital must remain at over 90 percent occupancy to break even, adding beds would have created operating losses for the institution—an option the team did not have available.

The new challenge became improving patient satisfaction given the increasing wait times for hospital beds. The team took the following eight actions:

1. Added a team of physicians to the ED to provide care to admitted patients as they awaited beds.
2. Created a labor-management joint team to improve patient flow on the inpatient units (with a goal of discharging patients within four hours of a discharge clearance note being written by a physician).
3. Created the ED Diplomat program, which is a daily 2:00 p.m. to 8:00 p.m. rotation of senior hospital leaders who meet each ED patient with a long stay, explain the wait, manage expectations, and give free hospital TV services and free parking when necessary.
4. Increased nurse and nurse aide staffing in the ED.

5. Ordered hospital beds to move patients from stretchers to more comfortable beds while they wait.
6. Began a program to provide food and telephones for patients in the ED.
7. Opened a discharge lounge for patients awaiting discharge to open up beds sooner.
8. Created housekeeping and transport SWAT teams to facilitate room turnovers on inpatient floors.

Most recent measurements show patient satisfaction in the ED has increased to 75 percent. However, it is premature to call this an upward trend.

Discussion Question

What more can this hospital do to address this problem—understanding that opening more inpatient beds would cost upwards of $1.5 million and put the already ailing institution into a negative financial position?

Reading List of Books
for Healthcare Managers

Bibliographic materials are scattered throughout the text. This section is devoted to a short list of management books chosen because they are (1) useful and (2) easy to read.

Berry, L. L., and K. D. Seltman. 2008. *Management Lessons from Mayo Clinic.* New York: McGraw Hill.

Bossidy, L., and R. Charan. 2002. *Execution: The Discipline of Getting Things Done.* New York: Crown.

Bridges, W. 1991. *Managing Transitions: Making the Most of the Change.* Reading, MA: Perseus Books.

Buckingman, M., and C. Coffman. 1999. *First, Break All the Rules: What the World's Greatest Managers Do Differently.* New York: Simon and Schuster.

Christensen, C. M. 1997. *The Innovator's Dilemma: When New Technologies Cause Great Firms to Fail.* Boston: Harvard University Press.

Collins, J. 2001. *Good to Great.* New York: HarperCollins.

Gray, J. A. M. 2004. *Evidence-Based Healthcare*, 2nd edition. New York: Churchill Livingstone.

Griffith, J. R. 1993. *The Moral Challenges of Health Care Management.* Chicago: Health Administration Press.

Kotter, J. P. 1996. *Leading Change.* Boston: Harvard Business School Press.

Kouzes, J. M., and B. Z. Posner. 2007. *The Leadership Challenge: How to Keep Getting Extraordinary Things Done in Organizations*, 4th edition. San Francisco: Jossey-Bass.

McAlearney, A. S. 2003. *Population Health Management: Strategies to Improve Outcomes.* Chicago: Health Administration Press.

O'Toole, J., and E. E. Lawler III. 2006. *The New American Workplace.* New York: Palmgrave McMillan.

Pointer, D. D., and J. E. Orlikoff. 2002. *Getting to Great: Principles of Health Care Organization Governance.* San Francisco: Jossey-Bass.

Porter, M. E., and E. O. Teisberg. 2006. *Redefining Health Care: Creating Value-Based Competition on Results.* Boston: Harvard Business School Press.

Salamon, J. 2008. *Hospital.* New York: Penguin Press.

Senge, P. M. 1990. *The Fifth Discipline: The Art and Practice of the Learning Organization.* New York: Doubleday Currency Publishers.

Studer, Q. 2003. *Hardwiring Excellence.* Gulf Breeze, FL: Fire Starter.

Index

Academic Emergency Medicine, 161

Academic medical centers: personal digital assistant (PDA) purchases by, 146–147; professional integration in, 293–294

Accelerating Change and Transformation in Organizations and Networks (ACTION), 8

Accountability, 357–418; application of, 357; case studies in, 377–418; commentary on, 357–361; customer-focused, 357; external demands for, 21–22, 26; for job responsibilities, 70–71; for knowledge transfer, 22; manager's perspective on, 378–379, 387–405; *versus* mutual adjustment, 379; and organizational performance, 357, 358–360; patient's perspective on, 377, 378, 379, 380–387; of physicians, 357, 377, 378; readings abut, 363–376; stakeholders' mutual agreements regarding, 379

Accreditation, of home health care organizations, 125

Accreditation Commission for Health Care, Inc., 125

Acquisition, of research evidence, 8, 14–16, 23

ACTION (Accelerating Change and Transformation in Organizations and Networks), 8

Acuity-adaptable rooms, 195, 196–197, 198, 199–201, 200–201

Adaptation, 295–353; case studies in, 317–353; to change, 251; commentary on, 297–298; in home health care industry, 318–328; readings about, 299–316; strategic cycling and, 299–316; in visiting nurse services, 317–328

"Adhocracy," 152

Advice, as research evidence source, 20

Advocates/advocacy, for patients' rights, 246, 378

Affirmative action programs, 409

Agency for Health Care Policy and Research, 93. *See also* Agency for Healthcare Research and Quality (AHRQ)

Agency for Healthcare Research and Quality (AHRQ): Accelerating Change and Transformation in Organizations and Networks (ACTION), 8; clinical practice guidelines, 93; as evidence-based management resource, 8, 12–13; Integrated Delivery System Research Network (IDSRN), 8; as management research evidence source, 20; as research evidence source, 15, 20

Agenda for Change, 92

Alternatives, selection of, 13

Ambulatory care, physicians' complaints about, 292

Ambulatory care networks, of Medicaid, 271–272

Ambulatory surgery centers, 4, 297, 367–368; adverse effects on hospitals, 221–222; as wholesale strategy, 224

American Cancer Society, 341–342

American College of Healthcare Executives (ACHE), website, 59–60

American Healthways, 187

American Hospital Association, 251; Healthy Communities movement, 243

American Management Association, website, 59–60

American Medical News, 188

Anecdotal evidence, 20

Anti-kickback laws, 224

Application, of research evidence, 8, 13, 18–19

Appreciative inquiry, 220, 230–231

Assessment, of research evidence, 8, 13, 16–17

Audit systems, 241, 242, 248

Authority, of managers, 264

Autonomy: of nurses, 215–216; of physicians, 223

Balanced scorecards, 83, 300, 358

Baldrige Health Care Criteria. *see* Malcolm Baldrige Health Care Criteria for Performance Excellence

Baptist Hospital, Inc., management practices: focus on patient and markets, 246, 247; human resources management, 250, 251; information management, 248–249; leadership, 241–242, 243; and organizational characteristics, 240

Behavioral healthcare, restricted health insurance coverage for, 410–411

Benchmarking, 86, 148, 309

Berwick, Donald, 79

Best practices, 155, 230

Billing process: patient-focused, 372; reengineering of, 372; for uninsured patients, 339

Billings, John Shaw, 295

Board of trustees: meetings of, 140; relationship with hospital CEOs, 378–379, 387–405

Bonuses, 242

Bottom-line management, 223

Bottom-up processes, positive deviance as, 230

Brown and Toland Medical Group, 189

Budgets: capital, 292; patient care directors' influence on, 116–124

Bureaucracy, 300; machine, 152; professional, 153

Burnout, 223, 236

"Burnout jobs," 205

Bush, George W., 363–364

California: healthcare pricing availability in, 369; physician group bankruptcies in, 185

California Cooperative Healthcare Reporting Initiative (CCHRI), Diabetes Continuous Quality Improvement Project, 191

California HealthCare Foundation, 371

Canadian Health Services Research Foundation, 9

Capital expenditures, as percentage of sales, 85

Capitation, 154; changes in, 305–306

Cardiac arterial bypass graft (CABG), patient's critique of, 380–387

Care continuum, 306

Career development. *See also* Professional development: executive, 251

CareScience, 98

Case management departments, promotions within, 352–353

Case managers, 21

Case Western Reserve University, 267

Catholic Health Initiative, management practices: focus on patients, 247; leadership, 241, 242; measurement and analysis, 248–249; organizational characteristics and, 240; process management, 252; values statement, 241

Cedars Lebanon Hospital, Los Angeles, 114–115

Celebration Health, 198

Center for Health Management Research (CHMR), 15, 18–21

Center on Budget and Policy Priorities, 162

Centers for Disease Control and Prevention (CDC), 160–161

Centers for Medicare & Medicaid Services: Conditions of Participation, 127; Core Measures Program, 351, 353; hospice and home health care regulations, 125, 126, 127; Hospital Compare website, 92; in-hospital mortality rate calculations of, 92; performance accountability standards of, 21; as research evidence source, 20; "7th Scope of Work" initiative, 248

Centralization, as organizational design, 177–183

Central Med Health System (CMHS), investment decision making process at, 340–347

Champions, 234–235

Change: adaptation to, 251; in medical technology, 297; organizational support for, 357, 358; in performance measurement, 90; understanding of, 6

Charge description masters (CDMs), 370

Charges, 365–366; analysis of, 370; definition of, 365, 366

Charity care. *See also* Uninsured patients: case studies in, 405–408; pricing of, 371, 372

Charts, organizational, 153, 179

Checklists, 99

Chief executive officers (CEOs), 357; and charity care, 405–408; patients' complaints to, 377, 378, 379, 380–387; performance evaluation of, 400–404; relationship with board of trustees, 378–379, 387–405

Children's Hospital, Columbus, Ohio, 115

Christensen, Clayton, 163

Chronic Care Model, 156

Chronic disease management. *See* Disease management programs

Citizens Healthcare Working Group, 160

Clara Maas Health System, continuous quality improvement initiative, 137–139

Clarian Health, 198

Cleveland Clinic Foundation, 322

Cleveland MetroHealth Medical Center, 321, 322, 326

Clinical practice, guidelines for, 93, 94

Clinical programs, investment decision making for, 341–346

Clinton administration, 174

Cochrane Collaborative: Consumer and Communication Review Group, 12–13; Effective Practice and Organization of Care Group, 8; as evidence-based management evidence source, 12–13; randomized clinical trial registry, 107; website, 23

Codman, E.A., 79

Collaboration, physician-hospital. *See* Professional integration

Colleagues, as research evidence source, 14

Commission on Accreditation of Rehabilitation Services, 125

Commoditization, of healthcare, 364

Communication: strategic planning-based, 304; structural dialogue, 232–235

Communities, hospitals' relationships with, 243, 298

Community surveys, 297

Compensation. *See also* Financial incentives; Income; Salaries: for disease management, 189; and evidence-based decision making, 23

Competencies, in healthcare management, 8–9

Competency Assessment Tool, 62–63

Competition: among healthcare organizations, 297; *versus* cooperation, 306; in cosmetic surgery industry, 349; in home health care industry, 318–328; physician-hospital, 227–229; strategic response to, 308

Competitor analysis, 310

Complaints: about ambulatory care, 292; from managers, 69–71; from patients, 247, 377, 378, 379, 380–387; standardized response process for, 247

Compliance, with post-discharge medication plans, 229–230

Comprehensive critical coronary care (CCC), 198

Computerized provider order entry (CPOE) systems, 108–109, 200; implementation failures, 114–115

Concierge medicine, 224

Confidentiality, of medical records, 249–250

Conflicts of interest, 408–409

Congestive heart failure, disease

management programs for, 183, 189–190

Consultants, 24; healthcare market share of, 216–217; as performance improvement team support, 248; as research evidence source, 14, 20

Consumer Reports, 360, 361

Consumers and Communication Review Group, 15

Contingency planning, 311

Continuous quality improvement (CQI), 137–139, 242, 243

Continuum of care, 153

Contracts, negotiation of, 215

Control, 81–147; case studies, 107–147; commentary on, 81–87; example, 81–82; loss of, 305; in performance measurement, 82–147; readings about, 89–105; as strategic planning outcome, 304; system of, 83–87

Controllers, 50–58

Convenient Care Association, 164

Convenient care clinics, 153–154, 159– 172, 225; concerns about, 163, 165; definition of, 159–160; growth of, 160; integration with traditional healthcare delivery, 165–167; and medical home model, 165; rationale for, 160–162; standards of, 164; uninsured patients' use of, 162

Cooperation, *versus* competition, 306

Coordination, organizational, 152–153

Corporate university model, 181–183

Cor Solutions, 192

Cosmetic surgery practice, changing focus of, 348–350

Cost. *See also* Healthcare costs: definition of, 365, 366; fixed, 85; per case, 85; per day, 85; per visit, 85; relationship to charges, 366; variable, 85

Cost control, management information system for, 116–124

Cost pricing, market-driven, 370

Cost sharing, 363, 366–367

Crisis management, 231–232

Crossing the Quality Chasm (Institute of Medicine), 357, 538

Cross-subsidies, for uninsured patients, 369–370

Cultural convergence, 235–236

Cultural organizational dimension, 20, 22–23, 25, 26

Cusano, Anthony, 229

Customers, of healthcare organizations, 305

"Dance of the blind reflex," 224, 225– 226, 227, 234

Databases, as research evidence source, 14, 15

Database searching, guidelines for, 15

Data collection: cost of, 90; as managerial skill, 5–6

Day care, medical, 292–293

"Death in the middle" phenomenon, 373

Decentralization, *versus* centralization, 176–183

Decentralized nursing stations, 195, 197, 199–200

Decision making. *See also* Evidence-based decision making: about clinical expansion investments, 340–346; about organizational design, 173–174; evaluation of, 359; harmful, 27; for organizational adaptation, 317; strategic planning-based, 304

Deductibles, increase in, 367

Defensive reasoning, 220, 226; appreciative inquiry response to, 230

Development. *See also* Career development; Professional development: managerial framework for, 6; organizational, 175–183; staff development programs, 23

Diabetes Control and Complications Trial, 193

Diabetes Healthways, 192

Diabetes management programs, 190– 193; commercial, 192–193

Dimensions, organizational, 24–26

Disability costs, as performance evaluation measure, 85

Discharge: follow-up telephone calls after, 297; medication plan compliance after, 229–231

Discharge planning: managers of, 352–

353; protocols for, 121

Discipline, organizational, 304

Discounts: in managed care, 370, 371; for uninsured patients, 371

Disease Management Association of America, 166, 187

Disease management programs, 156, 166, 187; case studies, 183–193; for congestive heart failure, 183, 189–190; definition, 187; for diabetes mellitus, 190–193; in-house programs, 188; overview, 186–187; physicians' views of, 188–190

Disease Management Purchasing Consortium and Advisory Council, 186

Disparity, in healthcare access, 351–352

Diversity, of hospital workforce, 251

Diversity training, 251

DM Vendor Profile, 186

Donations, to hospitals, 413–415

Drucker, Peter, 107

Effective Practice and Organization of Care Groups, 15

Ego costs, 18

Einstein, Albert, 163

Electronic medical records (EMRs), 85, 249; of convenient care clinics, 146, 165; of telephone medical services, 225

Electronic medical record system implementation, 107, 108–115; barriers to, 109, 110–114; case study, 107, 108–115; failure, 114–115; information systems departments' perspective on, 109–111; physicians' opposition to, 110–113, 114, 115

Emergency care departments: non-urgent care provided by, 160–161; overcrowding in, 160–161; patient satisfaction with, 329–330, 415–418; quality improvement in, 139; storefront clinics and, 225; uninsured patients' use of, 161, 339, 406, 407, 408; waiting times in, 139, 337, 338, 417

Emergency Medical Treatment and Active Labor Act (EMTALA), 222, 406

Emotional intelligence, 5

Empathy, 5

Employers, hospitals' relationships with, 247

End-of-life care, 290

Environment, organizational, 151

Environmental analysis, 60–62

Environmental context, of healthcare, 305–307

Environmental demands, 297

Environmental scanning, 246–247, 310

Ergonomics, 411–412

Errors: in medication administration, 86; patients' reporting of, 381–383, 386; in transactions, 82

Estes, Melinda, 269–270, 274, 276, 278

Ethical behavior, of hospitals, 242–243

Ethnic factors, in healthcare disparity, 351–352

Evidence-based decision making: acceptance of, 7–8; knowledge transfer study of, 19–21; as managerial competency, 8–9; models, 11–12; organizational guidelines for, 23; as process, 10–12; skills required for, 5–6; underutilization of, 19–21; Web-based information for, 8

Evidence-based health services management: applications of, 12–19; balanced scorecards in, 300; components of, 261; in core business transaction management, 12, 13; definition of, 10–12; objective/purpose of, 16; in operational management, 12, 13; organizational dimensions and, 24–26; reconsideration of, 7–10; strategic cycling model of, 299–316; strategic importance of, 21–22; in strategic management, 12, 13; strategies for increasing the use of, 20–26; systematic reviews of, 12–13

Evidence-based medicine: integrated with evidence-based health services management, 21; rationale for, 27

Evidence-based organizational design, 194–202; acuity-adaptable rooms, 195, 196–197, 198, 199–201; decentralized nursing stations, 195, 197, 199–200; financial implications of, 200–201; implementation challenges to, 199–200

Evidence-based quality improvement, 127–137

Evidence syntheses, 15–16

Expectations: about medication errors, 86; about organizational performance, 357, 358–360; about patients, 378; as control system component, 83, 86; of nurses, 215–216; of patients, 377–378; of physicians, 215, 216

Experimentation, 6

Experts, as research evidence source, 14

Faculty practice administration, 37–50

Federal agencies, healthcare research support from, 8

Federal government, healthcare oversight role of, 222

Federally qualified health centers (FQHC), 406, 407

Feedback, 81

Fee-for-service plans, 154

Financial incentives, for goal achievement, 242

Financial management, 3

Financial performance improvement, of orthopedic units, 116–124; ADC Census requirements and, 121, 123; discharge planning protocols in, 121; hours-per-patient day (HPPD) and, 121, 122; length-of-stay (LOS) reductions and, 117, 121, 123–124; monthly departmental variance reports in, 116–117, 118–120

5 Million Lives Campaign, 155

Focus, organizational, 84

Focus groups, 23, 297

Fraud, 306, 324

Freidson, Eliot, 213

Fringe benefit costs, as performance evaluation measure, 85

Funding, sources of, 298

Fundraising, 388, 393, 413–415

Geisinger Health System, 155, 165, 166

General Electric (GE), 4

Generative relationships, 311

Gerner, Brandon, 345

Globalization, 221, 222

Goal achievement: measurement of, 151; as organizational purpose, 151–152

Goal planning, for professional development, 63

Goals: comparison with performance, 252; as control system component, 83, 84–85; definition of, 84; formulation of, 357; management research and, 22; organizational, 3; as performance evaluation criterion, 83; prioritization of, 75–76; specification of, 85

Goal statements, 84–85

Google Scholar, 15

Group Health Cooperative of Puget Sound, 156

Harvard Business Review, 20, 163

Harvard Vanguard Medical, disease management program, 188

HCOs. *See* Healthcare organizations

Health Affairs, 20

Healthcare, continuous shifts in, 305–307

Healthcare access, disparity in, 351–352

Health Care Advisory Board, 20, 341–342

Healthcare costs: barriers to reduction of, 155–156; out-of-pocket, 366–367; as outsourcing cause, 221

Healthcare delivery system, deficiencies in, 160–161

Healthcare Financial Management Association, Patient Friendly Billing, 372

Health Care Financing Administration. *See also* Centers for Medicare & Medicaid Services, 92

Healthcare insurance coverage: behavioral/psychiatric care restrictions in, 410–411; consumer-driven plans, 367; cost-payment percentages of, 369, 370; deductibles, 367; payer-mix, 298; premiums, 367, 368

Healthcare Leadership Alliance, 8, 27

Healthcare organizations: funding sources, 298; goals of, 3; as research evidence source, 14, 15; types of, 4

Healthcare reform, 160

Healthcare report cards, 90, 94–95

Healthcare system: barriers to changes

in, 155–156; complexity of, 4; performance standards for, 21–22

HealthCast 2020: Creating a Sustainable Health System, 364, 365

Health Insurance Portability and Accountability Act (HIPAA), 249–250

Health Leadership Competency Model, 8–9

Health maintenance organizations (HMOs), 4; hospital-owned, 347–348; managers' conflicts of interest with, 408–409; Medicaid, 347–348; organizational design of, 154

Health Management Services, 192

Health Plan Employer Data and Information Set (HEDIS), 93

Health savings accounts (HSAs), 367

Heart failure patients: evaluation of care for, 90; hospital-specific mortality rates in, 92; minority-group, 351

Henry Ford Health System, 188, 246

Home health care: hospital-based, 320, 339; Medicare reimbursement for, 322, 324; monitoring of, 326; physician visits in, 327

Home health care organizations: accreditation of, 125; contracts with hospitals, 320–321; evidence-based quality management in, 124–137; performance data of, 124–137; regulation of, 125–126; response to collaborators and competitors, 318–328

Home Health Quality Initiative, 127

Hospice care: quality assessment and performance improvement in, 126, 127, 128; regulation of, 125

Hospital Compare website, 92

Hospital Corporation of America, 154

Hospitalist programs, 204–207

Hospitalists, 219, 222, 224–225; definition of, 224; effect on hospital costs and quality of care, 17, 18–19; in surgical services, 237

Hospitalization, patient's critique of, 380–387

Hospital-physician relationship. *See* Professional integration

Hospital report cards, 309

Hospitals. *See also* Inpatient care; *names of specific hospitals:* acuity-adaptable rooms, 195, 196–197, 198, 199–201; bad debts of, 406; charge description masters (CDMs) of, 370; charity care provided by, 405–408; community, 222; consumers' trust in, 365; contracts with home health care organizations, 320–321; donations to, 413–415; effect of outpatient facilities on, 221–222; healthcare disparity of, 351–352; mergers of, 27; mission, 81; reimbursement sources of, 367; services to uninsured patients, 405–408; specialty, 221–222, 224; uncompensated care provided for, 162; values, 81; vision, 81

Hours-per-patient day (HPPD), 121, 122

Hugo, Victor, 364

Human resources management, 250–251; professional development in, 62–63; role in organizational development, 177–183

Hypertension care, pay-for-performance plans for, 141–143

IDSRN (Integrated Delivery System Research Network), 8

Implementation, in strategic cycling planning, 311–312

Incentive systems, 83, 86–87

Incident reports, 85

Income, of physicians, 222

Independent physician association (IPA), organizational design implementation, 183–193

India: healthcare costs in, 155, 225; healthcare tourism in, 225

Industry-University Research Collaborative, 8

Inefficiency, 107

Inflation, 366

Information: as control system component, 83, 85; for performance measurement, 83; as power, 364–365

Information management teams, 248–249

Information systems: just-in-time, 87;

organizational design of, 210–212
Information technology (IT), 91; effect on organizational design, 154; role in performance measurement, 99–100
Injury prevention, 411–412
Innovation: disruptive, 163; process, 154
Inpatient care: hospitalists' role in, 224–225; *versus* outpatient care, 221–222
Institute for Healthcare Improvement, 20, 155, 252; Whole Systems Measures, 129–130
Institute of Medicine, Report of the Committee on Quality, 357, 358
Integrated Delivery System Research Network (IDSRN), 8
Integrated healthcare delivery designs, 153
Intensive care units (ICUs): electronic monitoring and reporting systems, 249; pediatric cardiac, 287–292
Intermountain Healthcare system: information management, 249; Institute for Healthcare Delivery Research, 248; Institute for Healthcare Improvement participation, 252; organizational characteristics and, 240; strategic planning, 246; TPS methodology use, 155
Internal analysis, for professional development planning, 61–63
Internet: as healthcare information source, 365; as performance indicator source, 129–130; as research evidence source, 14, 15, 20
Interventional cardiology programs, 222, 343–346
Interviewing, of faculty practice administrator candidates, 37–50
Investment decision making, 340–346, 340–347

Job changes, 72–75
Job descriptions, lack of, 68–69
Job responsibilities, lack of accountability for, 70–71
Jobs, managerial, characteristics of, 5
Job satisfaction, of nurses, 215–216
Joint Commission on the Accreditation of Healthcare Organizations (JCAHO),

20; Agenda for Change initiative, 92; Core Measure sets, 90, 92–93, 98; home health care accreditation by, 125; Key Measures, 248; as management research evidence source, 20; ORYX initiative, 92–93; performance accountability standards of, 2021; performance data requirements of, 92–93; as performance indicator source, 129
Joint ventures, 219
Journal articles: research evidence presentation in, 18; as research evidence source, 20
Journal clubs, 22–23
Journal of General Internet Medicine, 188
Journal of Healthcare Management, 62
Journal of Oncology Management, 341–342

Kaiser-Permanente, 154; disease management program, 188
Kizer, Kenneth, 213
Knowledge management, 248–250
Knowledge transfer: accountability structure for, 22; managers' participation in, 23–24; between researchers and managers, 19–21
Kurtzman, Ellen, 213

Leadership, Baldrige Healthcare Criteria for, 241–243
Lean production processes, 154
Leapfrog Group, 21
Learning, organizational, 251
Learning organizations, 177–178, 180
Length-of-stay (LOS), reductions in, 117, 121, 123–124, 204–205, 206
Les Miserables (Hugo), 364
Life Masters, 183, 184
Lift systems, staff's implementation of, 411–412
Linkage analysis, 311
Lovelace Clinic, disease management program, 188
Loyalty, of patients, 247
Lutheran Medical Center, Brooklyn, New York, 415–418

Malcolm Baldrige Health Care Criteria for Performance Excellence, 97–98, 240–257; focus on patients and markets, 246–248; focus on staff, 250–251; leadership, 241–243; measurement analysis and knowledge management, 248–250; organizational performance improvement, 256; process management, 251–256; strategic planning, 243–246

Mall clinics, 225. *See also* Convenient care clinics

Malpractice lawsuits, 378

Managed care. *See also* Health maintenance organizations (HMOs): discounts for, 370, 371; effect on reimbursement payments, 305–306; Medicaid, 360

Management: bottom-line, 223; strategic approach in, 5–6

Management information system, for staffing and cost control, 116–124

Management Mistakes in Healthcare (Hofmann and Perry), 8

Management research: factors affecting, 20; manager's participation in, 23–24, 26

Managers: authority of, 264; clinical outcome improvement participation, 219; complaints from, 69–71; conflicts of interest, 408–409; of discharge planning, 352–353; expectations about patients, 378; job resignation, 36, 68–69, 72–75; as minority-group members, 409–410; morale of, 69–71; organizational settings for, 4; perspective on accountability, 378–379, 387–405; power of, 263, 264; roles and responsibilities of, 3–4; self-image of, 3–4; underutilization of evidence-based decision making among, 19–21

Market assessments, 23

Marketing, competition *versus* cooperation in, 306

Market share: as performance evaluation measure, 85; relationship to organization's size, 216–217

Maryland Quality Indicators, 248

Matria, 192, 193

Mayo Clinic, 155, 360–361

McDonald's, 82

McKesson CareEnhance, 192

Medicaid: ambulatory care networks, 271–272; cost-payment percentages of, 369, 370; effect on healthcare system complexity, 4; HMO contracts, 270–271; HMOs, 347–348; managed care, 270–271, 347–348, 360; performance evaluation requirement of, 94

Medical advisory panel (MAP), of structural dialogue, 232–233

Medical records. *See also* Electronic medical records (EMRs): confidentiality of, 249–250

Medical supply manufacturers, healthcare market share of, 216–217

Medical technology, changes in, 297

Medicare: cost-payment percentages of, 369, 370; effect on healthcare system complexity, 4; effect on professional integration, 222; fraud associated with, 324; home health care performance monitoring by, 324, 326; home health care reimbursement by, 125, 322, 324; as hospital pricing information source, 367; performance evaluation requirement of, 94

Medicare Modernization Act of 2003, 126–237

Medicare Quality Improvement Community (MedQIC), 130

Medication errors, 198; expectations regarding, 86

Medication plans, post-discharge, 229–230

MEDLINE, 15

Mentors, loss of, 74

Merck & Co., Inc., 192

Mergers, of hospitals, 27

Metaphors, 231–232

MetroHealth System of Cleveland, 265–287; departmental reorganization, 274; financial status, 272–274; information systems, 274; Management Council of, 270, 278, 279–281; as Medicaid provider, 265, 270–271; medical leadership of, 276, 278; medical staff/management relationship, 268–270; mission statement, 267–268; organizational chart, 277; outcome measurement program, 274–275; overview of, 267–268; quality improvement department, 275, 282–283

Minnesota, healthcare pricing availability in, 369

Minority-group members: disparity in healthcare access, 351–352; as managers and professional staff, 251, 409–410

Mintzberg, Henry, 149, 152–153

Minute clinics, 4

Mission/mission statements: applications of, 241; definition of, 84; example, 81

Missouri PRO, 248

Mistakes, in healthcare management, 8, 27

Modern Healthcare, 20

Monthly departmental variance reports, 116–117, 118–120

Morale: of managers, 69–71; of staff, 250

Mortality rates, hospital-specific, 92

Motivation, 5; lack of, as error source, 82; as strategic planning outcome, 304

Multiculturalism, 409–410

Musculoskeletal injuries, prevention of, 411–412

Mutual adjustment, 379

Myocardial infarction patients: evaluation of care for, 90; hospital-specific mortality rates in, 92

National Association of Community Health Centers, Inc., 161

National Center for Healthcare Leadership, Health Leadership Competency Model, 8–9

National Center for Health Statistics, 160–161

National Healthcare Report Card, 90

National health insurance, 9, 174

National Hospice and Palliative Care Organization, 127, 218

National Hospital Ambulatory Medical Care Survey, 161

National Quality Forum, performance accountability standards of, 21

National Science Foundation, Industry-University Research Collaborative, 8

Needleman, Jack, 213

Negotiations: of contracts, 215; financial, 366

Neighborhood health centers, 4

New England Journal of Medicine, 20

New Hampshire, healthcare pricing availability in, 369

New York City, Medicaid managed care in, 360

New York State, healthcare costs in, 415

New Zealand, healthcare outcome improvement in, 235–236

North Mississippi Medical Center, 371

Nurse practitioners, 160, 163, 225

Nurses: attitudes toward acuity-adaptable rooms, 199, 201; attitudes toward healthcare managers, 3–4; consumers' trust in, 365; job satisfaction, 215–216; professional environment, 215–216; relationships with hospital CEOs, 390–391, 392, 394, 396; relationships with patient care directors, 287, 288–289, 291; role in financial performance, 116–124

Nursing, accountability-based practice model of, 242

Nursing homes: diversity management in, 409–410; skilled, 4

Nursing stations, decentralized, 195, 197, 199–200

Objectives: as control system component, 83, 84–85; determination of, 84–85; lack of specification of, 85; as performance evaluation criteria, 83; of physicians, nurses, and hospitals, 216; strategic planning support for, 304

Obstetrical-gynecological services, 346–347

Older adults, annual physician visits by, 161

Omnibus Budget Reconciliation Act, 360

Operating room staff, 222

Operational efficiency, 221

Operational management, 12, 13

Opportunities, identification of, 5

Opportunity costs, of research evidence applications, 18

Organizational culture, 20, 22–23, 26

Organizational design, 149–212; case studies of, 173–212; centralized, 177–183; commentary on, 151–158; decision making about, 173–174; definition of, 152; evidence-based, 194–202; healthcare delivery and, 154–155; for hospitalist program, 204–207; of information systems, 210–212; levels of, 173–174; for medical center restructuring, 202–204; readings about, 159–172; of rehabilitation services, 207–210; role of management in, 156–157; system-focused, 177–183; types of, 152; understanding of, 152–153; variation and innovation in, 154–156

Organizational development, centralized, 175–183

Organizational focus, 84

Organizational structure. *See also* Organizational design: determinants of, 174–178

Organizations: definition of, 151; goal achievement purpose of, 151–152

Orthopedic units, financial performance improvement in, 116–124; ADC Census requirements and, 121, 123; discharge planning protocols in, 121; hours-per-patient day (HPPD) and, 121, 122; length-of-stay (LOS) reductions and, 117, 121, 123–124; monthly departmental variance reports in, 116–117, 118–120

ORYX initiative, 92–93

Osteoporosis screening, 190

Outcome and Assessment Information Set (OASIS), 127, 324, 326

Out-of-pocket payment, for healthcare, 369, 372, 373

Outpatient care. *See also* Ambulatory surgery centers: growth in, 221–222

Outpatient imaging centers, 224

Outsourcing firms, healthcare market share of, 216–217

Overtime, as performance evaluation measure, 85

Patient advocates, 246

Patient care directors (PCDs): financial performance and responsibilities of, 116–124; of pediatric cardiac intensive care units, 287–292

Patient care guidelines, 7

Patients: advocacy for, 246, 378; complaints from, 377, 378, 379, 380–387; expectations of, 377–378; hospitals' relationships with, 246–248; managers' expectations about, 378

Patient satisfaction: with acuity-adapatable rooms, 198; with emergency department care, 329–330, 415–418; with inner-city hospitals, 415–418; as performance measure, 93–94; strategies for, 246–248; surveys of, 85, 297

Pay-for-call stipends, 222

Pay-for-performance plans: for hypertension care, 141–143; influence on quality goals, 96; legislation related to, 360; performance accountability standards of, 21

Payment, definition of, 366

Pediatric care directors, relationships of: with families, 287, 289–290; with nurses, 287, 288–289, 291; social workers, 288, 290–291

Performance: as Baldrige Health Care Criteria, 256; expectations of, 357, 358–360; managers' contributions to, 36; patients' control of, 378; required reporting of, 85

Performance data: analysis costs, 97, 98–99; comparative analysis of, 86, 90–92; costs related to, 90; from home health care organizations, 124–137; Joint Commission on the Accreditation of Healthcare Organizations requirements for, 92–93; publicly-available, 90; reliability of, 99; reporting of, 90–91, 91, 97

Performance data collection: costs of, 97, 98–99; point-of-service, 99

Performance data management

committees, 99, 100

Performance data warehouses, 99

Performance evaluation: goal-based, 83; of hospital CEOs, 400–404; measures for, 85; objectives-based, 83; stakeholders' expectations and, 357, 368–360

Performance expectations, 4–5

Performance improvement councils, 252

Performance improvement teams, 241–242, 244, 248, 252

Performance measurement/measures, 89–105; alignment with quality improvement, 132; challenges to, 89–91; changes in, 90; clinical performance, 131; comparative outcome-based, 90–93, 95; control in, 82–147; costs of, 98–99; customer satisfaction, 131; efficiency of, 98–99; evaluation of, 91–95; frequent reporting of, 241; healthcare processes-based, 93; for home health care, 127–137; influence of external stakeholders on, 95–97; as information source, 95; information technology use in, 99–100; meaningful systems in, 95–100; "measurement creep" prevention in, 100; multidimensional, 241; operational performance, 131; patient outcomes-based, 92–93; patient satisfaction-based, 93–94; questions for evaluation of, 97–98, 100; risk management, 131–132; sources of, 129–130; standardized, 90, 94; system wide, 99

Performance standards, for healthcare systems, 21–22

Personal digital assistants (PDAs), 109, 146–147

Personal experience, as research evidence source, 16, 20

Pfizer Health Solutions InformaCare, 192

Pharmaceutical companies, healthcare market share of, 216–217

Physician assistants, 160

Physician champions, 234–235

Physician-hospital relationship. *See* Professional integration

Physician liaison personnel, 247

Physicians: attitudes toward healthcare managers, 3–4; community hospitals and, 222; concierge, 224; consumers' trust in, 365; expectations of, 261–262; as hospital pricing information source, 367; income of, 222; job satisfaction of, 223; as managers, 263; morale of, 223; pay-for-call stipends for, 222; power of, 261; primary care, 165, 224–225; relationship with managers, 261–264; shortage of, 160, 161; wholesale strategies of, 223–224

Piney Woods Hospital, emergency department quality improvement initiative, 317–340, 329–339; community perception data, 339; comparative balance statement data, 330, 332; comparative income statement data, 330, 331; employee satisfaction survey data, 325, 327; financial performance analysis for, 338–339; patient satisfaction data, 335, 337, 338; physician satisfaction survey data, 335, 337–338; waiting time improvement, 337, 338

Plan-Do-Study-Act (PDSA) cycle, 129–130

Pneumonia patients, evaluation of care for, 90

Point-of-service data collection, 99

Point-of-service plans, 154

Porter, Zach, 317–340

Positive deviance strategy, 220, 227–229, 230

Positive reinforcement, 230

Power: information as, 364–365; of managers, 263, 264; of physicians, 261

Preferred provider organizations (PPOs), 4

Preventive care, 306; convenient care clinics' role in, 166; demand for, 162

Price, definition of, 365, 366

Price discounts, 357

Price elasticity, 373

Price transparency, 365–373; "death in the middle" phenomenon and, 373; definition of, 364; demand for, 363–364; effect on balance of power, 364–365; effect on healthcare

industry, 363–374; as healthcare commoditization, 364
PricewaterhouseCoopers, 364, 365, 367, 371
Pricing. *See also* Price transparency: analysis of, 370–371; effect of cost sharing on, 366–367
Pricing information: consumers' demand for, 367–368, 371, 372; relationship to quality, 368–369; sources, 365
Pricing structure, in healthcare, 363
Private-pay patients, 369, 370
Process changes, redesign of, 241–242
Process innovations, 154
Process management, 251–256
Process measures, for healthcare, 93
Professional development: Competency Assessment Tool for, 62–63; information sources for, 59–60; job changes and, 72–75; scenario analysis of, 64–6; strategic planning for, 58–68
Professional integration, 213–294; at academic medical centers, 293–294; appreciative inquiry strategy for, 220, 230–231; barriers to, 221–223; business models of, 223–226; case studies, 229–235, 261–294; commentary on, 215–217; cultural change and, 220; cultural convergence and, 235–236; "dance of the blind reflex" and, 224, 225–226, 227, 234; as financial collaboration, 227; marketplace considerations in, 216–217; in medical day care programs, 292; motivation for, 219–220; "mural dyslexia" and, 220; obstacles to, 227–229; in pediatric cardiac intensive care unit, 287–292; physicians' and nurses' expectations about, 215–216; physicians' involvement in, 236–237; positive deviance strategy for, 220, 227–229; readings on, 219–259; retail strategies for, 224–225; *versus* "silo mentality," 235; steps in, 236–237; structural dialogue strategy for, 220, 232–235; supportive strategies for, 226–229
Profit, as performance evaluation measure, 85

Promotions: within case management departments, 352–353; risk and benefits associated with, 76–78
Prospective payment systems, for home health care, 322, 324
Psychiatric care, restricted health insurance coverage for, 410–411
Psychiatric drug therapy, 297
PubMed, 15

Quality: consumer ratings of, 93–94; dimensions of, 129–130; poor, cost of, 82; professional criteria for, 83; relationship to pricing information, 368–369
Quality action teams (QATs), 138
Quality improvement: collaborative approach in, 90–91; continuous quality improvement (CQI), 137–139, 242, 243; customer-mindedness, 297; effect of performance measurement systems on, 91; eight-step decision-making model of, 11, 12; in emergency departments, 139; evidence-based management for, 127–137; in home health care organizations, 124–137; implication for performance data analysis, 86; monetary incentives and, 87
Quality improvement movement, 107
Quantitative assessment, of healthcare outcomes, 3
Question formulation. *See* Research question formulation

Racial factors, in healthcare disparity, 351–352
Radiation oncology services, proposed investment in, 340–346
Radiologists, 154; professional integration of, 222–223
Radiology tests, digital, 297
Rapid-sequence change processes, 233
Reasoning, defensive, 220, 226; appreciative inquiry response to, 230
Reengineering, 82, 156, 233, 372
Referrals, 224
Reform, of healthcare system, 160, 174

Regulations: compliance with, 306; as obstacle to professional integration, 222

Rehabilitation services, 207–210

Reimbursement, for healthcare: changes in, 305–306; lack of, 222

Research evidence: application of, 8, 13, 18–19; definitions of, 20; relevancy of, 15–16; sources of, 14–15; syntheses of, 15–16; systematic reviews of, 12–13

Research evidence presentation, 13, 17–18; accountability for, 22

Research evidence syntheses: applications of, 16–17; assessment of, 16–17; presentation in, 17–18; relevance, 15–16

Research question formulation, 13, 14

Research "rounds," 22–23

Research seminars, 22–23

Research services, specialized, 24

Residents, unionization of, 293–294

Resignation, from managerial positions, 36, 68–69, 72–75

Resource allocation, 219

Resource misallocation, 377

Resource scarcity, 151

Retail health clinics. *See* Convenient care clinics

Retail mall clinics. *See* Convenient care clinics

Retail strategies, 224–225

Risk aversity, 3

Risk management, 131–132; incident reports in, 85

Roberts, Gwen, 329–330

Robert Wood Johnson Foundation, 351; Expecting Success program, 155; Urgent Matters program, 155

Roles, of managers, 3–4; ambulatory health service program management, 50–58; case studies, 35–78; case studies of, 35–78; faculty practice administration, 37–50; prioritization of goals, 75–76; professional development planning, 58–68; risks and benefits associated with, 35–36, 72–78

"Rounds," research, 22–23

Ryan, Mary Jean, 256

St. Luke's Hospital, Kansas City, management practices: focus on patient satisfaction, 247; human resources, 251; leadership, 241; measurement and analysis, 248; organizational characteristics and, 240; patient advocacy program, 246; performance management process, 242

Salaries: of physicians, 215; requests for increase in, 72

Saratoga Institute, 250

Scenario analysis, for professional development, 64–66

Scenario-based planning, 311

Selective care, 219

Self-awareness, 5

Self-care, 156. *See also* Disease management programs

Self-image, of managers, 3–4

Self-referrals, 224

Self-regulation, 5

Seminars, research, 22–23

Service value chain, 242

Shareholder impact analysis, 310–311

Shareholders. *See also* Stakeholders: definition of, 310

Shewhart PDSA Quality Improvement Cycle, 11–12

Shinseki, Erik, 220

Shortell, Stephen M., 7

Sick time, as performance evaluation measure, 85

Sister Mary Jean Ryan, 256

Sisters of Mercy Health System, 96–97

Situational analysis, for emergency department quality improvement, 329–339; community perception data, 339; comparative balance statement data, 330, 332; comparative income statement data, 330, 331; employee satisfaction survey data, 325, 327; financial performance analysis for, 338–339; patient satisfaction data, 335, 337, 338; physician satisfaction survey data, 335, 337–338; waiting time improvement, 337, 338

Six Sigma, 86, 154

Size, of organizations, 216–217

Small area analyses, 91

Social skills, 5

Social workers, 288, 290–291

Spectrum Health, 369

SSM Health Care, management practices: corporate review process, 242–243; information management, 248–249; leadership, 241; organizational characteristics and, 240; performance improvement teams, 242–243; process management, 252

Staff. *See also* Nurses; Physicians: morale of, 250

Staff development programs, 23

Staffing, management information system for, 116–124

Staff turnover, as performance measure, 85

Stakeholder analysis, for professional development planning, 60–61

Stakeholders, 379; claims on healthcare organizations, 360–361; definition, 310; demands from, 3; external, 21; information requests from, 89; performance criteria and standards of, 21; and performance evaluation, 95–97, 357, 358–360; sharing of research evidence with, 23; and strategic planning, 306

Standardization: in healthcare, 82–83; in performance measurement, 90, 94

Standardized order sets, 114

Stanford University, 27

Stark Laws, 224

State health departments, home health care accreditation by, 125

Sternin, Jerry, 229, 230, 236

Storefront clinics, 225

Story-telling, 231–232

Strategic cycling, 299–316; benchmarking element, 309; contingency planning in, 311; as continuous process, 300, 307, 308; core message of, 299–300; elements of, 308–312; evidence-based management concept of, 300; executive summary of, 301–302; implementation phase, 311–312; learning concept of,

300; mission and values validation element, 309; overview of, 307–308; primary strategy development element, 310; prioritization in, 312; purpose of, 301; research and data analysis element, 309–310; scenario development in, 311; shareholder impact analysis element, 310–311; transitional evaluation, 312; vision development element, 309

Strategic decision making, evidentiary process in, 20

Strategic management, 12, 13, 358

Strategic organizational dimension, 24, 26

Strategic planning: adverse consequences of, 302–303; Baldrige Health Care Criteria for, 243–246; definition of, 243; in dynamic environments, 305–307; effectiveness of, 302; implementation stage of, 303; linear model of, 301; "masterpiece" plans in, 303; positive consequences of, 303–304; for professional development, 58–68; time horizons in, 300

Strategic tunnel vision, 303

Strengths/Weaknesses/Opportunities/Threats (SWOT) analysis, 309–310

Stricklin, Mary Lou, 318, 322, 327

Structural dialogue, 220, 232–235; medical advisory panels for, 232–233

Structural organizational dimension, 24–25, 26

Struk, Cynthia, 128–134

Sturtevant, Bonnie, 229–230

Superior Medical Group, 156

Support systems, for staff, 81

Surgical procedures. *See also* Ambulatory surgery centers: population-based utilization studies of, 91

Surveys: community, 297; of consumer expectations, 359; of patient satisfaction, 85, 297

SWOT (Strengths/Weaknesses/Opportunities/Threats) analysis, 309–310

Systematic reviews, relevance of, 15–16

System-focused organizational design, 177–183

Systems, defensive reasoning response to, 226

Systems thinking, 308

Technical organizational dimension, 25–26

Technology, for evidence-based design, 199–200

TelaDoc, 225

Telemedicine, 154, 225

Telephone calls, for post-discharge medication compliance, 229–230

Terminally-ill patients, medical day care for, 292–293

Thinking: analytical, 8–9; strategic, 5–6; system-focused, 177–183

Third-party payer system, 366

Tourism, healthcare-based, 225

Toyota Production System (TPS), 154, 155

Training programs, 251; centralized, 180–183

Transfer, of patients, 196, 197

Transparency. See Price transparency

Trauma centers, inner-city, 415–418

Trust, 365

Uninsured patients: convenient care clinic use, 162; cross-subsidies for, 369–370; emergency department use, 161, 339, 406, 407, 408; hospital costs and prices for, 370–371

Unionization: of healthcare workers, 215; of residents, 293–294

United Kingdom National Health Service: Delivery and Organization Programme, 9; Health Management Online, 9; National Library for Health, 9

United Kingdom Prospective Diabetes Study, 193

United States Clinical Preventive Services Task Force, 93

United States Department of Health and Human Services, 364

University Hospitals of Cleveland, 322

University of California at San Francisco, 27

University of Pennsylvania, disease management program, 188

Value compass, 83

Values: definition of, 84; example, 81

Values statements, applications of, 241

Variation, 82–83

Veterans' Administration, 154; hospital network of, 4

Virginia Mason Medical Center of Seattle, 155

Vision/vision statements: applications of, 241; definition of, 84; example, 81; formulation of, 357

Visiting Nurse Association, Cleveland, 317, 318–328; board of trustees, 319, 321; component services, 321–322, 326–327, 328; contracts with hospitals, 320–321; corporate operative structure, 325; effect of Medicare regulations on, 322, 324, 326; future priorities, 327; mission and value statements, 319; organizational chart, 322; relationships with collaborators and competitors, 318–328; reorganization of, 320–321

Visiting Nurse Association Health Care Partners of Ohio (VNAHPO), evidence-based quality improvement initiative, 127–137

Visiting Nurse Service of America, rehabilitation services of, 207–210

Visiting nurse services, 4

Voluntary Hospitals of America, 154

Wagner, Edward, 156

Waiting time, in emergency departments, 139, 337, 338, 417

Walker, Harry, 272

Walk-in clinics. See Convenient care clinics

Waterbury Hospital Health Center, 229–230

Water contamination, in hospitals, 231–232

White, Terry, 268–269, 270

Wholesale purchase, of healthcare, 357

Wholesale strategies, 223–224

Whole Systems Measures, for quality

improvement, 129–130
Wisconsin, healthcare pricing availability
    in, 369
Wisconsin Hospital Association
    Information Center, 369
Work, organization of, 154, 174

About the Editors

Anthony R. Kovner, PhD, is professor of public and health management at The Wagner School of Public Service at New York University, and director of the Master of Science in Management concentration for nurse leaders. Kovner is an organizational theorist by training, and his research interests include nurse leadership, evidence-based management, and non-profit governance. He has been a senior manager in two hospitals, a nursing home, a group practice, and a neighborhood health center, as well as a senior healthcare consultant for a large industrial union. Professor Kovner has written 11 books and 91 peer-reviewed articles, book chapters, and case studies. His other books include: *Health Services Management,* with Duncan Neuhauser (Health Administration Press 2004), *Health Care Management in Mind: Eight Careers* (Springer 2000) and *Health Care Delivery in the United States,* 9th edition, coeditor, with James Knickman (Springer 2008). In addition, he has been a consultant to the NewYork-Presbyterian Hospital, the Robert Wood Johnson Foundation, the W. K. Kellogg Foundation, Montefiore Medical Center, and the American Academy of Orthopedic Surgeons. He is a board member of the Lutheran Medical Center, and a fellow of the New York Academy of Medicine, and was director for more than 20 years of NYU/Wagner's program in health policy and management. Professor Kovner received his PhD in public administration from the University of Pittsburgh.

Ann Scheck McAlearney, ScD, is associate professor of health services management and policy at The Ohio State University's College of Public Health. Her current research projects are in the areas of organizational change and leadership development, information technology innovations in healthcare, quality improvement and patient safety, and access to care for individuals with cancer. Prior to returning to academics, Dr. McAlearney held positions and had consulting arrangements with various organizations, including Uni-Health, Monsanto Health Solutions, PacifiCare Health Systems, Merck & Co., UCLA Medical Center, Arthur Young & Company, the Congressional

Budget Office, and the World Health Organization. She is the author of *Population Health Management: Strategies to Improve Outcomes*, published by Health Administration Press, and the co-editor of *Improving Clinical Practice: Total Quality Management and the Physician*, published by Jossey-Bass.

Duncan Neuhauser, PhD, is the Charles Elton Blanchard, MD, Professor of Health Management, Department of Epidemiology and Biostatistics, Medical School, Case Western Reserve University. He holds secondary professorships in internal medicine, family medicine, and organizational behavior and is the co-director of the Health Systems Management Center at his university. For 15 years he was the editor of *Medical Care*. His other books include *Coming of Age*, 2nd edition (1994) (a 60-year history of the American College of Healthcare Executives), and, with Edward McEachern, MD, and Linda Headrick, MD, *Clinical IQ: A Book of Readings* (Joint Commission Press 1996). He is a member of the Institute of Medicine.

About the Contributors

Sofia Agoritsas is an administrator at Maimonides Medical Center in Brooklyn, New York.

Emily A. Allinder is the business manager at the Saint Luke's Surgical Institute of Saint Luke's Hospital in Kansas City, Missouri.

Thomas R. Allyn, MD, FACP, is chief of nephrology at Santa Barbara Cottage Hospital and chief executive officer of the Santa Barbara Artificial Kidney Center, LLC, in California.

Julie M. Anstine is the leadership and project facilitator for the Office of the Senior Vice President of The Ohio State University.

James Begun, PhD, is the James A. Hamilton Professor of Healthcare Management in the Division of Health Policy and Management at the University of Minnesota.

Nathan Burt is an administrative fellow at OhioHealth in Dublin, Ohio.

Claudia Caine is executive vice president and chief operating officer of the Lutheran Medical Center in Brooklyn, New York.

James Castiglione is a librarian at the Brooklyn College Library in New York.

Kenneth Cohn, MD, FACS, is a general surgeon and director at Cambridge Management Group.

J. Mac Crawford, RN, PhD, is an assistant professor at The Ohio State University in Columbus.

Jason Dopoulos is an investment banker specializing in healthcare organizations at Lancaster Pollard in Columbus, Ohio.

Kyle Dorsey is a student in The Ohio State University Master of Health Administration Program.

Leonard H. Friedman, PhD, is a professor of public health at Oregon State University in Corvallis.

John R. Griffith, FACHE, is the Andrew Pattullo Collegiate Professor in the Department of Health Management and Policy of the University of Michigan School of Public Health in Ann Arbor.

Randa S. Hall is co-chair of the Health Administration Case Competition at University of Alabama–Birmingham.

Denise Hamilton, CPA, is co-chair of the Health Administration Case Competition at University of Alabama–Birmingham.

Kathleen Heatwole, PhD, is vice president of planning and development at Augusta Health Care, Inc., in Fishersville, Virginia.

Gary Kalkut, MD, is the senior vice president and chief medical officer at Montefiore Medical Center in the Bronx, New York.

David A. Kaplan is administrator of the Department of Surgery at Mount Sinai Medical Center in New York.

Abhi Kasinadhuni is a research assistant in the College of Public Health at The Ohio State University.

Dean Q. Lin, FACHE, is CEO of CareWorks Convenient Healthcare and vice president of business development for Geisinger Health System in Danville, Pennsylvania.

Sandy Lutz is director of the Health Research Institute at Pricewaterhouse Coopers LLP.

Larry K. McReynolds is executive director of the Lutheran Family Health Center in Brooklyn, New York.

David G. Melman, JD, is vice president of legal and compliance for Standard Security Life Insurance Company of New York.

Helen S. Nunberg, MD, is a physician in Santa Cruz, California.

Breanne Pfotenhauer is a project manager for planning and business development at Nationwide Children's Hospital in Columbus, Ohio.

Daivd J. Reisman is administrative director of emergency services at Massachusetts General Hospital in Boston.

Sarah Mathews Roesch is employed at The Ohio State University's College of Public Health.

Thomas G. Rundall, PhD, is the Henry J. Kaiser Professor of Organized Health Systems at the University of California, Berkeley.

Rebecca L. Schmale, PhD, is vice president of organizational development at Ohio Health in Columbus.

Nicholas Schmidt is a planning analyst at Summa Health System in Akron, Ohio.

Paula H. Song, PhD, is an assistant professor of health services management and policy at The Ohio State University in Columbus.

Patrice L. Spath, RHIT, is president of Brown-Spath & Associates, a healthcare publishing and training company in Forest Grove, Oregon.

Cynthia Struk, PhD, RN, PNP, is vice president of process improvement and research for the Visiting Nurse Association in Cleveland, Ohio.

Jacob Victory is director of operational performance management for the Visiting Nurse Service of New York in New York City.

Erick Vidmar is a senior analyst at the Cleveland Clinic in Abu Dhabi, United Arab Emirates.

Jason A. Waibel is a 2006 graduate of The Ohio State University Master of Health Administration Program.

Brook Watts, MD, is director of inpatient quality improvement at Louis Stokes Cleveland Veteran's Affairs Medical Center in Ohio.

Jeffrey Weiss, MD, is medical director of Montefiore Medical Center and assistant professor of medicine at the Albert Einstein College of Medicine in the Bronx, New York.

Kenneth R. White, PhD, FACHE, is a professor of health administration and nursing and director of the Graduate Program in Health Administration at Virginia Commonwealth University in Richmond.